Oncogenes and Tumour Suppressors

EDITED BY

Gordon Peters

AND

Karen H. Vousden

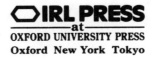

IRL PRESS
—at—
OXFORD UNIVERSITY PRESS
Oxford New York Tokyo

Oxford University Press, Great Clarendon Street, Oxford OX2 6DP

Oxford   New York

Athens   Auckland   Bangkok   Bogota   Bombay   Buenos Aires
Calcutta   Cape Town   Dar es Salaam   Delhi   Florence   Hong Kong
Istanbul   Karachi   Kuala Lumpur   Madras   Madrid   Melbourne
Mexico City   Nairobi   Paris   Singapore   Taipei   Tokyo   Toronto

and associated companies in
Berlin   Ibadan

Oxford is a trade mark of Oxford University Press

Published in the United States
by Oxford University Press Inc., New York

© Oxford University Press, 1997

A catalogue record for this book is available from the British Library

Library of Congress Cataloging in Publication Data
(Data available)
ISBN 0 19 963595 1 (Hbk)
ISBN 0 19 963594 3 (Pbk)

Typeset by Footnote Graphics, Warminster, Wilts
Printed in Great Britain by The Bath Press Ltd, Bath

Coventry University

Preface

It is now around 20 years since the first identification of a cellular oncogene, *c-SRC*, and about 10 years since the isolation of the prototypic tumour suppressor, the retinoblastoma protein, pRB. These key events heralded an age of discovery in which the genetic alterations commonly found in tumour cells were shown to impinge on a limited number of target genes. Through the study of such genes we have learned a great deal about how cell growth and differentiation is normally regulated and how these regulatory mechanisms go awry in cancer. It is therefore timely to take stock of some of the major developments and critical players in this field of research. To do this, we have commissioned an eminent team of researchers to summarize the current state of their particular fields of expertise. An exhaustive account of signal transduction and cell cycle regulation could fill many more pages than we have available and we have therefore had to restrict the range of genes and subject areas that are addressed in this volume, which we have divided into two parts entitled 'Oncogenes and signal transduction' and 'Tumour suppressors and cell cycle control'.

The first part deals with the so-called 'Oncogenes' — not special genes that cause cancer but normal cellular genes whose aberrant expression or function can contribute in some way to the development of neoplasia. As a general rule, the mutations/ alterations affecting these genes are dominant in that the oncogenic consequences can be manifest in the continued presence of the normal gene product. Indeed, in some instances it is simply the elevated or untimely expression of the normal gene product that is oncogenic. In others, the activity, regulation, or substrate specificity of the gene product is altered.

Much of the information about such genes has come from the study of animal retro-viruses. Since these viruses replicate by inserting a copy of their genome into that of the host cell, they are obligatory mutagens and can have dramatic effects on the structure and expression of genes at their sites of integration. In rare instances they go as far as capturing some of the cellular DNA and transducing it as part of their own genomes. These are the viral oncogenes (*v-ONCs*) whose altered function and high levels of expression are associated with very rapid tumour development in infected animals. Although there are no equivalents in humans, such acutely oncogenic agents have provided a wealth of information about the existence and function of oncogenes, and many of the same genes are implicated in human tumours where they are activated by different mechanisms, such as chromosomal rearrangements, gene amplification, or point mutation.

There are of the order of 100 known oncogenes as well as many close relatives that may also turn out to be important in tumorigenesis. The products of most of these genes fall into five broad functional categories: growth factors, growth factor recep-tors, cytoplasmic protein kinases, GTP-binding proteins, and transcription factors, each of which is dealt with in a separate chapter in part I. All of these genes contribute to the signal transduction mechanisms through which a cell senses its extracellular environment, and responds by altering its patterns of gene expression and undergoing cell division.

The cell division cycle provides the framework for part II, whose major themes are the tumour suppressor genes. In contrast to the activating mutations that afflict the proto-oncogenes, the critical lesions in tumour suppressor genes confer a loss or impairment of function. An obvious consequence is that mutated versions of these genes are recessive and tumorigenesis generally (although not always) requires the inactivation or silencing of the second allele. Two classical tumour suppressors, pRB and p53, dominate the discussion largely because of their pivotal roles both in tumorigenesis and in the processes that normally regulate the cell cycle. They are also the principal targets of a variety of DNA tumour viruses that encode proteins designed to abrogate the functions of both genes, a remarkable example of convergent evolution. As well as providing a paradigm for the interaction of oncogenes and tumour suppressors, such observations are relevant to human cancers associated with viral infections. The *RB* and *p53* genes also provide the benchmarks for other tumour suppressor genes implicated in inherited cancer syndromes. Tracing the inheritance of mutated alleles as well as sporadic alterations that affect these genes can have direct clinical relevance and it is only fitting that we include a chapter on the possible ways in which the knowledge accrued in the last two decades can be applied to clinical practice and the diagnosis and management of cancer.

In being selective, our choice of topics will undoubtedly rankle some whose interests appear under-represented. Nevertheless, we hope that we have succeeded in imparting some of the excitement of the field of research in a form that is accessible to the novice and informative to the initiated.

London
May 1997

G. P.
K. H. V.

Contents

3 Growth factor receptors in cell transformation   55

CARL-HENRIK HELDIN AND LARS RÖNNSTRAND

4 Oncogenic cytoplasmic protein tyrosine kinases 87

SERGE ROCHE AND SARA A. COURTNEIDGE

5 The RAS/RAF/ERK signal transduction pathway 121

SUSAN G. MACDONALD AND FRANK McCORMICK

6   Oncogenic transcription factors: FOS, JUN, MYC, MYB, and ETS   155

SUZANNE J. BAKER AND TOM CURRAN

Part II   TUMOUR SUPPRESSORS AND CELL CYCLE CONTROL

7 Mammalian cell cycle control   189

JONATHON PINES

8 The retinoblastoma gene product and its relatives   233

NICHOLAS B. LA THANGUE

9 The tumour suppressor gene p53   261

SUMAN B. GANGOPADHYAY, JACINTH ABRAHAM, YUN PING LIN, AND
SAM BENCHIMOL

Contributors

JACINTH ABRAHAM

The Ontario Cancer Institute/Princess Margaret Hospital and Department of Medical Biophysics, University of Toronto, 610 University Avenue, Toronto M5G 2M9, Canada.

SUZANNE J. BAKER

Department of Developmental Neurobiology, St. Jude Children's Research Hospital, 332 North Lauderdale, Memphis, TN 38105, USA.

SAM BENCHIMOL

The Ontario Cancer Institute/Princess Margaret Hospital and Department of Medical Biophysics, University of Toronto, 610 University Avenue, Toronto M5G 2M9, Canada.

DONALD M. BLACK

Cancer Molecular Genetics Research Group, Beatson Institute for Cancer Research, Switchback Road, Glasgow, UK.

SARA A. COURTNEIDGE

SUGEN Inc., 515 Galveston Drive, Redwood City, CA 94063, USA.

TOM CURRAN

Department of Developmental Neurobiology, St. Jude Children's Research Hospital, 332 North Lauderdale, Memphis, TN 38105, USA.

SUMAN B. GANGOPADHYAY

The Ontario Cancer Institute/Princess Margaret Hospital and Department of Medical Biophysics, University of Toronto, 610 University Avenue, Toronto M5G 2M9, Canada.

JOHN K. HEATH

School of Biochemistry, University of Birmingham, Edgbaston, Birmingham B15 2TT, UK.

CARL-HENRIK HELDIN

Ludwig Institute for Cancer Research, Box 595, Biomedical Center, S-751 24, Uppsala, Sweden.

STEPHAN IMREH

Microbiology and Tumour Biology Center (MTC), Karolinska Institute, S-171 77 Stockholm, Sweden.

GEORGE KLEIN

Microbiology and Tumour Biology Center (MTC), Karolinska Institute, S-171 77 Stockholm, Sweden.

NICHOLAS B. LA THANGUE
Division of Biochemistry and Molecular Biology, Davidson Building, University of Glasgow, Glasgow G12 8QQ.

YUN PING LIN
The Ontario Cancer Institute/Princess Margaret Hospital and Department of Medical Biophysics, University of Toronto, 610 University Avenue, Toronto M5G 2M9, Canada.

SUSAN G. MACDONALD
Onyx Pharmaceuticals, 3031 Research Drive, Richmond, CA 94806, USA.

FRANK McCORMICK
Onyx Pharmaceuticals, 3031 Research Drive, Richmond, CA 94806, USA.

HARDEV PANDHA
ICRF Oncology Unit, Department of Clinical Oncology, Royal Postgraduate Medical School, Hammersmith Hospital, London W12 0NN, UK.

JONATHON PINES
The Wellcome/CRC Institute, and the Department of Zoology, Tennis Court Road, Cambridge CB2 1QR, UK.

SERGE ROCHE
CJF9207 INSERM faculté de Pharmacie, Ave Ch. Flahaut 34060 Montpellier, France.

LARS RÖNNSTRAND
Ludwig Institute for Cancer Research, Box 595, Biomedical Center, S-751 24, Uppsala, Sweden.

KAROL SIKORA
ICRF Oncology Unit, Department of Clinical Oncology, Royal Postgraduate Medical School, Hammersmith Hospital, London W12 0NN, UK.

LASZLO SZEKELY
Microbiology and Tumour Biology Center (MTC), Karolinska Institute, S-171 77 Stockholm, Sweden.

KLAS G. WIMAN
Microbiology and Tumour Biology Center (MTC), Karolinska Institute, S-171 77 Stockholm, Sweden.

Abbreviations

Throughout the text, we have elected to use capital letters to denote genes and their products, irrespective of their species of origin. While this contravenes the convention used for example to distinguish homologues in *Homo sapiens* and *Mus musculus*, this uniformity seems less confusing in the context of a general discussion. Nevertheless, genes are denoted in italics and the corresponding products in plain text. Since many of the genes symbols in common use are neither acronyms nor abbreviations, we have made little attempt to explain their derivations either here or in the text.

AIDS	acquired immune deficiency syndrome
ALL	acute lymphoblastic leukaemia
ALV	avian leukosis virus
AML	acute myelocytic leukaemia
A-MuLV	Abelson murine leukaemia
AP-1	activator protein 1
APC	adenomatous polyposis coli
APL	acute promyelocytic leukaemia
ATF	activating transcription factor 1
BDNF	brain-derived neurotrophic factor
BL	Burkitt's lymphoma
BWS	Beckwith–Wiedemann syndrome
CAD	carbomyl-P-synthetase/aspartate transcarbamylase/dihydroorotase
CBF	core binding factor
CBP	CREB-binding protein
CDK	cyclin-dependent kinase
CEA	carcino-embryonic antigen
CGH	comparative genomic hybridization
CKI	casein kinase I
CKII	casein kinase II
CLL	chronic lymphocytic leukaemia
CML	chronic myelogenous leukaemia
CNTF	ciliary neurotrophic factor
CRE	cyclic AMP response element
CREB	cyclic AMP response element binding protein
CSF1	colony stimulating factor-1
DCIS	ductal carcinoma *in situ*
DDS	Denys–Drash syndrome
DM	double minute chromosome
DNA-PK	double-stranded DNA activated protein kinase

EBNA	EBV-encoded nuclear antigen
EBV	Epstein–Barr virus
EGF	epidermal growth factor
ER	oestrogen receptor
FAK	focal adhesion kinase
FAP	familial adenomatous polyposis coli
FeLV	feline leukaemia virus
FGF	fibroblast growth factor
FISH	fluorescence *in situ* hybridization
GADD	growth arrest and DNA damage inducible gene
GAP	GTPase activating protein
G6PD	glucose-6 phosphate dehydrogenase
G-CSF	granulocyte colony stimulating factor
GH	growth hormone
GM-CSF	granulocyte colony stimulating factor
HBEGF	heparin binding epidermal growth factor
HBV	hepatitis B virus
HGF	hepatocyte growth factor
HIV	human immunodeficiency virus
HLH	helix–loop–helix
HPV	human papilloma virus
HSR	homogeneously staining region
HSV	herpes simplex virus
HTLV	human T cell leukaemia virus
HVA	herpesvirus aeteles
HVS	herpesvirus saimiri
IGF	insulin-like growth factor
IL	interleukin
INK4	inhibitor of CDK4
JAK	Janus kinase
LCL	lymphoblastoid cell line
LIF	leukaemia inhibitory factor
MAR	matrix attachment region
MCK	muscle creatine kinase
MCL	mantle cell lymphoma
M-CSF	macrophage colony stimulating factor (CSF-1)
MHC	major histocompatibility complex
MPC	mouse plasmacytoma
MPF	maturation promoting factor
MuLV	murine leukaemia virus
NDF	Neu differentiation factor
neoR	neomycin phosphotransferase
NFκB	nuclear factor kappa-B
NGF	nerve growth factor

NMR	nuclear magnetic resonance
NT	neurotrophin
ODC	ornithine decarboxylase
PALA	N-phosphonacetyl-L-aspartate
PCR	polymerase chain reaction
PDGF	platelet-derived growth factor
PKC	protein kinase C
PI3K	phosphatidylinositol-3'-kinase
PLC	phospholipase C
PSA	prostate-specific antigen
PTP-1D	phosphyotyrosine phosphatase 1D
RSV	Rous sarcoma virus
SCF	stem cell factor
SH2	SRC-homology domain 2
SH3	SRC-homology domain 3
SRE	serum response element
SRF	serum response factor
SSV	sarcoma virus
STAT	signal transducer and activator of transcription
TBP	TATA-binding protein
TCF	ternary complex factor
TFIID, H, I	transcription factor IID etc.
TGFα	transforming growth factor alpha
TGFβ	transforming growth factor beta
TNF	tumour necrosis factor
TPA	tetradecanoylphorbol 13-acetate
UBC	ubiquitin conjugating enzyme
VEGF	vascular endotheila growth factor
WAGR	Wilms – aniridia – genital abnormalities-mental retardation
WHV	woodchuck hepatitis virus
WT	Wilms' tumour

Part I

ONCOGENES AND SIGNAL TRANSDUCTION

1 | Mechanisms of oncogene perturbation

STEPHAN IMREH, LASZLO SZEKELY, KLAS G. WIMAN, and GEORGE KLEIN

1. DNA tumour virus oncogenes

Viruses have been implicated for a long time as possible aetiologic agents in the genesis of human and animal tumours. Isolation of various DNA and RNA viruses that induced tumours in experimental animals led to the belief that all of them carry genetic elements, oncogenes, that are responsible for tumour induction. However, it became apparent that the oncogenes of the RNA tumour viruses have been acquired from the host cell genome, were not necessary for viral replication, and were maintained in the virus stocks under sustained selection for tumorigenicity. In contrast the oncogenic DNA viruses were found to encode proteins that are essential for viral replication and are also responsible for tumour induction. Viruses of different types are believed to contribute to the aetiology of approximately 15% of all human tumours (1).

Due to the presence of virally-encoded proteins that are required for the maintenance of neoplastic growth, DNA virus-induced tumours tend to elicit a strong immune response in immunocompetent hosts. Normally, this protects the host, but tumours may develop as a consequence of congenital, iatrogenic, infectious or experimental immunosuppression and/or chronic growth stimulation by other cofactors. Three tumour types arise particularly frequently in immunocompromised humans: lymphomas, skin tumours, and Kaposi sarcoma. DNA viruses are definitely involved in the first two and suspected in the third. The lymphomas and immunoblastomas are often associated with Epstein–Barr virus (EBV), the skin tumours with human papillomaviruses (HPV). Kaposi sarcoma is particularly prone to appear in HIV-infected persons, but is essentially restricted to the homosexual risk group. This has been taken to indicate that another, unknown virus is involved, transmitted preferentially by homosexual contact, and perhaps facilitated by the HIV-induced immunosuppression, as in other opportunistic infections. The agent responsible for Kaposi sarcoma is not definitely known, but recent evidence has focused interest on an EBV-related herpesvirus, HHV8.

1.1 Papovaviruses

The known oncogenic DNA viruses belong to the papova-, adeno-, herpes-, and hepadna- virus families (reviewed in refs 2 and 3). Both genera of papovaviruses, the papillomaviruses and the polyomaviruses, have members with tumorigenic potential. These are relatively small (40–55 nm), non-enveloped viruses with double-stranded circular DNA genomes that code for six to nine polypeptides. The expression of the viral genome can be divided into early and late events (i.e. before and after viral DNA synthesis). Due to the small size of the virus genome, the papovaviruses have to rely on the host DNA synthesis machinery to replicate the viral DNA. Proteins from the early region can trigger resting cells to enter into S phase (see Chapter 7 for a discussion of the cell cycle) and are responsible for transformation. Depending on the type and differentiation state of the infected cell, transformation is manifest in a number of ways, including morphological changes, increased saturation density, loss of contact inhibition, ability to grow in an anchorage-independent manner or in multiple layers, reduced growth factor requirement *in vitro*, and an ability to form tumours upon inoculation into immunodefective hosts. Viral transforming proteins can increase the lifespan of the infected cells *in vitro*, occasionally leading to escape from senescence and the acquisition of unlimited proliferative capacity, commonly referred to as immortalization.

Papillomaviruses have been identified in mammals, birds, and reptiles and there are more than 70 different HPV types that can induce warts of the skin, the genital organs, and the upper aerodigestive tract. Although most HPV types give rise to benign lesions, the 'high risk' viruses, such as HPV16 and 18 are believed to be involved in the aetiology of cervical and anogenital carcinomas. Their transforming function is associated with the early proteins E6 and E7 (see below).

Polyomaviruses cause inapparent infections in their natural hosts but are tumorigenic in new-born or immunodeficient rodents. The lack of tumorigenicity in the wild is due to the efficient immune surveillance against the transformed cells. The two best known members of this genus are *Polyomavirus muris* ('polyomavirus') and *Polyomavirus macaque* (simian virus 40 or SV40). The early proteins of these viruses are called tumour (T) antigens, and are further defined as large (LT), middle (MT), and small (ST). The polyomavirus early region encodes three T antigens (LT, MT, and ST) whereas SV40 encodes two (LT and ST). The transforming and immortalizing functions of polyomavirus are mediated by the MT and LT antigens respectively, in contrast to SV40 where both functions are associated with the LT antigen. Both polyoma and SV40 LT antigens are multifunctional nuclear proteins that regulate viral DNA replication and transcription.

Both viruses are able to transform a variety of cell types of epithelial and mesenchymal origin *in vitro* and *in vivo*. Expression of SV40 LT from tissue-specific promoters in transgenic mice allowed the generation of several mouse strains that develop tumours in the target organ in a highly predictable fashion. Due to its relatively indiscriminate transforming ability, SV40 LT has also been used as an experimental tool to establish permanent cell lines from tissues that do not readily grow *in vitro*. While rodent cells are easily immortalized by SV40, human cells are quite refractory. Cells from patients with congenital chromosome fragility syndromes, such as Ataxia telangiectasia, Bloom syndrome, and Fanconi anaemia are more easily transformable, suggesting that additional genetic changes are required.

Polyomavirus hominis-1 (BK virus) and *-2* (JC virus) are widely present in the human population. Although both viruses are able to induce tumours in new-born hamsters, no association has been found with any human tumour. As with SV40, a single LT protein is responsible for the transforming activity of these viruses.

1.2 Adenoviruses

Adenoviruses are non-enveloped 70–90 nm particles with linear double-stranded DNA genomes that encode 20–30 polypeptides. Several of these viruses are common human pathogens causing upper respiratory tract infections, pneumonia, kerato-conjunctivitis, and infant gastroenteritis. They are not associated with any human malignancy but can induce tumours in new-born rodents and can transform non- or semi-permissive target cells. The E1A and E1B proteins, encoded by the early region, are responsible for the transformation (see below).

1.3 Herpesviruses

Herpesviruses are large (120–200 nm) enveloped viruses with double-stranded DNA genomes that encode more than 60 proteins. The best studied oncogenic herpes virus is Epstein–Barr virus (EBV) which is present in more than 90% of all human populations. Infection usually occurs in early childhood, with no apparent symptoms, whereas primary infection at later ages may induce a self-limiting lymphoproliferative disease, infectious mononucleosis. EBV infects resting B lymphocytes and transforms them into proliferating immunoblasts that can grow into immortal lymphoblastoid cell lines (LCLs) in culture. Nine virally-encoded proteins are expressed in the LCLs, the EBV-encoded nuclear antigens (EBNAs 1–6) and the membrane proteins (LMP1, 2a, and 2b). The concerted action of six viral genes (EBNAs 1, 2, 3, 5, and 6 and LMP1) is required for B cell immortalization. Although the exact roles of these genes remain unclear, EBNA1 binds to origins of viral DNA replication, is required for the maintenance of the viral DNA as an episome, and has a transcriptional transactivating function. EBNA2 and EBNA6 are transcriptional regulators of several cellular and viral promoters and may initiate the G0–G1 transition in EBV-infected primary B cells. LMP1 can transform established lines of rodent fibroblasts and immortalized human keratinocytes, can increase the expression of B cell activation markers and adhesion molecules on B lymphoblasts, can co-operate with EBNA2 to induce CD23, and can protect cells from apoptosis by inducing expression of BCL2.

It is an interesting paradox that although EBV is arguably the most potent immortalizing agent known, it is only rarely pathogenic in the human host. EBV-infected B cells that express the full set of EBNAs and LMPs elicit a vigorous T cell response in healthy individuals. However, in immunocompromised individuals, such as AIDS patients, organ transplant recipients, and individuals with certain congenital T cell deficiencies, EBV may induce immunoblastic lymphomas. EBV has also been isolated from several human malignancies although the role of the virus in the pathogenesis of these diseases remains to be elucidated. For example, 97% of the Burkitt lymphomas (BL) that occur in the high endemic tropical forest regions are EBV-positive. In contrast, only around 20% of sporadic BL and 30% of AIDS-associated BL carry the virus. Nasopharyngeal carcinoma (NPC) is regularly associated with the virus, irrespective of its ethnic origin and approximately half of all Hodgkin's lymphomas as well as certain forms of T cell lymphoma are EBV-positive. Other recently identified EBV-carrying tumours include gastric lymphoepitheliomas, adenocarcinomas, and leiomyosarcomas.

A number of herpesviruses are associated with malignancy in other species. For example, New World primates have their own lymphotropic herpesviruses, such as *Herpesvirus saimiri* (HVS) and *Herpesvirus ateles* (HVA), that target T rather than B cells. These viruses cause no disease in their natural hosts, the squirrel and spider monkey, respectively, but induce rapidly growing T cell lymphomas or lymphocytic leukaemias if injected into closely related New World primates. HVS and HVA can immortalize normal T cells of susceptible species (4). The highly contagious avian herpesvirus, Marek's disease virus (MDV), induces malignant lymphomas in chickens. The virus replicates productively in many different cell types but only the latent infection of T lymphocytes results in cell transformation. Few viral proteins are detected in MDV-induced LCLs, but one of them, called MEQ was recently identified as a transcriptional activator. It contains an amino terminal basic-leucine zipper domain similar to the JUN/FOS family of proteins (see Chapter 6) and a proline-rich carboxy terminal domain that resembles the product of the WT1 (Wilms' tumour) tumour suppressor protein (ref. 5; and Chapter 10).

1.4 Hepatitis viruses

Convincing epidemiological evidence shows that hepatitis B virus (HBV) is involved in the aetiology of primary hepatocellular carcinoma (HCC) in humans. The estimated 200–300 million chronic carriers of the virus have a 100-fold increased risk of developing HCC than non-carriers. HBV belongs to the hepadnaviridae family which are small (40–50 nm) enveloped viruses with a circular, partially double-stranded DNA genome. Infection of hepatocytes regularly leads to necrosis followed by multiple nodular hyperplasia and cirrhosis. Although the induction of regenerative hyperplasia might be involved in the initiation of HCC, HBV may have a more direct role (6). Thus, HBV-positive carcinoma cells carry integrated viral genomes and it is possible that activation of adjacent cellular genes may contribute to the development of the malignancy. The woodchuck hepatitis virus (WHV), a close relative of HBV, has been shown to integrate in the immediate neighbourhood of the *MYC* and *N-MYC* genes (7, 8). In human HCC, there have been isolated cases where HBV was found integrated into specific genes (9, 10). HBV-encoded proteins may also contribute to cell transformation and both the surface antigen (HBsAg) and the 17 kDa viral transactivator protein, pX, have been linked to the development of hepatocellular adenomas and carcinomas in transgenic mice (11, 12). Moreover, viral integration can lead to rearrangements of the viral genes that alter the functions of the encoded proteins. For example, pX sustains frequent carboxy terminal truncations when expressed from the integrated viral genome (13).

2. Cellular targets of DNA tumour viruses

Identification of the viral transforming proteins and their cellular partners led to unexpected discoveries of major importance not only for cancer research but for cell biology as a whole. Oncogenes of the DNA tumour viruses may interfere with almost all levels of the growth-regulating signal transduction pathways. Some of them can simulate the action of growth hormones, as exemplified by the bovine papilloma virus E5 protein that is able to bind to PDGF and EGF receptors (14). Others can mimic activated growth factor receptors, such as the EBV-encoded LMP1 protein that binds to and activates a factor associated with the tumour necrosis factor (TNF) receptor (15). The transforming protein of polyomavirus, MT, can activate growth signal transmitting tyrosine kinases such as SRC, YES, or LCK (16, 17; and Chapter 4). LCK is also activated by TIP, the product of HVS ORF-1 (18). Since some transforming gene products interact with nuclear proteins that have sequence-specific DNA binding activity, they may indirectly modulate the expression of growth regulatory genes. This is exemplified by the binding of EBNA2 and EBNA6 to the Jκ recombination signal-binding protein CBF1 (19, 20). Curiously, HVS also encodes a protein related to D-type cyclins (called v-cyclin) which can form an active complex with the cyclin-dependent kinase CDK6 (21; see Chapter 7).

The viral transforming proteins also interact with growth inhibitory proteins (Fig. 1). The most frequently mutated gene in human tumours, p53, was first found through the binding of its protein product (p53) to the LT protein of SV40 (22). Later p53 was shown to form molecular complexes with the 55 kDa E1B protein of adenoviruses and the E6 protein of papillomaviruses (23, 24). As discussed elsewhere (see Chapter 9) p53 is activated by DNA damaging and oxidizing agents and induces growth arrest and/or apoptosis. Different DNA tumour viruses have evolved different strategies to overcome its effect. SV40 LT inhibits the DNA binding activity of p53 to specific target sites (25) whereas adenovirus E1B does not affect the DNA binding but interferes with the transactivation function of p53 (26). In contrast, papillomavirus E6 induces ubiquitin-mediated degradation of p53 (27).

The same viruses also encode proteins that target another important tumour suppressor, the retinoblastoma gene product, pRB (Fig. 1 and Chapter 8). Thus, SV40 LT, adenovirus E1A, and papillomavirus E7 associate with pRB through a common amino acid motif, LxCxE (28–30). These three independently evolved viral proteins also interfere with the functions of the pRB-related proteins p107 and p130. This is a remarkable case of convergent evolution. Binding leads to the dissociation of the molecular complexes composed of the pRB family members and transcriptional regulatory proteins of the E2F family (31). In current models of cell cycle control, E2F activity is required for cells to initiate DNA synthesis (see Chapter 7). Some of these viral proteins also interact with and inhibit the function of p300 and the related CBP, a co-activator of the transcription factor CREB (32).

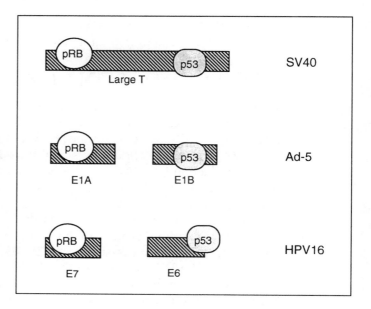

Fig. 1 Binding of DNA tumour virus oncoproteins to the products of the *RB* and *p53* tumour suppressor genes. The SV40 large T antigen binds to both pRB and p53. Similarly the E1A and E1B products of human adenovirus-5 and the E7 and E6 products of the oncogenic subtypes of HPV (for examples HPV16 and HPV18) bind to pRB and p53 respectively. The consequences are discussed in detail in Chapters, 7, 8, and 9

In addition to the activation of oncogenes and inactivation of tumour suppressors, some DNA tumour viruses also encode proteins that protect the target cells from apoptosis. This may prevent the elimination of cells that carry latently replicating viruses and may counteract premature cell death prior to the completion of lytic replication. The anti-apoptotic effect of the virus may be mediated through the up-regulation of cellular BCL2, as exemplified through the effect of the EBV-encoded LMP1 protein (33), or by the expression of a viral BCL2 homologue, such as the 19 kDa adenovirus E1B protein or the EBV encoded BHRF1 (34).

3. Retroviral transduction of cellular oncogenes

Cellular proto-oncogenes were first discovered through the study of RNA tumour viruses, now usually referred to as retroviruses (for an overview, see ref. 35). The retroviral genome consists of two genetically identical single-stranded RNA molecules, 8–10 kb in size. In general, retroviruses carry three genes, *gag* that encodes the major viral nucleocapsid proteins, *pol* that encodes the reverse transcriptase responsible for converting the viral RNA genome into double-stranded DNA, and *env* that encodes the viral envelope glycoproteins. Studies of Rous sarcoma virus (RSV) and other rapidly transforming (so-called 'acute') retroviruses revealed that their genomes carried additional sequences required for efficient transformation of cells. The transforming gene of RSV, *SRC*, was localized to a region near the 3' end of the viral genome. Complimentary DNA corresponding to the viral *SRC* gene, *v-SRC*, was found to hybridize to DNA from all vertebrate animals tested (36). These experiments allowed the identification of the cellular *SRC* gene, *c-SRC*, which is discussed in Chapter 4. Other retroviruses were subsequently shown to carry transforming genes

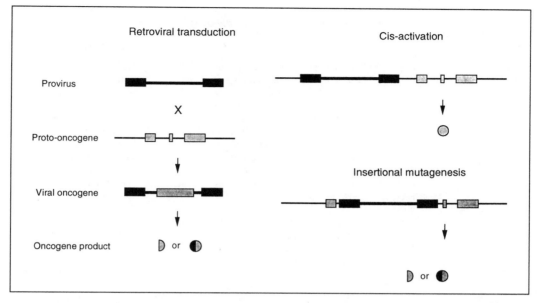

Fig. 2 Retroviral activation of cellular proto-oncogenes. The proviral DNA of a typical non-acute retrovirus is depicted in black (flanked by two long terminal repeats) and the cellular target gene as shaded boxes, each representing a coding exon. Acutely transforming retroviruses are formed via recombination between viral and cellular sequences such that a portion of the cellular gene becomes captured (transduced) within the viral genome. The transforming proteins encoded by these viruses are often fusions of viral and cellular sequences. Non-acute retroviruses activate cellular proto-oncognes by integrating adjacent to or within the target gene. These are distinguished as 'cis-activation' (in which the normal gene product is expressed at elevated levels) or 'insertional mutagenesis', where the cellular gene product is structurally altered.

or oncogenes, all of which have cellular counterparts. This led to the conclusion that the viral oncogenes have been captured from cellular DNA during transcription of proviral DNA and assembly of the virus particle, a process referred to as transduction (see Fig. 2).

RSV is unique among the acute retroviruses in that it carries all three genes needed for viral replication (*gag, pol,* and *env*) in addition to the oncogene, *v-SRC*. RSV is therefore both replication-competent and able to efficiently transform cells. In other known acute retroviruses, the viral oncogene has been incorporated at the expense of coding information required for viral replication (Fig. 2), and as a consequence, these viruses can only replicate together with helper viruses that provide the missing protein or proteins.

Whereas the viral oncogenes can efficiently transform cells, their cellular counterparts, the proto-oncogenes, are unable to do so under normal circumstances. Therefore, there must be essential differences between the viral and cellular oncogenes. First, the viral oncogenes are driven by the strong constitutive promoter in the retroviral long terminal repeat (LTR). As a consequence, they are usually expressed at significantly higher levels than the corresponding cellular proto-oncogenes, controlled by their

Table 1 Oncogenes activated by retroviral transduction

Gene	Virus	Type of protein
ABL	Abelson murine leukaemia virus	Tyrosine kinase
AKT	AKT8 murine leukaemia virus	Serine/threonine kinase
CRK	CT10 avian sarcoma virus	SH2–SH3 adaptor
ERBA	ES4 avian erythroblastosis virus	Hormone receptor
ERBB	ES4 avian erythroblastosis virus	Growth factor receptor
ETS	E26 avian erythroblastosis virus	Transcription factor
FES	Gardner Arnstein feline sarcoma virus	Tyrosine kinase
FGR	Gardner Rasheed feline sarcoma virus	Tyrosine kinase
FMS	McDonough feline sarcoma virus	Growth factor receptor
FOS	FBJ murine osteosarcoma virus	Transcription factor
FPS	Fujinami avian sarcoma virus	Tyrosine kinase
JUN	Avian sarcoma virus-17	Transcription factor
KIT	Hardy–Zuckerman feline sarcoma virus	Growth factor receptor
MOS	Moloney murine sarcoma virus	Serine/threonine kinase
MYB	Avian meyeloblastosis virus	Transcription factor
MYC	Avian myelocytomatosis virus	Transcription factor
RAF	3611 murine sarcoma virus	Serine/threonine kinase
H-RAS	Harvey murine sarcoma virus	GTP/GDP binding
K-RAS	Kirsten murine sarcoma virus	GTP/GDP binding
REL	Avian reticuloendotheliosis virus	Transcription factor
ROS	UR2 avian sarcoma virus	Growth factor receptor
SEA	S13 avian erythroblastosis virus	Growth factor receptor
SIS	Simian sarcoma virus	Growth factor
SRC	Rous avian sarcoma virus	Tyrosine kinase
YES	Y73 avian sarcoma virus	Tyrosine kinase

natural promoters, and do not respond to cellular control mechanisms that would normally regulate their transcription. In addition, many viral oncogenes carry point mutations, truncations, or deletions in the coding sequence that change the biochemical properties of their protein products. Table 1 lists some of the oncogenes that have been transduced by retroviruses.

4. Activation of oncogenes by retroviral insertion

In contrast to the oncogene-carrying acute retroviruses that induce tumours *in vivo* within weeks after infection and transform cells *in vitro*, the 'chronic' or 'non-acute retroviruses', such as avian leukosis virus (ALV), feline leukaemia virus (FeLV), mouse mammary tumour virus (MMTV), and other replication-competent retroviruses, induce tumours *in vivo* with a long latency and do not usually transform cells in tissue culture. In addition, the chronic retroviruses do not induce tumours at the site of inoculation, unlike the acute retroviruses, but act at a distant site or systemically. The tumours that arise are clonal or oligoclonal, i.e. they derive from a single or a few infected cells. The chronic retroviruses do not carry any oncogene. Then how do these viruses cause tumours?

Table 2 Oncogenes activated by retroviral insertion

Gene	Virus	Type of protein
MYC	Avian leukosis virus	Transcription factor
MYC	Murine leukaemia virus	Transcription factor
MYC	Feline leukaemia virus	Transcription factor
N-MYC	Murine leukaemia virus	Transcription factor
WNT1	Mouse mammary tumour virus	Growth factor
WNT3	Mouse mammary tumour virus	Growth factor
FGF3	Mouse mammary tumour virus	Growth factor
FGF4	Mouse mammary tumour virus	Growth factor
FGF8	Mouse mammary tumour virus	Growth factor
ERBB	Avian leukosis virus	Growth factor receptor
MYB	Murine leukaemia virus	Transcription factor
MYB	Avian leukosis virus	Transcription factor
PIM1	Murine leukaemia virus	Serine/threonine kinase
PIM2	Murine leukaemia virus	Serine/threonine kinase
SPI1	Spleen focus forming virus	Transcription factor
FLI1	Friend murine leukaemia virus	Transcription factor
FMS	Murine leukaemia virus	Growth factor receptor
EVI1	Murine leukaemia virus	Transcription factor
CCND1	Murine leukaemia virus	Cyclin
CCND2	Murine leukaemia virus	Cyclin
LCK	Murine leukaemia virus	Tyrosine kinase
BMI1	Murine leukaemia virus/feline leukaemia virus	Transcription factor
PAL1/GFI1	Murine leukaemia virus	DNA binding protein

As first demonstrated in B cell lymphomas caused by ALV, the development of tumours after infection with chronic retroviruses may be due to proviral integration in the vicinity of a cellular oncogene, leading to deregulated expression of that gene (Fig. 2 and refs 37 and 38). The strong promoter/enhancer in the retroviral LTR is bidirectional and can drive transcription not only of the viral genes but of adjacent cellular genes as well. Thus, initiation of transcription in the retroviral LTR may produce an mRNA that contains both viral and cellular sequences or the mere presence of the virus in adjacent DNA can activate the expression of the target gene (Fig. 2). A rare cell that has acquired a provirus next to the c-MYC proto-oncogene, for instance, may thus express significantly elevated levels of MYC and therefore outgrow its neighbours and eventually form a tumour. The longer latency required for tumour formation by the chronic retroviruses presumably reflects two important differences from the acute retroviruses. First, proviral integration occurs more or less at random. Since tumorigenic integration must occur at a specific site, heavy bombardment of many cells with numerous virus particles is required before a proper hit can be scored. Secondly, tumours will appear only after clonal expansion of the rare cell that has sustained the tumorigenic integration. Table 2 lists cellular onco-genes that have been shown to be activated by proviral insertion (reviewed in refs 39–41). Although several of these genes were also identified in acute retroviruses (Table 1), it is important to stress that the analysis of tumours induced by non-acute retroviruses also led to the identification of novel genes through the characterization of tumour-specific restriction fragments containing both viral and cellular sequences, commonly known as provirus tagging (41). The *INT1* gene (now known as *WNT1*), activated by MMTV proviral insertion in mouse mammary tumours, was the first proto-oncogene identified using provirus tagging (42, 43). *INT2* (now *FGF3*) was identified by using the same strategy (44, 45). Both encode growth factors but belong to different gene families (46; and see Chapter 2). The *PIM1* locus, on the other hand, was identified as a common proviral integration site in T cell lymphomas induced by murine leukaemia virus (MuLV) and encodes a serine/threonine kinase (47). More recently, provirus tagging has been applied to transgenic mice that already carry an activated oncogene in an attempt to identify genes that collaborate in tumorigenesis (reviewed in ref. 41). Examples include the *BMI1, PAL1,* and *BLA1* genes that evidently encode proteins that co-operate with *MYC* in lymphomagenesis (48, 49).

5. Cytogenetic mechanisms of oncogene activation

It is now apparent that many of the cellular proto-oncogenes identified in retrovirally-induced tumours in animal models are also implicated in tumours with no viral aetiology. In this section we consider the evidence for oncogene activation by chromosomal translocation, gene amplification, or point mutation.

5.1 Historical perspective

In view of the abnormal cell divisions that could be frequently observed in tumour tissue (50), Boveri postulated, originally over 100 years ago, that cancer could be due to chromosomal aberrations (51). After a period of ignorance, the first systematic comparison of chromosomes prepared from tumour versus normal tissue and from metastatic versus primary tumour tissue was made by Andres (52). Since mitotic abnormalities were extremely frequent in all malignant specimens, he concluded that they occur at random and that chromosome anomalies are not a cause but a consequence of malignant growth.

The concept of tumour progression was originally proposed by Rous (53) and its 'rules' formulated by Foulds (54, 55). It describes the development of cancer as a clonal evolution where a series of mutations generate successive subclones with a gradually increasing proliferative potential, favouring emancipation of the cells from the growth control of the host. It was later shown that some of these changes become visible at the chromosomal level. The earliest observation of this type came from the discovery of the Philadelphia chromosome (56). Moreover, inherited chromosome fragility syndromes (Bloom syndrome, Fanconi anaemia, Ataxia telangiectasis, and Xeroderma pigmentosa) with a high frequency of spontaneous chromosome aberrations (57) were found to be associated with various malignancies (lymphomas in particular) and it was clear that the chromosome aberrations preceded the progression to a cancerous stage. The development of chromosome banding (58) subsequently led to the identification of the *Ig/MYC* translocations in human and rodent B cell-derived tumours, quickly followed by the discovery of numerous other tumour-associated rearrangements that can be observed at the microscopic level.

5.2 Chromosomal translocations involving the immunoglobulin genes

A recurring theme among the chromosomal translocations observed in tumour cells is that one of the translocation partners is either an immunoglobulin (*Ig*) gene or a T cell receptor (*TCR*) gene. The likely reason is that these loci undergo rearrangement in the normal course of B cell or T cell development and it is generally assumed that the translocations result from illegitimate exchanges by the recombinases that execute the physiological rearrangements of these genes. The net effect is that cellular genes of various types come under the influence of regulatory elements from the constitutively active *Ig* or *TCR* loci, such that their protein products, whether intact or mutated, are aberrantly active.

5.2.1 Translocations involving *MYC*

Translocations of the *Ig* and *MYC* genes have been observed in B cell-derived tumours of man, rat, and mouse. It is the only translocation that has been detected in three species, leading to tumour development in the same lineage (59, 60). These translocations are exclusive to B cell tumours, the only known exception being a single macrophage–monocyte line, KT-10 (61). Virtually all cases of Burkitt lymphoma (BL), a B cell-derived, immunoglobulin-producing tumour, carry one of three alternative translocations involving the *MYC* gene on chromosome 8q24 and either the *Ig* heavy chain gene on chromosome 14 or the light chain genes on chromosomes 2 or 22. As discussed above, EBV is an important cofactor in BL, and there is a correlation between the EBV carrying status and the *Ig/MYC* breakpoints in BL. In EBV-negative BLs, the translocation breakpoints occur closer to the *MYC* gene than in the EBV-positive cases. A possible explanation would be that greater distances between the genes can be tolerated because EBV contributes in some way to the survival and/or proliferation of the cell carrying the translocation.

In the translocations observed in endemic BL, the *MYC* gene usually remains intact, with translocation breakpoints scattered up to 350 kb 5′ of the gene (62). In sporadic BL on the other hand, the breakpoints cluster in the non-coding exon 1 and intron 1 regions of *MYC*. The *IgH* breakpoints can vary but have a main cluster in the switch region (63–65). *IgH* and *MYC* are oppositely oriented on the chromosome with the 5′ end of *IgH* telomeric on 14q and the 5′ end of *MYC* centromeric on 8q. Since the most common form of reciprocal translocation involves the exchange of two terminal chromosome fragments, the most likely combination juxtaposes *IgH* and *MYC* head to head, with transcription proceeding in opposite directions (66). In the variant translocations of BL, however, *MYC* remains in place on 8q24 and the *IgK* or *IgL* loci are translocated to a region downstream of *MYC*, called *PVT1* (plasmacytoma variant translocation; see below). Human *PVT1* comprises a transcriptional unit starting

57 kb from *MYC* and extending over a 140 kb region (67). In the t(2;8) translocation, *IgK* regulatory elements are juxtaposed to *MYC* whereas in t(8;22), *IgL* is linked to chromosome 8 about 300 kb 3' of *MYC*, thereby disrupting the *PVT1* transcriptional unit (68). Both the light chain genes therefore end up downstream and in the same orientation as *MYC* (69).

Malignant non-Hodgkin's lymphomas are frequent in HIV-positive patients and the tumours often carry translocations identical with BL. Both typical t(8;14) and variant t(2;8) and t(8;22) translocations have been recorded. The molecular architecture corresponds with that of endemic BL (usually in EBV-positive cases) or with sporadic BL (mostly in EBV-negative cases) (70).

Around 95% of mouse plasmacytomas (MPC), which are differentiated B cell-derived plasma cell tumours of the peritoneal cavity, carry one of three translocations involving chromosome 15D2, the location of murine *MYC*. The typical t(12;15) translocation corresponds to *IgH/MYC*, the t(6;15) variant to *IgK/MYC*, and the t(15;16) variant to *MYC/IgL* (71, 72). These variant translocations were found to occur in a region between 80 and 360 kb 3' of *MYC* for which the name *PVT* was coined (for plasmacytoma variant translocation). The orientations of the genes involved in typical and variant translocations are identical in MPC and BL. In the typical MPC translocation, the *MYC* breakpoints cluster at the 5' end of the gene within the non-coding first exon and intron; the coding exons remain intact. Since the *IgH* breakpoints occur predominantly in the switch region in these plasma cell tumours, the recombination enzymes must have acted on both chromosomes, leading to one legitimate rearrangement and one illegitimate rearrangement. Recently our group has found a *IgK/N-MYC*, t(6;12)(C2;B1) in an MPC suggesting that the translocation may have occurred during the early phase of B cell development, when *N-MYC* is open for transcription and therefore presumably translocation (73, 74). If so, the translocation has not interfered with the continued differentiation of the cell.

Immunocytomas arise spontaneously in the Louvain strain of rat. These are plasma cell tumours originating from the ileocecal lymph nodes and carry a t(6;7)(q3.2;q3.3) translocation that juxtaposes *IgH* and *MYC* (75, 76).

The *Ig/MYC* translocations lead to the constitutive activation of *MYC* in the tumours of all three species, with concomitant down-regulation of the normal allele. The most likely interpretation is that the constitutively expressed MYC protein prevents the programmed exit of cells from the cell cycle. This would be in line with the idea that BL cells are phenotypically similar to germinal centre centroblasts or centrocytes. Under normal circumstances, they would presumably have entered a resting G0 stage, awaiting the activating antigen that would trigger surface immunoglobulin expression. Similarly plasma cells normally end up in a G0-like state, but if one of the *MYC* alleles becomes subordinate to regulatory elements from the Ig locus, it remains active and keeps the cell cycling in spite of its phenotype.

5.2.2 Immunoglobulin translocations with other genes

The precedents set by the *Ig/MYC* translocations led to the characterization of several other breakpoints, originally designated *BCL1*, *BCL2*, etc, all involving the immuno-

Table 3 Oncogenes activated by chromosomal translocation

Translocation	Affected genes	Disease
t(8;14)(q24;q32)	*MYC–IgH*	Burkitt's lymphoma
t(2;8)(p12;q24)	*IgK–MYC*	Burkitt's lymphoma
t(8;2)(q24;q11)	*MYC–IgL*	Burkitt's lymphoma
t(11;14)(q13;q32)	*CCND1–IgH*	Mantle cell lymphoma
t(11;22)(q13;q11)	*CCND1–IgL*	Mantle cell lymphoma
t(14;18)(q32;q21)	*BCL2–IgH*	Follicular lymphoma
t(2;18)(p12,q21)	*IgK–BCL2*	Follicular lymphoma
t(18;22)(q21;q11)	*BCL2–IgL*	Follicular lymphoma
t(3;14)(q27;q32)	*BCL6–IgH*	Non-Hodgkin lymphoma
t(3;22)(q27;q11)	*BCL6–IgL*	Non-Hodgkin lymphoma
t(8;14)(q24;q11)	*MYC–TCR* α/δ	T-ALL
t(1;14)(p32;q11)	*TAL1–TCR* α	T-ALL
t(7;9)(q35;q34)	*TCR* β*-TAL2*	T-ALL
t(1;7)(p34;q35)	*LCK–TCR* β	T-ALL
t(11;14)(p15;q11)	*RBTN1–TCR* α	T-ALL
t(11;14)(p13;q11)	*RBTN2-TCR* α/δ	T-ALL
t(7;11)(q35;p13)	*TCR* β*-RBTN2*	T-ALL
t(10;14)(q24;q11)	*HOX11–TCR* α	T-ALL
t(7;10)(q35;q24)	*TCR* β*-HOX11*	T-ALL
t(7;19)(q35;p13)	*TCR* β*-LYL1*	T-ALL
t(9;22)(q34;q11)	*BCR–ABL*	CML, ALL, CML
t(6;9)(p23;q34)	*DEK–CAN*	AML
t(4;11)(q21;q23)	*MLL*	Childhood ALL, AML
t(1;19)(q23;p13)	*PBX–E2A*	Pre-B ALL
t(17'19)(q22;p13)	*HLF–E2A*	Pro-B All
t(5;12)(q33;p13)	*PDGFR* β*-TEL*	CMML
t(15;17)(q22;q21)	*PML–RARA*	PML, APL
inv10(q11.2;q21)	*RET–D10S170*	Papillary thyroid cancer
t(12;16)(q13;p11)	*CHOP/TLS–FUS*	Myxoid liposarcoma, rhabdomyosarcoma
t(11;22)(q23;q12)	*FLI1–EWS*	Ewing's sarcoma
t(21;22)(q13;q12)	*ERG–EWS*	Ewing's sarcoma
t(12;22)(q13;q12)	*ATF1–EWS*	Melanoma of soft parts

globulin heavy chain locus on chromosome 14 or one of the light chain loci (77, 78; and see Table 3).

The t(11;14)(q13;q32) translocation (alias *BCL1*) is characteristic of a subtype of non-Hodgkin's lymphoma now classified as mantle-cell lymphoma (MCL) but 10–15% of B-CLL cases also carry this translocation (79). There are many parallels with BL in terms of the breakpoints between the joining and variable regions of *IgH*, the rare variants involving light chain genes, and breakpoints both upstream and downstream of the target gene (80). However, it was several years before the target gene was identified as *CCND1* (cyclin D1) since it lies some 120 kb downstream of the original *BCL1* breakpoint (81). The functions of cyclin D1 are discussed in Chapter 7.

The t(14;18)(q32;q21) translocation involves the so-called *BCL2* locus on chromosome 18 and the target gene bears the same name (82). The translocation is typical of follicular lymphoma (85%) but is also present in around 20% of diffuse B cell lymphomas (83). B-CLLs also show high BCL2 expression but only 10% of them carry a translocation. Again, rare variant translocations have been observed involving the immunoglobulin light chain gene. *BCL2* encodes the prototype of a family of proteins involved in regulating apoptosis and since BCL2 has been shown to be protective against programmed cell death (84), then deregulated expression would be consistent with sustained proliferation and tumorigenesis.

Abnormalities of the long arm of chromosome 3 have been described in many B and T cell-derived tumours. In some cases of non-Hodgkin lymphomas (NHL), the 3q translocations were found to involve the immunoglobulin loci (85–87) and cloning of the breakpoint at 3q27 led to the identification of *BCL6* (*LAZ3*). *BCL6/LAZ3* encodes a zinc-finger protein sharing homology with several transcription factors (88, 89). The 3q27 region participates in several other rearrangements with chromosomes 2, 4, 7, 14, and 22 (90). In a major study of 244 lymphoid tumours, *BCL6* rearrangements were found in 45% of diffuse large cell lymphomas (DLCL) and 35.5% of diffuse lymphomas with a large cell component (DLLC) but not in B- and T-ALLs, B- and T-CLLs, and multiple myelomas (91).

5.3 Chromosomal translocations involving the T cell receptor genes

There are four *TCR* genes designated α, β, γ, and δ that map to chromosomes 14q11.2, 7q32-q35, 14q11.2, and 7p15 respectively. As the T cell receptors are known to rearrange by mechanisms similar to those used by the immunoglobulin genes, it is not surprising that reciprocal translocations involving one of the *TCR* genes are observed in T cell leukaemias (see Table 3). The translocations are believed to occur at the onset of the *TCR* rearrangement in pre-T stage and have breakpoints in the J and D segments of the α, β, and δ genes; no translocation has yet been found involving the *TCR* γ gene (78). In virtually every case, the target gene is brought under the influence of the relatively well characterized *cis*-acting regulatory sequences of the *TCR* gene (92).

In contrast to B cell neoplasms, where a relatively small number of proto-oncogene partners are involved, the *TCR* translocations have multiple partners many of which encode transcription factors (see Table 3). These include *MYC*, translocated with the *TCR* α/δ locus in the t(8;14)(q24;q11) translocation in T-ALL (93). Another prominent example is the *TAL1* gene (also known as *SCL* and *TCL5*) which is a basic helix–loop–helix protein (see Chapter 6) affected by the t(1;14)(p32;q11) translocation (reviewed in ref. 94). Interestingly, in up to 26% of childhood T-ALLs, the *TAL1* gene has undergone ~ 90 kb deletions that are not detectable at the cytogenetic level (95). These eliminate exon 1, and a similar result is achieved in the t(1;14) translocation where the breakpoint in *TAL1* occurs within the first intron (94). *TAL2* was identified because of its sequence homology to *TAL1* and subsequently found to be translocated with *TCR* β in rare cases of T-ALL. Another relative of *TAL*, designated *LYL1*, is activated by the t(7;19)(q35;p13) translocation (96). It is assumed that the deleted or rearranged TAL and LYL proteins activate a set of target genes that are not normally expressed in T cells.

A similar explanation is likely to apply to the *RBTN/TTG* genes on chromosome 11p which were identified because of their involvement in translocations with the *TCR* α/δ locus (97, 98). The RBTN proteins or rhombotins contain a cysteine-rich LIM motif that is thought to adopt a zinc-finger structure and to contribute to protein–protein interactions, for example with TAL1 and TAL2 (99, 100). Continuing the transcription factor theme, the homeobox gene *HOX11* on chromosome 10q24 has been shown to participate in translocations with either the *TCR* α gene, t(10;14), or the *TCR* β gene, t(7;10) (94). The breakpoints occur at variable distances centromeric (5′) of *HOX11* and expression of the gene is only detectable in T-ALLs that carry the translocation (94).

Interestingly, the T-ALL cell line HSB-2 carries a t(1;7)(p34;q35) translocation that involves the *TCR* β gene and *LCK* (101), which encodes a SRC-family protein tyrosine kinase (Chapter 4). The *LCK* gene maps within the same chromosomal band as *TAL1* (1p32) and its product, p56, is expressed by thymocytes and peripheral T cells, and is one of the proteins involved in the initiation of TCR signal transduction (102). It is also activated by proviral insertion in thymomas induced by Moloney murine leukaemia virus (see ref. 41).

5.4 Translocations resulting in oncogenic fusion proteins

5.4.1 BCR–ABL and the Philadelphia translocation

The first example of a tumour-specific cytogenetic marker was the Philadelphia chromosome, Ph1, present in virtually all cases of CML (56). The typical translocation, t(9;22)(q34;q11) occurs in about 90% of cases with the remainder generally showing either simple variants, linking the 22q11 region with a different chromosome, or more complex variants involving a third chromosome (103). In all forms of Ph1, the *ABL* proto-oncogene on chromosome 9 is fused to the *BCR* (breakpoint cluster region) gene on chromosome 22 (reviewed in ref. 104) and in the fraction of cases with an apparently normal karyotype, the translocation can be detectable at the molecular level by Southern blotting, PCR, or FISH (105–107).

ABL encodes a tyrosine kinase (see Chapter 4) and was first identified within a transforming retrovirus (see Table 1) where it becomes fused to viral *gag* sequences. The t(9;22) translocation juxtaposes *BCR* and *ABL* in a 5′ to 3′ configuration, again resulting in chimeric product. Although the breakpoints on chromosome 22 are relatively clustered, those on chromosome 9 are distributed over about 50 kb and can occur upstream or downstream of the 1A exon of *ABL*. In about 95% of CML, RNA splicing generates a transcript that fuses *BCR* sequences to exon 2 of *ABL* resulting in a 210 kd BCR–ABL fusion protein (p210) lacking the normal amino terminus of ABL.

In the remaining cases and in most Ph1-positive ALLs, the breakpoint occurs more proximally in the *BCR* gene resulting in a shorter fusion protein, p185 (108). Both fusion proteins are constitutively active tyrosine kinases and show increased activity relative to c-ABL. It is important to note that in contrast to the *Ig/MYC* translocations, the normal *ABL* allele is not down-regulated in Ph1-positive cells and a normal 145 kDa protein is expressed as well as the fusion protein (109, 110).

5.4.2 The 11q23 breakpoint cluster

Several lymphoblastic and myeloblastic leukaemias have cytogenetically visible rearrangements affecting chromosome 11q23. The most frequent and first described abnormality is the t(4;11)(q21;q23) translocation in childhood ALL, but approximately 90% of infantile monoblastic AMLs, 70% of infantile ALLs, and 60% of infantile AMLs have different 11q23 abnormalities. Although they all involve 11q23, as many as 40 different chromosome segments may participate in these exchanges (111; and J. Rowley, personal communication). Most of them seem to be reciprocal translocations as judged by FISH analyses (112, 113).

The common gene on chromosome 11q23 has been called *MLL* (for mixed lineage leukaemia or myeloid/lymphoid leukaemia) but is also known as *ALL1*, *HRX*, or *HTRX1*, the latter names deriving from the homologies with the *Drosophila* trithorax gene (*TRX*) (78, 111). MLL and TRX contain a series of zinc-finger motifs and the possibility that MLL is a mammalian homeobox gene regulator might explain its involvement in malignancies derived from so many different haematopoietic lineages. The *MLL* breakpoints are clustered in an 8.3 kb region between exons 8 and 11 and in all cases studied so far, the translocations generate fusion proteins that retain essentially the same region of MLL (114–117). Removal of the amino terminus of MLL may therefore be more important than the gene to which it is fused.

5.4.3 The *PML1–RARA* translocation in acute promyelocytic leukaemia

The acute form of promyelocytic leukaemia (APL) is associated with a t(15;17)(q21;q11–22) translocation which juxtaposes the retinoic acid receptor α gene (*RARA*) on chromosome 17q and a previously unknown gene on chromosome 15 called *PML1* (94, 118). Breaks in the receptor gene occur within the first intron and there are two major breakpoint clusters in *PML1*, generating different PML1–RARα fusion proteins, designated L and S. Although both of the derivative chromosomes have the potential to generate a product, it is unclear whether the reciprocal fusion, in which the amino terminus of the receptor is joined to the carboxy terminus of PML1, plays any role in APL. In normal cells PML1 is localized in discrete subnuclear bodies, designated PODs (for PML-related oncogenic domains) but this pattern is disrupted in APL cells. However, treatment with retinoic acid can relocalize the PML1–RARα fusion protein to the PODs (119). Interestingly, retinoic acid is known to induce clinical remission in PML patients presumably by promoting the differentiation of the leukaemic cells beyond the promyelocytic stage (120, 121). Although the function of PML1 has yet to be elucidated, its structure suggests that it will play some role in transcriptional regulation.

5.4.4 Other gene fusions

Around 30% of pre-B acute lymphoblastic leukaemias (pre-B-ALL) have a translocation, t(1;19) (q23;p13), that fuses the homeobox gene *PBX* on chromosome 1 with part of the *E2A* gene on chromosome 19. The latter encodes bHLH transcription factors and takes its name from the E2 enhancer domain in the immunoglobulin kappa gene. A fusion protein is generated in which the bHLH region of E2A is replaced by the homeodomain of PBX (77, 122, 123). In pro-B-ALL, the t(17;19) translocation fuses E2A with the bZIP protein HLF creating a chimeric transcription factor (124, 125).

A number of translocations observed in solid tumours also create hybrid transcription factors. These are exemplified by the rearrangements of the *EWS* gene which was originally identified because of its involvement in the t(11;22) translocation found in Ewing's sarcoma (126, 127). *EWS*, located on chromosome 22q12, is a highly conserved gene that encodes a 656 amino acid protein with three glycine-rich segments and a domain homologous to RNA-binding proteins. In Ewing's sarcoma, the amino terminal region of EWS, including the glycine-rich domain, is fused to the DNA binding domain of FLI1, an ETS-related transcription factor that was first identified as a target for proviral insertion in erythroleukaemias (see Table 2). The functional consequences of this fusion are discussed in Chapter 6. Several distinct translocations have also been observed involving EWS and other ETS-related proteins, such as ERG in t(21;22) and ETV1 in t(7;22), as well as fusions to the DNA binding domains of other types of transcription factors, such as ATF1 and WT1 (78, 128).

The same theme prevails in translocations detected in three types of mesenchymal tumour: myxoid liposarcoma (MLPS), synovial sarcoma, and rhabdomyosarcoma (129). In MLPS, the t(12;16) translocation fuses *CHOP* on 12q13.1 to the amino terminal domain of a gene called *TLS* (translocated in liposarcoma), also known as *FUS* (130–132). *CHOP* is a transcription factor that is induced by DNA damage and can cause growth arrest by blocking the interaction between DNA and CEBP-like transcription factors. *TLS* is highly homologous with *EWS*. In the chimeric protein, only the leucine zipper domain of *CHOP* is retained and rather than acting as a transcription inhibitor the fusion protein becomes a transcriptional activator (78). *TLS* has also been shown to fuse with *ERG* in AML suggesting that its effect is not lineage restricted.

Further involvement of the ETS-family is apparent in chronic myelomonocytic leukaemia where the t(5;12)(q33;p13) translocation results in a fusion between the tyrosine kinase domain of platelet-derived growth factor receptor β (*PDGFRβ*) on chromosome 5 and a novel *ETS*-like gene *TEL*, on chromosome 12 (78, 133). The break on chromosome 5 eliminates the first 1766 nucleotides of the normal PDGFRβ transcript and the ETS-domain of TEL is lost upon translocation (Chapter 6). *TEL* has also been shown to participate in translocations with *ABL* (134).

One final example that illustrates the diversity of chromosomal translocations is the fusion of the *c-RET* proto-oncogene to a regulatory subunit of a protein kinase due to a paracentric inversion of chromosome 10 in papillary thyroid carcinoma (135).

5.5 Oncogene activation by gene amplification

Oncogene amplification has been frequently detected in human tumours and in cultured cancer cells. It is more characteristic of solid tumours and relatively rare in lymphoid malignancies. DNA amplification was first observed cytogenetically as double minute chromosomes (DMs) or homogeneously staining regions (HSRs), but nowadays direct DNA analyses (Southern blotting) or molecular cytogenetic methodologies such as fluorescence *in situ* hybridization (FISH) and comparative genomic hybridization (CGH) can be applied (see ref. 136). DMs are episomal forms of amplified DNA that generally lack centromeres and are unequally distributed between daughter cells at mitosis. Under the microscope they appear as pairs of isodiametric extrachromosomal bodies stainable with all chromatin dyes. There are exceptions to this rule when centromeric segments participate in the amplification process (137, 138) but in general the number of DMs in a given population of cells can vary between metaphases and with passage number. In contrast, HSRs are chromosomally integrated forms of amplified DNA. They represent either the replacement of the normal chromosome banding pattern with an extended region of homogeneous staining or the insertion of such a region into an otherwise normally banded chromosome. DMs and HSRs tend to be mutually exclusive and are potentially interchangeable manifestations of the amplified DNA. Thus, DMs can potentially integrate into distant chromosomal sites to generate heritable HSRs.

Benner *et al.* (139) reviewed published cytogenetic analyses of tumours taken directly from patients to determine the percentage of DMs versus HSRs and to compare this ratio with data found in human tumour cell lines. Of the 200 human tumours reviewed, 91% contained DMs only, 6.5% contained HSRs, and 2.5% contained both. In 109 cell lines, 60.6% contained DMs, 26.6% contained HSRs, and 18% contained both. In epithelial solid neoplasia DMs and HSRs were found in 40% of breast adenocarcinomas, 17% of NSCLC, 18% of stomach and oesophagus, and 15% of uterine carcinomas.

Since DNA amplification does not occur in normal cells, it is generally assumed that the amplified DNA is maintained as a result of selection. One of the best examples would be the amplification of drug resistance genes, such as DHFR; the amplification is only maintained as long as the selective pressure is on (i.e. in the continued presence of the drug). This suggests that oncogene amplification must convey a selective advantage on the tumours in which it occurs, otherwise it would be lost (140). For example, we have observed *MYC* amplification in a rare and highly malignant (leukaemic) form of human plasma cell tumour that is not apparent in solid plasmacytomas (141). Similarly, in the mouse osteosarcoma cell line, SEWA, which carries an amplification of *MYC* (reviewed in ref. 137), there is a positive correlation between the degree of *MYC* amplification and tumorigenicity *in vivo* (142). Cells selected for growth as solid tumours *in vivo* (as opposed to ascites) or for adherent growth *in vitro* contained substantially fewer copies of the *MYC* amplicon (143).

The overwhelming majority of oncogene amplifications found so far in human tumours affect the *MYC* family (144). In small cell lung cancer (SCLC) for example, all three members of the *MYC* family, *c-*, *N-*, and *L-MYC*, can be involved and *MYC* amplification is associated with a more invasive and more metastatic phenotype (145). Another well studied example is the amplification of *N-MYC* in neuroblastoma, the most frequent solid tumour in childhood. Amplification of *N-MYC* is associated with the late stages of neuroblastoma and with poor prognosis (146). It appears to be the paternal allele of *N-MYC* that is preferentially amplified suggesting that genomic imprinting might have some role in influencing neuroblastoma progression (147).

Some neuroblastomas have been found to have DMs containing sequences from chromosome 12q13–14 rather than *N-MYC*. A likely target would be the human homologue of *MDM2* (mouse double minute), which was originally identified because of its presence on a DM, and whose product associates with and negatively regulates p53 (see Chapter 9). Indeed, amplification of this region of chromosome 12 is relatively common in gliomas and sarcomas (80, 148). However, not all examples of the amplification involve *MDM2* and recent evidence also implicates the gene encoding the cyclin-dependent kinase CDK4 (80).

Uncertainty over which amplified gene is the most significant is a recurrent theme as many of the amplification units observed in human tumours encompass several candidate oncogenes. A typical example would be the amplification unit on chromosome 11q13 that occurs in breast cancer, squamous cell carcinoma of the head and neck, lung, and oesophagus, and in bladder tumours (reviewed in ref. 149). The amplification often extends for over 1.5 megabase pairs of DNA and includes two bona fides oncogenes, *FGF3* and *FGF4*, that are targets for retroviral insertion in MMTV-induced mouse mammary tumours (see Table 2). It also includes the *BCL1* locus that is translocated in B cell lymphomas (see Table 3) and its target oncogene *CCND1* (cyclin D1), as well as the *EMS1* gene that encodes the human homologue of cortactin (149). Current evidence suggests that *CCND1* is the critical player on the amplified DNA, since unlike *FGF3* and *FGF4*, its expression is increased as a consequence of amplification.

The other major targets for amplification are the genes encoding the EGF receptor (*ERBB1/HER1*) and the related *ERBB2/HER2* (see Chapter 3). Both genes are amplified in breast cancer as well as other major malignancies but *ERBB2* has attracted a great deal of interest, partly because of its association with ER-negative breast cancers and poor prognosis and partly as a potential target for therapy (150).

6. Point mutations

The classic example of oncogene activation by point mutation is that of the *H-*, *K-*, and *N-RAS* oncogenes. The activating mutations are generally single amino acid substitutions at positions 12, 13, and 61 that give rise to mutant RAS proteins with reduced intrinsic GTPase activity compared to the wild-type protein (see Chapter 5). Such mutations occur at a high frequency in a large variety of human tumours, including carcinoma of the colon, pancreas, and bladder, as well as melanomas, and various types of leukaemia (151). Interestingly, the same mutations occur in tumours induced experimentally with chemical carcinogens (152) suggesting a potential link between *RAS* mutations and environmental insults.

Although point mutations are more commonly associated with loss of function mutations in tumour suppressor genes (see Chapter 10), there are two other notable examples of activating point mutations in a cellular proto-oncogene. The first is the so-called *NEU* gene which sustains point mutations in chemically-induced neuroblastomas in the rat (153). *NEU* is in fact the rat homologue of the *ERBB2/HER2* gene and the mutation in the transmembrane domain activates the receptor. The second example also involves a tyrosine kinase receptor, encoded by the *RET* gene (Chapter 3). Mutations in *RET* are associated with both inherited and sporadic forms of endocrine tumours, such as medullary thyroid cancer, Hirschsprung disease, and multiple endocrine neoplasia types 2A and 2B (154).

7. Concluding remarks

It is now generally accepted that single changes in multiple genes participate in the evolution of the neoplastic phenotype. However, in considering the variety of mechanisms that can activate cellular oncogenes and inactivate tumour suppressors, it is important to stress that the selection is for the phenotype and not the mechanisms that give rise to it. Thus, one of the remarkable and encouraging features of the field is the extent to which the same or similar genes are implicated in tumours of different types, of different aetiology, or from different species. An example would be the convergence of DNA tumour virus oncoproteins on the pRb and p53 pathways (Fig. 1). Another would be the fact that oncogenes originally discovered within the genomes of animal retroviruses, such as *RAS*, *MYC*, and *ABL* (Table 1) are directly implicated in human cancers where they are activated by point mutation, gene amplification, and chromosome translocation. Similarly, several of the new genes identified at sites of retroviral integration (Table 2) feature prominently among the targets of chromosomal abnormalities and in the modern age of molecular cytogenetics, such abnormalities continue to provide a rich source of information on the location and identity of oncogenes and tumour suppressors (Table 3).

Many of the events that activate cellular oncogenes are simple accidents of fate, such as the randomness of retrovirus integration, mistakes in the replicative strategy of the virus, or in the recombinases responsible for gene rearrangements. Others may reflect environmental insults or genetically inherited traits that make certain individuals more susceptible to such errors. But despite their accidental nature, the various aberrations discussed in this chapter highlight three major ways in which a normal gene can become 'oncogenic'. The simplest is where an otherwise normal gene is expressed at an inappropriately high level, for example as a result of DNA amplification. The second is where an otherwise normal gene is expressed in an inappropriate cell type, for example as a consequence of translocation to an active chromosomal locus. The third is where the function of the gene product is perturbed. There are of course many variations to this latter theme, ranging from simple point mutations to gene fusions, from altered activity to altered substrate specificity, and more.

It therefore appears that the molecular findings have fully vindicated Leslie Foulds' description of tumour progression in the late 1950s (54). He spoke about progression as a series of changes in several 'unit characteristics' that were capable of assorting independently of each other, with the result that progression could proceed along several pathways, in different tumours of the same kind. The proviral insertions, gene amplifications, chromosomal translocations, and other perturbations described in this chapter therefore constitute real examples of such 'unit characteristics' whose biochemical and physiological consequences are discussed in other chapters.

References

1. zur Hausen, H. (1991) Viruses in human cancers. *Science*, **254**, 1167.
2. Klein, G. (1980) Viral oncology. Raven Press, New York.
3. Tooze, J. (1980) Molecular biology of tumor viruses. Cold Spring Harbor Laboratory, Cold Spring Harbor, New York.
4. Del Prete, G., De Carli, M., D'Elios, M. M., Fleckenstein, I. M., Fickenscher, H., Fleckenstein, B., *et al.* (1994) Polyclonal B cell activation induced by herpesvirus saimiri-transformed human CD4+ T cell clones. Role for membrane TNF-alpha/TNF-alpha receptors and CD2/CD58 interactions. *J. Immunol.*, **153**, 4872.
5. Jones, D., Lee, L., Liu, J. L., Kung, H. J., and Tillotson, J. K. (1992) Marek disease virus encodes a basic-leucine zipper gene resembling the *fos/jun* oncogenes that is highly expressed in lymphoblastoid tumors. *Proc. Natl. Acad. Sci. USA*, **89**, 4042.
6. Robinson, W. S. (1994) Molecular events in the pathogenesis of hepadnavirus-associated hepatocellular carcinoma. *Annu. Rev. Med.*, **45**, 297.
7. Hsu, T., Moroy, T., Etiemble, J., Louise, A., Trepo, C., Tiollais, P., *et al.* (1988) Activation of *c-myc* by woodchuck hepatitis virus insertion in hepatocellular carcinoma. *Cell*, **55**, 627.
8. Wei, Y., Ponzetto, A., Tiollais, P., and Buendia, M. A. (1992) Multiple rearrangements and activated expression of *c-myc* induced by woodchuck hepatitis virus. *Res. Virol.*, **143**, 89.
9. Dejean, A., Bougueleret, L., Grzeschik, K. H., and Tiollais, P. (1986) Hepatitis B virus DNA integration in a sequence homologous to v-erb-A and steroid receptor genes in a hepatocellular carcinoma. *Nature*, **322**, 70.
10. Wang, J., Zindy, F., Chenivesse, X., Lamas, E., Henglein, B., and Brechot, C. (1992) Modification of *cyclin A* expression by hepatitis B virus DNA integration in a hepatocellular carcinoma. *Oncogene*, **7**, 1653.
11. Chisari, F. V., Klopchin, K., Moriyama, T., Pasquinelli, C., Dunsford, H. A., Sell, S., *et al.* (1989) Molecular pathogenesis of hepatocellular carcinoma in hepatitis B virus transgenic mice. *Cell*, **59**, 1145.

12. Koike, K., Moriya, K., Iino, S., Yotsuyanagi, H., Endo, Y., Miyamura, T., *et al.* (1994) High-level expression of hepatitis B virus *HBx* gene and hepatocarcinogenesis in transgenic mice. *Hepatology*, **19**, 810.

13. Wei, Y., Etiemble, J., Fourel, G., Vivitski-Trepo, L., and Beundia, M. A. (1995) Hepadna virus integration generates virus-cell cotranscripts carrying 3′ truncated X genes in human and woodchuck liver tumors. *J. Med. Virol.*, **45**, 82.

14. Nilson, L. A. and DiMaio, D. (1993) Platelet-derived growth factor receptor can mediate tumorigenic transformation by the bovine papillomavirus E5 protein. *Mol. Cell. Biol.*, **13**, 4137.

15. Mosialos, G., Birkenbach, M., Yalamanchili, R., VanArsdale, T., Ware, C., and Kieff, E. (1995) The Epstein–Barr virus transforming protein LMP1 engages signaling proteins for the tumor necrosis factor receptor family. *Cell*, **80**, 389.

16. Courtneidge, S. A. and Smith, A. E. (1983) Polyoma virus transforming protein associates with the product of the *c-src* cellular gene. *Nature*, **303**, 435.

17. Kornbluth, S., Sudol, M., and Hanafusa, H. (1987) Association of polyoma middle-T antigen with *c-yes* protein. *Nature*, **325**, 171.

18. Biesinger, B., Tsygankov, A. Y., Fickenscher, H., Emmrich, F., Fleckenstein, B., Bolen, J. B., *et al.* (1995) The product of the Herpesvirus saimiri open reading frame 1 (tip) interacts with T cell-specific kinase p56lck in transformed cells. *J. Biol. Chem.*, **270**, 4729.

19. Grossman, S. R., Johannsen, E., Tong, X., Yalamanchili, R., and Kieff, E. (1994) The Epstein–Barr virus nuclear antigen 2 transactivator is directed to response elements by the J kappa recombination signal binding protein. *Proc. Natl. Acad. Sci. USA*, **91**, 7568.

20. Ling, P. D., Hsieh, J. J., Ruf, I. K., Rawlins, D. R., and Hayward, S. D. (1994) EBNA-2 upregulation of Epstein–Barr virus latency promoters and the cellular CD23 promoter utilizes a common targeting intermediate CBF1. *J. Virol.*, **68**, 5375.

21. Jung, J. U., Stager, M. and Desrosiers, R. C. (1994) Virus-encoded cyclin. *Mol. Cell. Biol.*, **14**, 7235.

22. Lane, D. and Crawford, L. (1979) T-antigen is bound to a host protein in SV40-transformed cells. *Nature*, **278**, 261.

23. Sarnow, P., Ho, Y. S., Williams, J., and Levine, A. J. (1982) Adenovirus E1b-58kD tumor antigen and SV40 large tumor antigens are physically associated with the same 54 kD cellular protein in transformed cells. *Cell*, **28**, 387.

24. Werness, B. A., Levine, A. J., and Howley, P. M. (1990) Association of human papillolmavirus types 16 and 18 E6 proteins with p53. *Science*, **248**, 76.

25. Farmer, G., Bargonetti, J., Zhu, H., Friedman, P., Prywes, R., and Prives, C. (1992) Wild-type p53 activates transcription *in vitro*. *Nature*, **358**, 83.

26. Yew, P. R., Liu, X., and Berk, A. J. (1994) Adenovirus E1b oncoprotein tethers a transcriptional repression domain to p53. *Genes Dev.*, **8**, 190.

27. Scheffner, M., Werness, B. A., Huibregste, J. M., Levine, A. J., and Howley, P. M. (1990) The E6 oncoprotein encoded by human papillomavirus types 16 and 18 promotes the degradation of p53. *Cell*, **63**, 1129.

28. DeCaprio, J. A., Ludlow, J. W., Figge, J., Shew, J. Y., Huang, C. M., Lee, W. H., *et al.* (1988) SV40 large tumor antigen forms a specific complex with the product of the retinoblastoma susceptibility gene. *Cell*, **54**, 275.

29. Whyte, P., Buchkovich, K. J., Horowitz, J. M., Friend, S. H., Raybuck, M., Weinberg, R. A., *et al.* (1988) Association between an oncogene and an anti-oncogene: the adenovirus E1A proteins bind to the retinoblastoma gene product. *Nature*, **334**, 124.

30. Munger, K., Werness, B. A., Dyson, N., Phelps, W. C., Harlow, E., and Howley, P. M. (1989) Complex formation of human papillomavirus E7 proteins with the retinoblastoma tumor suppressor gene product. *EMBO J.*, **8**, 4099.

31. Chellappan, S., Kraus, V. B., Kroger, B., Munger, K., Howley, P. M., Phelps, W. C., *et al.* (1992) Adenovirus E1A, simian virus 40 tumor antigen, and human papillomavirus E7 protein share the capacity to disrupt the interaction between transcription factor E2F and the retinoblastoma gene product. *Proc. Natl. Acad. Sci. USA*, **89**, 4549.

32. Lundblad, J. R., Kwok, R. P. S., Laurance, M. E., Harter, M. L., and Goodman, R. H. (1995) Adenoviral E1A associated protein p300 as a functional homologue of the transcriptional co-activator CBP. *Nature*, **374**, 85.

33. Henderson, S., Rowe, M., Gregory, C. D., Croom-Carter, D., Wang, F., Longnecker, R., *et al.* (1991) Induction of *bcl-2* expression by Epstein–Barr virus latent membrane protein 1 protects infected B-cells from programmed cell death. *Cell*, **65**, 1107.

34. Chiou, S. K., Tseng, C. C., Rao, K., and White, E. (1994) Functional complementation of the adenovirus E1B 19-kilodalton protein with *Bcl-2* in the inhibition of apoptosis in infected cells. *J. Virol.*, **68**, 6553.

35. Varmus, H. (1989) An historical overview of oncogenes. In *Oncogenes and the molecular origins of cancer* (ed. R. A. Weinberg). Cold Spring Harbor Laboratory, Cold Spring Harbor, New York.

36. Stehelin, D., Varmus, H. E., Bishop, J. M., and Vogt, P. K. (1976) DNA related to the transforming gene(s) of avian sarcoma viruses is present in normal avian DNA. *Nature*, **260**, 170.

37. Hayward, W. S., Neel, B. G., and Astrin, S. M. (1981) Activation of a cellular *onc* gene by promoter insertion in ALV-induced lymphoid leukosis. *Nature*, **290**, 475.

38. Payne, G. S., Bishop, J. M., and Varmus, H. E. (1982) Multiple arrangements of viral DNA and an activated host oncogene in bursal lymphomas. *Nature*, **295**, 209.

39. Clurman, B. E. and Hayward, W. S. (1988) Insertional activation of proto-oncogenes previously identified a viral oncogenes. In *Cellular oncogene activation* (ed. G. Klein). Marcel Dekker, Inc., New York.

40. Peters, G. (1990) Oncogenes at viral integration sites. *Cell Growth Diff.*, **1**, 503.

41. Jonkers, J. and Berns, A. (1996) Retroviral insertional mutagenesis as a strategy to identify cancer genes. *Biochim. Biophys. Acta*, **1287**, 29.

42. Nusse, R. and Varmus, H. E. (1982) Many tumors induced by the mouse mammary tumor virus contain a provirus integrated in the same region of the host genome. *Cell*, **31**, 99.

43. Nusse, R., van Ooyen, A., Cox, D., Fung, Y. K. T., and Varmus, H. (1984) Mode of proviral activation of a putative mammary oncogene (*int-1*) on mouse chromosome 15. *Nature*, **307**, 131.

44. Peters, G., Brookes, S., Smith, R., and Dickson, C. (1983) Tumorigenesis by mouse mammary tumor virus: evidence for a common region for provirus integration in mammary tumors. *Cell*, **33**, 367.

45. Dickson, C., Smith, R., Brookes, S., and Peters, G. (1984) Tumorigenesis by mouse mammary tumor virus: proviral activation of a cellular gene in the common integration region int-2. *Cell*, **37**, 529.

46. Peters, G. (1991) Inappropriate expression of growth factor genes in tumors induced by mouse mammary tumor virus. *Semin. Virol.*, **2**, 319.

47. Cuypers, H. T., Selten, G., Quint, W., Zijlstra, M., Robanus Maandag, E., Boelens, W., *et al.* (1984) Murine leukemia virus-induced T-cell lymphomagenesis: integration of proviruses in a distinct chromosomal region. *Cell*, **37**, 141.

48. Haupt, Y., Alexander, W. S., Barri, G., Klinken, S. P., and Adams, J. M. (1991) Novel zinc finger gene implicated as *myc* collaborator by retrovirally accelerated lymphomagenesis in *Eμ-myc* transgenic mice. *Cell*, **65**, 753.

49. van Lohuizen, M., Verbeek, S., Scheijen, N., Wientjens, E., van der Gulden, H., and Berns, A. (1991) Identification of cooperating oncogenes in *Eμ-myc* transgenic mice. *Cell*, **65**, 737.

50. Arnold, J. (1879) Beobachtungen über kernteilungen in der zellen der geschwülste wichows. *Arch. Pathol. Anat.*, **78**, 279.

51. Boveri, T. (1914) Zur frage der enstehung maligner tumoren. Gustva Fischer Verlag, Jena.

52. Andres, A. (1932) Zellstudien an Menschenkrebs, der chromosomale bestand in primärtumor und in der metastase. *Z. Zellforsch. Mikrosk. Anat.*, **16**, 88.

53. Rous, P. and Beard, J. W. (1935) The progression to carcinoma of virus induced rabbit papilloma (Shope). *J. Exp. Med.*, **62**, 523.

54. Foulds, L. (1954) The experimental study of tumor progression: a review. *Cancer Res.*, **14**, 327.

55. Klein, G. and Klein, E. (1985) Evolution of tumours and the impact of molecular oncology. *Nature*, **315**, 190.

56. Nowell, P. C. and Hungerford, D. A. (1960) Chromosome studies on normal and leukemic human leukocytes. *J. Natl. Cancer Inst.*, **25**, 85.

57. German, J. (1969) Chromosome breakage syndromes. *Birth Defects*, **5**, 117.

58. Caspersson, J., Zech, L., Johansson, C., and Modest, E. J. (1970) Identification of human chromosomes by DNA binding fluorescing agents. *Chromosoma*, **30**, 215.

59. Klein, G. (1983) Specific chromosomal translocations and the genesis of B-cell derived tumors in mice and men. *Cell*, **32**, 311.

60. Klein, G. (1993) Multistep evolution of B-cell derived tumors in humans and rodents. *Gene*, **135**, 189.

61. Imreh, S., Wang, Y., Panda, C. K., Babonits, M., Axelson, H., Silva, S., *et al.* (1994) Hypersomy of chromosome 15 with retrovirally rearranged *c-myc*, loss of germline *c-myc* and *IgK/c-myc* juxtaposition in a macrophage-monocytic tumour line. *Eur. J. Cancer*, **30A**, 994.

62. Joos, S., Falk, M. H., Lichter, P., Haluska, F. G., Henglein, B., Lenoir, G. M., *et al.* (1992) Variable breakpoints in Burkitt lymphoma cells with chromosomal t(8;14) translocation separate *c-myc* and the *IgH* locus up to several hundred kb. *Hum. Mol. Genet.*, **1**, 625.

63. Pelicci, P. G., Knowles, D. M., Magrath, I., and Dalla-Favera, R. (1986) Chromosomal breakpoints and structural alterations of the *c-myc* locus differ in endemic and sporadic forms of Burkitt's lymphoma. *Proc. Natl. Acad. Sci. USA*, **83**, 2984.

64. Saglio, G., Grazia Borello, M., Guerassio, A., Sozzi, G., Serra, A., *et al.* (1993) Preferential clustering of chromosomal breakpoints in Burkitt lymphomas and L3 type acute lymphoblastic leukemias with a t(8;14) translocation. *Genes Chrom. Cancer*, **8**, 1.

65. Shiramizu, B. and Magrath, I. (1990) Localization of breakpoints by polymerase chain reactions in Burkitt's lymphoma with t(8;14) translocation. *Blood*, **75**, 1848.

66. Dalla-Favera, R., Bregni, M., Erikson, J., Patterson, D., Gallo, R. C., and Croce, C. M. (1982) Human *c-myc* onc gene is located on the region of chromosome 8 that is translocated in Burkitt lymphoma cells. *Proc. Natl. Acad. Sci. USA*, **79**, 7824.

67. Shtivelman, E., Henglein, B., Groitl, P., Lipp, M., and Bishop, J. M. (1989) Identification of a human transcription unit affected by the variant chromosomal translocations 2;8 and 8;22 of Burkitt lymphoma. *Proc. Natl. Acad. Sci. USA*, **86**, 3257.

68. Zeidler, R., Joos, S., Delecluse, H. J., Klobeck, G., Vuillame, M., Lenoir, G. M., *et al.* (1994) Breakpoints of Burkitt's lymphoma t(8;22) translocations map within a distance of 300 kb downstream of *MYC*. *Genes Chrom. Cancer*, **9**, 282.

69. Klein, G. (1989) Multiple phenotypic consequences of the *Ig/Myc* translocation in B-cell-derived tumors. *Genes Chrom. Cancer*, **1**, 3.

70. Gauwerky, C. E. and Croce, C. M. (1993) Chromosomal translocations in leukemia. *Semin. Cancer Biol.*, **4**, 333.

71. Ohno, S., Babonits, M., Wiener, F., Spira, J., and Klein, G. (1969) Non-random chromosome changes involving *Ig* gene chromosomes Nos 12 and 6 in pristane induced mouse plasmacytomas. *Cell*, **16**, 1001.

72. Potter, M. and Wiener, F. (1992) Plasmacytogenesis in mice: model of neoplastic development dependent upon chromosomal translocations. *Carcinogenesis*, **13**, 1681.

73. Silva, S., Wang, Y., Babonits, M., Axelson, H., Wiener, F., and Klein, G. (1992) An exceptional mouse plasmacytoma with new *Kappa/N-myc* T(6;12)(C1;B) translocation expresses *N-myc* but not *c-myc*. *Curr. Top. Microbiol. Immunol.*, **182**, 251.

74. Axelson, H., Wang, Y., Silva, S., Mattei, M. G., and Klein, G. (1994) Juxtaposition of N-myc and Ig kappa through a reciprocal t(6;12) translocation in a mouse plasmacytoma. *Genes Chrom. Cancer*, **11**, 85.

75. Wiener, F., Babonits, M., Spira, G., Klein, G., and Bazin, H. (1982) Non-random chromosomal changes involving chromosome 6 and 7 in spontaneous rat immunocytomas. *Int. J. Cancer*, **29**, 431.

76. Pear, W., Ingvarsson, S., Steffen, D., Münke, M., Francke, U., Bazin, H., *et al.* (1986) Multiple chromosomal rearrangements in a spontaneously arising t(6;7) rat immunocytoma juxtapose *c-myc* and immunoglobulin heavy chain sequences. *Proc. Natl. Acad. Sci. USA*, **83**, 3676.

77. Korsmeyer, S. J. (1992) Chromosomal translocations in lymphoid malignancies reveal novel proto-oncogenes. *Annu. Rev. Immunol.*, **10**, 785.

78. Rabbitts, T. H. (1994) Chromosomal translocations in human cancer. *Nature*, **372**, 143.

79. Harris, N. L., Jaffe, E. S., Stein, H., Banks, P. M., Chan, J. K. C., Cleary, M. L., *et al.* (1994) A revised European–American classification of lymphoid neoplasms: a proposal from the international lymphoma study group. *Blood*, **84**, 1361.

80. Hall, M. and Peters, G. (1996) Genetic alterations of cyclins, cyclin-dependent kinases, and Cdk inhibitors in human cancer. *Adv. Cancer Res.*, **68**, 67.

81. Withers, D. A., Harvey, R. C., Faust, J. B., Melnyk, O., Carey, K., and Meeker, T. C. (1991) Characterization of a candidate *bcl-1* gene. *Mol. Cell. Biol.*, **11**, 4846.

82. Tsujimoto, Y., Finger, L., Yunis, J. J., Nowell, P. C., and Croce, C. M. (1984) Cloning the chromosome breakpoint of neoplastic B-cells with the t(14;18) chromosome translocation. *Science*, **226**, 1097.

83. Yunis, J. J., Frizzera, G., Oken, M. M., McKenna, J., Theologides, A., and Arnesen, M. (1987) Multiple recurrent genomic defects in follicular lymphoma: a possible model for cancer. *N. Engl. J. Med.*, **316**, 79.

84. Hockenbery, D., Nunez, G., Milliman, C., Schreiber, R. D., and Korsmeyer, S. J. (1990) Bcl-2 is an inner mitochondrial membrane protein that blocks programmed cell death. *Nature*, **348**, 334.

85. Offit, K., Jhanwar, S., Ebrahim, S. A. D., Filippa, D., Clarkson, F. B. D., and Chaganti, R. S. K. (1989) t(3;22)(q27;q11): a novel translocation associated with diffuse non-Hodgkin's lymphoma. *Blood*, **74**, 1876.

86. Bastard, C., Tilley, H., Lenormand, B., Bigorgne, C., Boulet, D., Kunlin, A., *et al.* (1992) Translocations involving band 3q27 and Ig gene regions in non-Hodgkin lymphoma. *Blood*, **79**, 2527.

87. Ohno, H., Akasaka, T., Ohmura, K., Nakamura, T., Gohma, I., Masuya, M., *et al.* (1994) Non-Hodgkin's lymphomas with chromosomal translocations involving 3q27 band and immunoglobulin gene loci: report of two cases. *Cancer Genet. Cytogenet.*, **72**, 33.

88. Kerckaert, J. P., Deweindt, C., Tilly, H., Quief, S., Lecocq, G., and Bastard, C. (1993) *LAZ3*, a novel zinc-finger encoding gene, is disrupted by recurring chromosome 3q27 translocations in human lymphomas. *Nature Genet.*, **5**, 66.

89. Ye, B. H., Lista, F., Lo Coco, F., Knowles, D. M., Offit, K., Chaganti, R. S. K., *et al.* (1993) Alterations of a zinc finger-encoding gene, *BCL-6*, in diffuse large-cell lymphoma. *Science*, **262**, 747.

90. Bernard, O. A. and Berger, R. (1995) Molecular basis of 11q23 rearrangements in hematopoietic malignant proliferation. *Genes Chrom. Cancer*, **13**, 75.

91. Lo Coco, F., Ye, B. H., Lista, F., Corradini, P., Offit, K., Knowles, D. M., *et al.* (1994) Rearrangements of the *BCL6* gene in diffuse large cell non-Hodgkin's lymphoma. *Blood*, **83**, 1757.

92. Leiden, J. M. (1993) Transcriptional regulation of T cell receptor genes. *Annu. Rev. Immunol.*, **11**, 539.

93. Shima, E. A., Le Beau, M. M., McKeithan, T. W., Minowada, J., Showe, L. C., Mak, T. W., *et al.* (1986) Gene encoding the a chain of the T-cell receptor is moved immediately downstream of *c-myc* in a chromosomal 8;14 translocation in a cell line from a human T-cell leukemia. *Proc. Natl. Acad. Sci. USA*, **83**, 3439.

94. Nichols, J. and Nimer, S. D. (1992) Transcription factors, translocations and leukemia. *Blood*, **80**, 2953.

95. Brown, L., Cheng, J.-T., Chen, Q., Siciliano, M. J., Crist, W., Buchanan, G., *et al.* (1990) Site-specific recombination of the *tal-1* gene is a common occurrence in human T-cell leukemia. *EMBO J.*, **9**, 3343.

96. Mellentin, J. D., Smith, S. D., and Cleary, M. L. (1989) *lyl-1*, a novel gene altered by chromosomal translocations in T cell leukemia, codes for a protein with a helix–loop–helix DNA binding motif. *Cell*, **58**, 77.

97. McGuire, E. A., Hockett, R. D., Pollock, K. M., Bartholdi, M. F., O'Brien, S. J., and Korsmeyer, S. J. (1989) The t(11;14)(p15;q11) in a T cell acute lymphoblastic leukemia cell line activates multiple transcripts including *Ttg*-1, a gene encoding a potential zinc finger protein. *Mol. Cell. Biol.*, **9**, 2124.

98. Boehm, T., Foroni, L., Kaneko, Y., Perutz, M. F., and Rabbitts, T. H. (1991) The rhombotin family of cysteine-rich LIM-domain oncogenes: distinct members are involved in T-cell translocations to human chromosomes 11p15 and 11p13. *Proc. Natl. Acad. Sci. USA*, **88**, 4367.

99. Sanchez-Garcia, I. and Rabbitts, T. H. (1994) The LIM domain: a new structural motif found in zinc-finger-like proteins. *Trends Genet.*, **10**, 315.

100. Wadman, I., Li, J., Bash, R. O., Forster, A., Osada, H., Rabbitts, T. H., *et al.* (1994) Specific *in vivo* association between the bHLH and LIM proteins implicated in human T cell leukemia. *EMBO J.*, **13**, 4831.

101. Burnett, R. C., David, J. C., Harden, A. M., Le Beau, M. M., Rowley, J. D., and Diaz, M. O. (1991) The *LCK* gene is involved in the t(1;7)(p34;q34) in the T-cell acute lymphoblastic leukemia derived cell line HSB-2. *Genes Chrom. Cancer*, **3**, 461.

102. Chan, A. C., Desai, D. M., and Weiss, A. (1994) The role of protein tyrosine kinases and protein tyrosine phosphatases in T-cell antigen receptor signal. *Annu. Rev. Immunol.*, **12**, 555.

103. Sessarego, M., Martinelli, G., Chiamenti, A., Defferrari, R., Fugazza, G., Bruzzone, R., *et al.* (1993) Molecular analysis of six variant Philadelphia chromosome translocations in chronic myeloid leukemia. *Cancer Genet. Cytogenet.*, **67**, 50.

104. Heisterkamp, N., Stephenson, J. R., Groffen, J., Hansen, P. F., de Klein, A., Bartram, C. R., *et al.* (1983) Localization of the *c-abl* oncogene adjacent to a translocation break point in chronic myelogenous leukemia. *Nature*, **306**, 239.

105. Telenius, H., Carter, N. P., Bebb, C. E., Nordenskjold, M., Ponder, B. A., and Tunnacliffe, A. (1992) Degenerate oligonucleotide-primed PCR: general amplification of target DNA by a single degenerate primer. *Genomics*, **13**, 718.

106. Tkatchuk, D. C., Westbrook, C. A., Andeeff, M., Donlon, T. A., Cleary, M. L., Suryanarayan, K., *et al.* (1990) Detection of *bcr–abl* fusion in chronic myelogenous leukemia by *in situ* hybridization. *Science*, **250**, 559.

107. Zhang, J., Meltzer, P., Jenkins, R., Guan, X. Y., and Trent, J. (1993) Application of chromosome microdissection probes for elucidation of *BCR–ABL* fusion and variant Philadelphia chromosome translocations in chronic myelogenous leukemia. *Blood*, **12**, 3356.

108. Kurzrock, R., Gutterman, J. U., and Talpaz, M. (1988) The molecular genetics of Philadelphia chromosome-positive leukemias. *N. Engl. J. Med.*, **319**, 990.

109. Konopka, J. B., Watanage, S. M., Singer, J. W., Collins, S. J., and Witte, O. N. (1985) Cell lines and clinical isolates derived from Ph1-positive chronic myelogenous leukemia patients express c-abl proteins with a common structure alteration. *Proc. Natl. Acad. Sci. USA*, **82**, 1810.

110. Rowley, J. D., Aster, J. C., and Sklar, J. (1993) The clinical applications of new diagnostic technology on the management of cancer patients. *J. Am. Med. Assoc.*, **270**, 2331.

111. Rowley, J. D. (1993) Rearrangements involving chromosome band 11q23 in acute leukemia. *Semin. Cancer Biol.*, **4**, 377.

112. Cherif, D., derSarkissian, H., Derre, J., Tokino, T., Nakamura, Y., and Berger, R. (1992) The 11q23 breakpoint in acute leukemia with t(11;19)(q23;P13) is distal to those t(4;11), t(6;11) and t(9;11). *Genes Chrom. Cancer*, **4**, 107.

113. Kobayashi, H., Espinosa, R., Thirman, M. J., Gill, H. J., Fernald, A. A., Diaz, M. O., *et al.* (1993) Heterogeneity of breakpoints of 11q23 rearrangements in hematologic malignancies identified with fluorescence *in situ* hybridization. *Blood*, **82**, 547.

114. Ziemin-Van Der Poel, S., McCabe, N. R., Gill, H. J., Espinosa, R. I., Patel, Y., Harden, A., *et al.* (1991) Identification of a gene, *MLL*, that spans the breakpoint in 11q13 translocations associated with human leukemias. *Proc. Natl. Acad. Sci. USA*, **88**, 10735.

115. Djabali, M., Selleri, L., Parry, P., Bower, M., Young, B. D., and Evans, G. A. (1992) A trithorax-like gene is interrupted by chromosome 11q23 chromosomal translocations in acute leukemias. *Cell*, **71**, 691.

116. Gu, Y., Nakamura, T., Alder, H., Prasad, R., Canaani, O., Cimino, G., *et al.* (1992) The t(4;11) chromosome translocation of human acute leukemias fuses the ALL-1 gene, related to Drosophila trithorax, to the AF-4 gene. *Cell*, **71**, 701.

117. Tkatchuk, D. C., Kohler, S., and Cleary, M. L. (1992) Involvement of a homolog of Drosophila trithorax by 11q23 chromosomal translocations in acute leukemias. *Cell*, **71**, 691.

118. Gillard, E. F. and Solomon, E. (1993) Acute promyelocytic leukemia and the t(15;17) translocation. *Semin. Cancer Biol.*, **4**, 359.

119. Weis, K., Rambaud, S., Lavau, C., Jansen, J., Carvalho, T., Carmo-Fonseca, M., *et al.* (1994) Retinoic acid regulates aberrant nuclear localization of PML-RARa in acute promyelocytic leukemia cells. *Cell*, **76**, 345.

120. Huang, M. E., Ye, Y. C., Chen, S. R., Chai, J. R., Lu, J. X., Zhoa, L., *et al.* (1988) Use of all-trans retinoic acid in the treatment of acute promyelocytic leukemia. *Blood*, **72**, 567.

121. Castaigne, S., Chomienne, C., Daniel, M. T., Ballerini, P., Berger, R., Fenaux, P., *et al.* (1990) All-trans retinoic acid as a differentiation therapy for acute promyelocytic leukemia: I Clinical results. *Blood*, **76**, 1704.

122. Kamps, M. P., Murre, C., Sun, X. H., and Baltimore, D. (1990) A new homeobox gene contributes the DNA binding domain of the t(1;19) translocation protein in pre-B ALL. *Cell*, **60**, 547.

123. Nourse, J., Mellentin, J. D., Galili, N., Wilkinson, J., Stanbridge, E., Smith, S. D., *et al.* (1990) Chromosomal translocation t(1;19) results in synthesis of a homeobox fusion mRNA that codes for a potential chimeric transcription factor. *Cell*, **60**, 535.

124. Hunger, S. P., Ohyashiki, K., Toyama, K., and Cleary, M. L. (1992) HLF, a novel hepatic bZIP protein, shows altered DNA-binding properties following fusion to E2A in t(17;19) acute lymphoblastic leukemia. *Genes Dev.*, **6**, 1608.

125. Inaba, T., Roberts, W. M., Shapiro, L. H., Jolly, K. W., Raimondi, S. C., Smith, S. D., *et al.* (1992) Fusion of the leucine zipper gene HLF to the E2A gene in human acute B-lineage leukemia. *Science*, **257**, 531.

126. Delattre, O., Zucman, J., Plougastel, B., Desmaze, C., Melot, T., Peter, M., *et al.* (1992) Gene fusion with an ETS DNA-binding domain caused by a chromosome translocation in human tumours. *Nature*, **359**, 162.

127. Delattre, O., Zuchman, J., Melot, T., Garau, X. S., Zucker, J. M., Lenoir, G., *et al.* (1994) The Ewing family of tumors—a subgroup of small-round-cell tumors defined by specific chimeric transcripts. *N. Engl. J. Med.*, **331**, 294.

128. Jeon, I.-S., Davis, J. N., Braun, B. S., Sublett, J. E., Roussel, M. F., Denny, C. T., *et al.* (1995) A variant Ewing's sarcoma translocation (7;22) fuses the *EWS* gene to the ETS gene *ETV1*. *Oncogene*, **10**, 1229.

129. Heim, S. and Mitelman, F. (1987) Cancer cytogenetics. Alan R. Liss, New York.

130. Aman, P., Ron, D., Mandahl, N., Fioretos, T., Heim, S., Arheden, K., *et al.* (1992) Rearrangement of the transcription factor gene *CHOP* in myxoid liposarcomas with t(12;16) (q13;p11). *Genes Chrom. Cancer*, **5**, 278.

131. Crozat, A., Aman, P., Mandahl, N., and Ron, D. (1993) Fusion of *CHOP* to a novel RNA-binding protein in human myxoid liposarcoma. *Nature*, **363**, 640.

132. Rabbitts, T. H., Forster, A., Larson, R., and Nathan, P. (1993) Fusion of the dominant negative transcription regulator *CHOP* with a novel gene *FUS* by translocation t(12;16) in malignant liposarcoma. *Nature Genet.*, **4**, 175.

133. Golub, T. R., Barker, G. F., Bohlnader, S. K., Hiebert, S. W., Ward, D. C., Bray-Ward, P., *et al.* (1994) Fusion of the *TEL* gene on 12p13 to the AML1 gene on 21q22 in acute lymphoblastic leukemia. *Proc. Natl. Acad. Sci. USA*, **92**, 4917.

134. Papadopoulos, P., Ridge, S. A., Boucher, C. A., Stocking, C., and Wiedemann, L. M. (1995) The novel activation of ABL by fusion to and ets-related gene TEL. *Cancer Res.*, **55**, 34.

135. Bongarzone, I., Butti, M. G., Coronelli, S., Borello, M. G., Santoro, M., Mondellini, P., *et al.* (1994) Frequent activation of ret protooncogene by fusion with a new activating gene in papillary thyroid carcinomas. *Cancer Res.*, **54**, 2979.

136. Kallioniemi, O. P., Kallioniemi, A., Sudar, D., Rutovitz, D., Gray, J. W., Waldman, F., *et al.* (1993) Comparative genomic hybridization: a rapid new method for detecting and mapping DNA amplification in tumors. *Semin. Cancer Biol.*, **4**, 41.

137. Levan, G., Stahl, F., and Wettergren, Y. (1992) Gene amplification in the murine SEWA system. *Mutation Res.*, **276**, 285.

138. Hammond, D., Hancock, B., and Goyns, M. H. (1994) Identification of a subclass of double minute chromosomes containing centromere-associated DNA. *Genes Chrom. Cancer*, **10**, 139.

139. Benner, S. E., Wahl, G. M., and von Hoff, D. D. (1991) Double minute chromosomes and homogeneously staining regions in tumours taken directly from patients versus in human tumor cell lines. *Anticancer Drugs*, **2**, 11.

140. Schwab, M., Klempnauer, K. H., Varmus, H., and Bishop, J. M. (1986) Rearrangement at the 5′ end of amplified *c-myc* in human COLO 320 cells is associated with abnormal transcription. *Mol. Cell. Biol.*, **6**, 2752.

141. Sümegi, J., Hedberg, T., Björkholm, M., Godal, T., Mellstadt, H., Nilsson, M. G., *et al.* (1985) Amplification of the c-myc oncogene in human plasma-cell leukemia. *Int. J. Cancer*, **36**, 367.

142. Martinsson, T. F., Stahl, P., Pollwein, A., Wenzel, A., Levan, A., Schwab, M., *et al.* (1988) Tumorigenicity of SEWA murine cells correlates with degree of *c-myc* amplification. *Oncogene*, **3**, 437.

143. Minarovits, J., Steinitz, M., Boldog, F., Imreh, S., Wirschubsky, Z., Ingvarsson, S., *et al.* (1990) Differences in *c-myc* and *pvt-1* amplification SEWA sarcoma sublines selected for adherent or no-adherent growth. *Int. J. Cancer*, **45**, 514.

144. Schwab, M. (1993) Amplification of *N-myc* as a prognostic marker for patients with neuroblastoma. *Semin. Cancer Biol.*, **4**, 13.

145. Makela, T. P., Saksela, K., and Alitalo, K. (1992) Amplification and rearrangement of *L-myc* in human small cell lung cancer (review). *Mutation Res.*, **276**, 307.

146. Brodeur, G. M., Azar, C., Brother, M., Hiemstra, J., Kaufman, B., Marshall, H., *et al.* (1992) Neuroblastoma. Effect of genetic factors on prognosis and treatment. *Cancer*, **70**, 1685.

147. Cheng, J. M., Hiemstra, J. L., Schneider, S. S., Naumova, A., Cheung, N. K., Cohn, S. L., *et al.* (1993) Preferential amplification of the paternal allele of the *N-myc* gene in human neuroblastomas. *Nature Genet.*, **4**, 191.

148. Collins, V. P. (1993) Amplified genes in human gliomas. *Semin. Cancer Biol.*, **4**, 27.

149. Fantl, V., Smith, R., Brookes, S., Dickson, C., and Peters, G. (1993) Chromosome 11q13 abnormalities in human breast cancer. *Cancer Surveys*, **18**, 77.

150. Hynes, N. E. (1993) Amplification and overexpression of the *erbB-2* gene in human tumors: its involvement in tumor development, significance as a prognostic factor, and potential as a target for cancer therapy. *Semin. Cancer Biol.*, **4**, 19.

151. Bos, J. L. (1989) *ras* oncogenes in human cancer: a review. *Cancer Res.*, **49**, 4682.

152. Zarbl, H., Sukumar, S., Arthur, A. V., Martin-Zanca, D., and Barbacid, M. (1985) Direct mutagenesis of Ha-*ras*-1 oncogenes by *N*-nitroso-*N*-methylurea during initiation of mammary carcinogenesis. *Nature*, **315**, 382.

153. Bargmann, C. I., Hung, M.-C., and Weinberg, R. A. (1986) Multiple independent activations of the *neu* gene by point mutation altering the transmembrane domain of p185. *Cell*, **45**, 649.

154. Ponder, B. A. J. (1995) Mutations of the RET proto-oncogene in multiple endocrine neoplasia type 2. *Cancer Surveys*, **25**, 195.

2 | Growth factors

JOHN K. HEATH

1. Introduction

Growth factors are extracellular polypeptide mediators of intercellular signalling. They exert their action by binding to specific receptors expressed by target cells, thereby initiating signal transduction processes inside the cell. Depending upon the nature of the target cell and the identity of the specific signalling mechanisms involved, changes in cell behaviour ensue. These can include the induction of cell differentiation, migration, death or survival, as well as activation or inhibition of cell multiplication (reviewed in ref. 1). The significance of growth factors in the context of oncogenesis is therefore that they have the property of evoking precisely those cellular responses that are subverted in the course of oncogenic transformation and tumorigenesis. Abnormal expression of growth factors, and consequential activation of cell signalling is therefore a potentially significant mechanism of oncogenic transformation.

Although it is clear that growth factors could play a direct role in the malignant phenotype, it is important to appreciate that growth factors may also play very significant indirect roles in tumour growth *in vivo*. Continued increase in tumour mass and consequential disease progression requires not only that the tumour cells continue to multiply but that they are prevented from dying or undergoing terminal differentiation. Certain growth factors are strong inducers of endothelial cell proliferation and chemotaxis and may therefore act by promoting tumour angiogenesis (enhanced vascularization) with consequential reduction in tumour necrosis and increased tumour burden (2, 3). Metastatic dissemination of tumour cells is a significant clinical feature of naturally occurring cancers. Certain growth factors have the ability to induce both chemotaxis and cell migration as well as the expression of enzymes involved in extracellular matrix destruction (4), both of which are prerequisites for metastatic dispersal. Finally, although attention is often focused on the expression of growth factors by tumour cells themselves, it is equally possible that growth factors expressed by stromal cells may play an important role in tumour biology.

1.1 Growth factor dissemination

Growth factors have traditionally been distinguished from classical endocrine hormones on the basis of their mechanism of dissemination and means of access to the target cell. Whereas endocrine hormones are secreted from a limited number of specialized glands and delivered to their target cell through the general circulation, most growth factors are expressed locally and exert their action within the same tissues. Moreover, an important feature of some growth factors is that they are released from cells in a latent or inactive form and require activation before their biological effects can occur. In other words, growth factor activity is tightly regulated in both time and space. This concept has been elaborated by distinguishing several different modes of delivery (Fig. 1).

Paracrine action refers to the situation where growth factors are expressed by cells within a tissue and act upon cells in their immediate environment. This is often brought about by specialized mechanisms which restrict diffusion of growth factors within a tissue. A common example would be association of the growth factor with components of the extracellular matrix (see below). A more specialized version of paracrine action is termed juxtacrine action. In this situation, growth factors are expressed either as a transmembrane form or tightly associated with the expressing cells. In juxtacrine action the growth factor can only signal when the expressing cells and the responding cell are in physical apposition.

Autocrine action refers to the situation in which the expressing cell and the responding cell are one and the same, leading to auto-stimulation of cell multiplication. Autocrine control mechanisms have often been implicated in the growth of tumour cells as well as in other pathophysiological situations (reviewed in ref. 5).

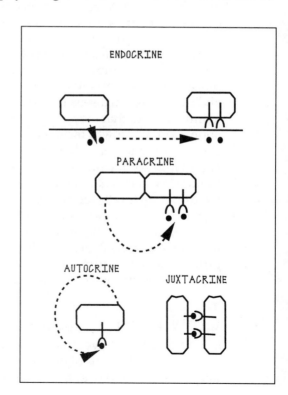

Fig. 1 Schematic representation of different types of growth factor dissemination. Endocrine cells release growth factors into the circulation where they are carried to a distant site. Paracrine cells release growth factors which act upon other cells in the immediate vicinity. Autocrine cells express growth factors which act upon themselves. Juxtacrine cells express growth factors in a membrane bound form which act on cells in physical contact.

There is very good evidence (reviewed below) that induction of autocrine control circuits by expression of a growth factor in a responsive cell type can lead to transformed behaviour *in vitro* and malignant growth *in vivo*. Autocrine action has accordingly been invoked to explain those situations in which activation of growth factor expression has been clearly associated with the onset of malignancy.

1.2   Regulatory networks

Aside from their controlled delivery to responding cells, another key feature of growth factor action is their assembly into regulatory networks. There is abundant evidence from many experimental systems that growth factors act by inducing the expression of a variety of different genes in a cell type-specific manner. Amongst the genes induced by growth factors may be other growth factors, or growth factor activators such as proteases. Couple this to the multifunctionality of growth factors and the varying responses of different cell types and it will be apparent that it is possible to create quite sophisticated control circuits within tissues composed of more than one cell type. Indeed it is more than likely that, *in vivo*, the action of any one growth factor is dependent upon the prior or concurrent action of others. In the context of tumour biology, therefore, it is important not only to consider growth factors expressed by the tumour cells themselves but the entire regulatory context in which the cells exist.

2.   Growth factor superfamilies

The number of agents that could be classified as growth factors has been rapidly rising over the last few years and it is certain that the current list is by no means complete. As increasing numbers of growth factors have been identified some important general themes have become apparent. First, growth factors can be grouped into families of molecules which are related at some level by their primary amino acid sequence. A more subtle grouping of growth factor families has emerged as their three-dimensional structures have been determined. It is becoming apparent that growth factors that share little similarity in primary sequence or biological function may, in fact, exhibit strong similarities in terms of tertiary structure. At the present time there are perhaps six or seven 'superfamilies' of growth factors based upon either known or predicted structural criteria (see Fig. 2), although this number will probably rise as new structures are determined.

2.1   The fibroblast growth factor family

The fibroblast growth factor (FGF) family currently comprises nine members, designated FGF1 to FGF9 (6). The prototype members of the family, FGF1 (formerly acidic FGF) and FGF2 (basic FGF) were originally discovered as activities present in pituitary or brain extracts which would induce the multiplication of fibroblast and vascular endothelial cells in culture (7). FGFs 1 and 2 were purified by virtue of their

ability to bind with high affinity to the sulfated polysaccharide heparin (8). This interaction with heparin proves to be a characteristic feature of all members of the FGF
family and is discussed further below. The crystal structures of both FGF1 and FGF2
have been determined (9). The two structures are remarkably similar and exhibit a

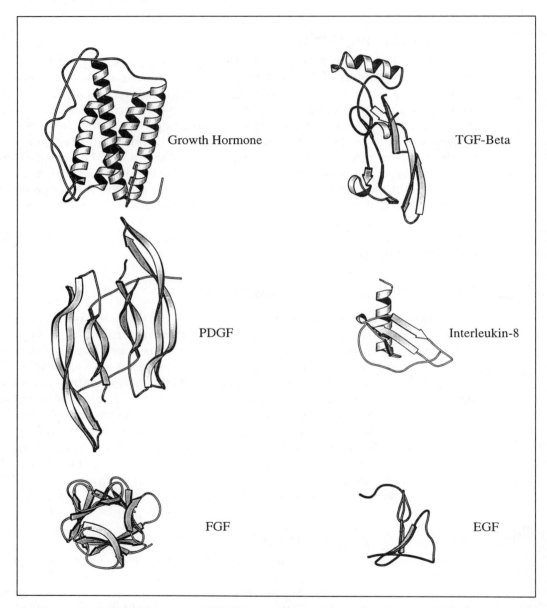

Fig. 2 The three-dimensional structures of prototype members of some growth factor superfamilies. Drawings
were made with MOLSCRIPT from published coordinates.

novel 12 stranded beta trefoil topology (Fig. 2). This characteristic structure is shared with the apparently unrelated growth factor interleukin-1 (1).

Following the initial identification of FGFs 1 and 2, further members of the family (defined by sequence homology) have been identified by a variety of independent routes. *FGF3* was identified as a gene (designated *INT2*) located at a common proviral integration site in tumours induced by mouse mammary tumour virus (MMTV; see Chapter 1 and ref. 10). FGF3 is a 239 amino acid polypeptide which shares 44% homology to FGF2 (11). The genomic localization of *FGF3* is very close to another member of the family, *FGF4*. The *FGF4* gene (originally called *HST1* or *kFGF*) encodes a 206 amino acid polypeptide with 40% homology to human FGF2 (12, 13). *FGF4* was initially isolated from Kaposi sarcoma and human stomach tumour DNA because of its capacity to induce the transformed phenotype when expressed in 3T3 mouse fibroblasts (12, 13). The *FGF5* gene was also cloned from human tumour DNA by virtue of its ability to induce cell transformation in 3T3 cells (14). However, it should be stressed that it is the normal forms of *FGF4* and *FGF5* DNA that induce transformation. The *FGF6* gene (also called *HST2*) was cloned by virtue of its homology to *FGF4* by DNA cross-hybridization (15). FGF7 (previously known as keratinocyte growth factor) differs from other members of the FGF family in that it exhibits a specific mitogenic effect on cell types of epithelial origin and was originally purified on the basis of this activity (16). FGF8 (androgen-induced growth factor) was isolated as a secreted agent responsible for the androgen-induced growth of steroid-dependent mouse mammary tumour cell lines and also identified as a target for proviral integration in MMTV-induced mammary tumours (17). The most recent addition to the family is FGF9 (glia-activating factor) which was purified and subsequently cloned from a human glioma cell line (18).

One of the characteristic features of the FGFs is their interaction with extracellular heparan sulfates in the form of glycosaminoglyans, such that their dissemination *in vivo* is tightly constrained by physical association with extracellular matrix components. The relationship between dissemination and biological activity is especially close in the case of FGFs since, at least in some cases, heparan appears to be required for the biological activity of the growth factor. The best illustration of this involves the use of cell lines which are genetically deficient in the metabolism of glycosaminoglycans. If these cells are transfected with a cloned FGF receptor gene they are unable to respond to exogenous FGF unless exogenous heparans are provided (19). This suggests that heparan acts to either promote the formation of a complex between the FGF ligand and its receptor (20) or induces some structural change in the ligand, such as dimerization (21), which promotes interaction with the receptor. These effects of heparin are relatively specific since they require sulfated polysaccharides of defined length and sequence (22, 23). FGF-binding oligosaccharide sequences can be found associated with a variety of core proteoglycans including syndecans and perlecan (24) as well as specific isoforms of CD44 (25). There is additionally some evidence that the expression of specific FGF-interacting oligosaccharides is subject to developmental and physiological regulation (26).

A surprising feature of FGFs 1 and 2 is that they lack classical secretory signal sequences and thus appear unable to be secreted from the cell by conventional means. This represents an extreme form of control over dissemination since it would appear that they cannot be made available to a responding cell unless released by cell lysis or some other mechanism. This could be significant in considering the possible roles of FGFs 1 and 2 *in vivo* and can be illustrated by a transgenic mouse model of dermal fibrosarcoma which develops in a pathway comprised of at least three stages: mild fibromatosis, aggressive fibromatosis, and fibrosarcoma. The latter two stages are highly vascularized when compared with both the normal dermis and the initial mild lesion. Analysis of cell cultures derived from biopsies of these lesions has revealed that FGF2 is synthesized in all three stages but there is a change in the localization of FGF2 from its normal cell-associated state to extracellular release in the latter two stages, which is concomitant both with the neovascularization seen *in vivo* and with the enhanced tumorigenicity of these cell lines. Thus, in this multistep tumorigenesis pathway there appears to be a discrete switch to the angiogenic phenotype that correlates with the release of FGF2 (27).

2.2 The epidermal growth factor family

Epidermal growth factor (EGF) was one of the first growth factors to be discovered. Injection of mouse submaxillary gland extracts into new-born mice was found to result in accelerated maturation of various epithelia, leading to premature eyelid opening and incisor eruption (28). EGF isolated from mouse submaxillary glands is a 6 kDa polypeptide with mitogenic actions on a wide variety of epithelial cells (29), as well as on 3T3 fibroblasts in culture. Transforming growth factor alpha (TGFα) was identified as an activity present in the culture supernatants of virally transformed leukaemia cells which had the property of competing with EGF for binding to its cell surface receptor (30). The molecular cloning and characterization of TGFα revealed a protein with homology to EGF and which exhibited considerable overlap in biological functions (reviewed in ref. 31). Both EGF and TGFα are expressed as transmembrane proteins from which the mature peptide is released by proteolysis (32, 33). The solution structures of EGF and TGFα determined by NMR techniques (34) reveal a canonical fold (Fig. 2), or module, that can be identified in many different proteins, most of which are devoid of mitogenic activity. This indicates that the receptor recognition functions of the EGF family have evolved from a core structural framework which can be employed for other purposes. Amphiregulin was purified as a growth inhibitor from the culture supernatants of phorbol ester treated human breast adenocarcinoma cells (35). Although amphiregulin shares considerable sequence homology with the mature forms of TGFα it also has an extended amino terminus, rich in basic residues, which interacts strongly with heparan sulfates (35). Various studies indicate that interaction with heparan sulfate is not only required for the biological activity of amphiregulin *in vitro* but also plays a role in correct processing and folding of the nascent amphiregulin protein (36, 37). More recently a number of novel EGF-like ligands have been identified (reviewed in ref. 38) including betacellulin (39), a growth factor secreted by experimentally induced pancreatic tumour cells, and heparin binding epidermal growth factor (HBEGF; see ref. 40). HBEGF is synthesized as a transmembrane protein (41) in which form it can act as the receptor for tetanus toxin. Thus, the biologically active ligand can either be presented to a responding cell in the form of a membrane-bound juxtacrine agent or be released from the cell membrane by proteolysis. HBEGF also contains regions rich in basic amino acids which tether the molecule in the extracellular matrix via association with heparan sulfate proteoglycans (42). More recently, a subgroup of the EGF family of ligands has been identified, known variously as 'heregulins' or 'neuregulins' (43, 44). These ligands interact with receptors closely related to the prototype EGF receptor and are widely expressed in both normal and malignant tissue, particularly in tissues of neural origin (45). The tumorigenic potential of TGFα has been examined by forced expression in transgenic mice in different tissues (46–48). These experiments show that TGFα is able to induce metaplasia and overgrowth in many epithelial tissues; on rare occasions these abnormal growths develop into frank neoplasia. This suggest that ectopic activation of EGF family members in tumours may be a predisposing but not determinative feature of malignant disease.

2.3 The platelet-derived growth factor family

Platelet-derived growth factor (PDGF) was one of the first growth factors to be isolated, as a major mitogen in human platelets (49). PDGF is a disulfide-linked dimer formed from two chains, PDGF-A (50) and PDGF-B (51), which give rise to three possible forms: AA and BB homodimers and AB heterodimers. The X-ray crystallographic structure of PDGF-BB has been determined (52; and Fig. 2) and shown to belong to the cystine knot family which also includes the transforming growth factor beta (TGFβ) and nerve growth factor (NGF) families (53). Since PDGF-A and PDGF-B exhibit different receptor binding specificities (see Chapter 3), the combinatorial assembly of different PDGF dimers can, in principle, yield growth factors with quite distinct biological specificities. In addition PDGF-A can be expressed in two distinct forms based upon alternative splicing of exon 6. This exon encodes a retention motif which, when present, causes the protein to become tightly associated with the producing cell (54) probably by association with glycosaminoglycans. This is another excellent example of the use of mechanisms that control growth factor dissemination. PDGF is also a striking example of a paracrine acting agent: during embryogenesis and in certain adult tissues, PDGF ligands and receptors are often found to be expressed in adjacent cell types within a tissue (55). PDGF appears to have the potential for quite broad ranging biological effects and can be shown to induce cell multiplication, chemotaxis, and inhibition of cell death in different biological systems *in vitro*.

Ectopic PDGF expression is one of the clearest examples of an autocrine mechanism of malignant transformation. The *v-SIS* oncogene associated with the acutely transforming retrovirus, simian sarcoma virus (SSV), was found to encode the PDGF-B chain (Chapter 1; and ref. 51). The formation of malignant tumours induced upon infection by SSV was clearly associated with the aberrant expression of PDGF-B encoded by the viral genome. These studies have been extended to show that, in some but certainly not all cell types, forced expression of PDGF results in cell transformation. Crucial to the autocrine model, in these *in vitro* experiments it has also been possible to demonstrate reversal of transformed parameters using various types of inhibitors of PDGF-B/receptor interaction (56). Since ectopic expression of PDGF is a frequent feature of certain types of tumour, such as glioblastoma, osteosarcoma, and meningioma, it is accordingly likely that PDGF-driven autocrine control circuits may have some role in naturally occurring tumours.

PDGF is the prototype member of an expanding family of growth factors exhibiting significant sequence homology. In terms of tumour biology, perhaps the most significant member of the family is vascular endothelial cell growth factor (VEGF; ref. 57). Unlike PDGF, VEGF has a very specific biological function: it is a specific growth factor for vascular endothelial cells. Like PDGF, VEGF is expressed as a disulfide-linked dimer and there are 'long' or 'short' forms, generated by alternative splicing, that are matrix bound or released respectively (58). As a result of specific effects on endothelial cell migration and multiplication, VEGF is a very potent and specific promoter of angiogenesis (59). VEGF is widely expressed by different types of tumours and there is now good evidence that VEGF expression is closely related to the extent of tumour vascularization since blockage of VEGF expression or signalling in tumour cell lines results in decreased vascularization and reduced tumour growth (60, 61). A very important feature of VEGF expression is that it is strongly induced by hypoxia (62) which is likely to occur in the centre of solid tumours. The increase in VEGF expression induced by hypoxia may then lead to angiogenesis, release from hypoxia, and promotion of tumour growth.

2.4   The WNT family

The WNT family of growth factors currently comprises 12 members. As discussed in Chapter 1, mammalian *WNT* genes were discovered on the basis of their association with virally-induced mammary tumours since integration of a provirus in the vicinity of the prototype family member *WNT1* (formerly called *INT1*) is a frequent event in MMTV-induced mammary carcinogenesis (63, 64). By analogy with *FGF3* and *FGF8*, it seems probable that activation of *WNT1* gene expression following proviral integration is a predisposing event in the formation of this class of mammary tumours. This can be demonstrated by the fact that forced expression of *WNT1* in the mammary gland of transgenic animals results in the formation of adenocarcinomas. The tumorigenic effects of *WNT1* activation appear to co-operate synergistically with members of the FGF family since infection of these *WNT1* transgenic mice with MMTV leads to accelerated mammary tumorigenesis with the *FGF8* gene being identified as a frequent site of insertion (65). Conversely, infection of *FGF3* transgenic mice with MMTV leads to accelerated induction of malignant mammary tumours with the *WNT1* gene being identified as a frequent site of viral integration (66). These experiments clearly show that *WNT* gene expression can be an important mediator of mammary carcinogenesis in an experimental setting although it is currently less clear how relevant these findings are to mammary carcinomas in humans.

The discovery of *WNT1* led to the identification of additional *WNT* genes and it has become apparent that the *WNT* family in general is highly conserved throughout evolution (including invertebrates) and that they have particularly significant roles in intercellular signalling during embryonic development (reviewed in ref. 64). Nothing is currently known of the three-dimensional structure of the WNT family, although sequence considerations suggest that they may comprise a unique growth factor superfamily with a novel three-dimensional fold. An important feature of *WNT* gene products is that they are tightly associated with the expressing cell and until recently it has proved difficult to obtain WNT protein in a soluble form (67). The action of *WNT* genes *in vivo* is therefore likely to be juxtacrine in nature. WNT signalling also displays intriguing parallels with mechanisms of cell adhesion in that both genetic evidence from *Drosophila* and overexpression experiments in *Xenopus* indicate that catenins, a class of cytosolic proteins associated with the cadherin-type homotypic cell adhesion molecules, act as a focus for WNT-mediate intracellular signalling (68, 69), and that catenins also associate with the tumour suppressor gene *APC* (69; and Chapter 10). This suggests that WNT signalling and homo-and heterotypic cell adhesion may be closely connected mechanistically and that altered function of these mechanisms may contribute to tumour formation or invasion.

2.5 Transforming growth factor beta family

The transforming growth factor beta (TGFβ) family is one of the largest groups of growth factors currently defined, represented by over 40 gene products with a wide variety of biological activities (reviewed in ref. 70). The prototypic member TGFβ1 was discovered as an activity present in the culture medium of virally transformed cells which, in collaboration with TGFα, a member of the EGF family, was able to induce many aspects of the transformed phenotype in fibroblast cell lines (71). TGFβ1 is a disulfide-linked dimer which is expressed in a latent form in association with a specific TGFβ binding protein (72). The release of biologically active TGFβ therefore requires breakdown of the latent complex (73). The latent TGFβ complex is often found associated with the extracellular matrix (74) and activated TGFβ dissemination is mediated by association with the non-signalling receptors betaglycan and endoglin (75). TGFβ1 therefore represents another example of paracrine action mediated by extracellular matrix association.

The X-ray crystallographic structure indicates that TGFβ1 is a member of the 'cystine knot' family with structural features reminiscent of PDGF (76; see Fig. 2). This is a surprising finding since TGFβs and other cystine knot family members exhibit quite distinct biological activities and interact with different classes of signalling receptor. Additional TGFβ family members have been cloned from a wide variety of species and display an immense diversity of biological functions, many of which are executed during embryonic stages of development. The TGFβ family can be grouped into a number of subfamilies based on sequence homologies. These include the activin, bone morphogenetic protein, Mullerian inhibitory substance, and nodal families (70). The proteins most closely related to TGFβ1 in both sequence and biological activity, TGFβ2 and TGFβ3, are major mediators of cell multiplication *in vivo* and *in vitro*.

TGFβ is a remarkable agent in that it can exert both positive and negative regulatory effects on cell proliferation depending upon the identity of the target cell type (reviewed in ref. 77). As was clear from the discovery of TGFβ1, its biological functions are often dependent upon the 'context' in which it acts and in particular the concurrent presence of other mitogenic agents. TGFβ is, in particular, a potent growth inhibitor of both epithelial and endothelial cell types. In the context of malignant cell proliferation, therefore, TGFβ1 could be considered as a significant suppressor of tumour cell growth. There is some support for this hypothesis in that mammary carcinogenesis in transgenic mice harbouring a predisposing *TGFα* transgene is suppressed when the animals are crossed with mice expressing active TGFβ1 under the control of a mammary-specific promoter (78).

These and related findings have led to the idea that escape from TGFβ-mediated growth suppression may be a significant mechanism of oncogenesis, especially in tumours of epithelial origin (79, 80). This idea has found powerful support from the identification of mutations in the TGFβ receptor II gene in human colon carcinoma cell lines with associated high rates of microsatellite instability (81). Moreover, a series of gastric tumour cell lines which exhibit resistance to TGFβ-induced growth arrest also exhibit a variety of different mutations in TGFβ receptors (82). These data are also consistent with information from animal models in which keratinocytes derived from animals with a disrupted *TGFβ1* gene exhibited accelerated carcinogenesis compared to wild-type when challenged with a tumour initiating stimulus in the form of the *H-RAS* oncogene (83). Finally, inactivating mutations in a gene implicated in TGFβ-mediated intracellular signalling, *DPC4*, have also been found at high frequency in pancreatic carcinoma cell lines (84; and Chapter 10).

TGFβ has characteristic and widespread effects on extracellular matrix deposition (85). Exposure of many different cell types to TGFβ results in enhanced matrix deposition which is brought about by suppression of matrix degrading proteases, induction of matrix degrading protease inhibitors, and induction of extracellular matrix structural components (86). The pathophysiological consequences of this property are that release of activated TGFβ is often associated with fibrosis and scarring. The consequences in terms of tumour biology may be complex but it seems probable that TGFβ-mediated induction of matrix deposition may act to inhibit tumour metastasis and spread.

2.6 Scatter factor/hepatocyte growth factor

Metastatic dissemination of tumour cells probably involves activation of cell motility to facilitate the invasive process. There is accordingly great interest in growth factors which induce chemotaxis or cell migration (so-called motogens). 'Scatter factor', as the name implies, was identified as an activity which induced scattering or motility in mammary epithelial cells. Molecular cloning of scatter factor revealed it to be identical to hepatocyte growth factor (HGF), a growth factor for adult liver cells (87). More recently a related scattering agent, macrophage-stimulating protein, has been cloned and found to be closely related to HGF (88). These two molecules therefore represent founders of a new growth factor family. The three-dimensional structure of HGF is currently unknown but it is of interest that HGF exhibits sequence homology to the protease plasminogen, including three copies of a 'kringle' domain and one copy of a serine protease-like domain (87). HGF is expressed in a latent pro-form and is activated by proteolytic cleavage by a urokinase-like enzyme (89). HGF, like many other agents discussed in this chapter, also associates specifically with the extracellular matrix by binding to heparan sulfate proteoglycans (90) and is therefore a predominantly paracrine effector. This is supported by numerous studies in which HGF and its cognate receptor, encoded by the *MET* proto-oncogene, are found expressed in adjacent cell layers; the ligand is predominantly expressed by mesenchymal cells and the receptor by epithelial populations (91).

The tumorigenic potential of HGF has been evaluated by transfecting epithelial and fibroblast cells lines with the appropriate vectors, the objective being to create an autocrine control circuit (92). The transfected cells were found to undergo profound morphological and behavioural changes and exhibit enhanced tumorigenicity in animal models. These findings contrast with the action of HGF on malignant colon carcinoma cells where application of exogenous HGF *in vitro* induced morphogenesis and suppressed invasive behaviour *in vivo* (93). Such differences illustrate the potential significance of the responding cell type in understanding the action of any particular growth factor.

2.7 The insulin-like growth factors

In certain respects, the insulin-like growth factors (IGFs) represent exceptions to some of the generalizations discussed above. Their principal biological role is the control of body mass during fetal and neonatal life (94). They were originally isolated as agents that mediated the effects of growth hormone on skeletal tissue growth. Two IGFs are currently known, IGFI and IGFII, both of which exhibit structural similarity to insulin (95) and can be placed in the insulin superfamily of hormones. Unlike many of the growth factors discussed in this chapter, IGFs can be viewed as endocrine agents and can be found in plasma and other body fluids. IGFI and IGFII differ principally in their timing of action during fetal and neonatal development. IGFII is expressed by many different tissues and can be found at high levels in fetal blood but the levels decline after birth and remain low throughout adult life except under conditions of stress or trauma. IGFI, by contrast, is expressed at low levels during fetal life but rises during postnatal life under the control of growth hormone. IGFI is almost exclusively expressed by the liver. Although this classical endocrine behaviour may seem quite distinct from other growth factors considered here, the IGFs in circulation are not in a free state but associate with a family of specific IGF-binding proteins (IGF-BPs). The exact biological function of IGF-BPs is not clear but an IGF/IGF-BP complex is inactive. In addition, some IGF-BPs exhibit strong affinity with extracellular matrix components and their affinity for IGFs is reduced upon binding to matrix (96). It is possible, therefore, that a major function of the IGF-BPs is to induce paracrine signalling by physical sequestration of the IGFs into the extracellular matrix.

At first sight the essentially anabolic role of IGFs would seem to have little to do with the process of carcinogenesis. It has become clear, however, that IGFs may play a significant auxiliary role in tumour growth by suppression of apoptosis. The first indications for this effect came from the induction of apoptosis by overexpression of the *MYC* oncogene in fibroblasts. The apoptotic effects of MYC could be rescued by exposure to IGFs (97). This suggested that, *in vivo*, IGFs may facilitate tumour growth by suppression of apoptosis. This has been elegantly tested by intercrossing transgenic mice with an SV40 LT-dependent predisposition to pancreatic β cell carcinomas with mice homozygous for a disruption in the *IGFII* gene. It was found that the double mutant mice exhibit roughly the same frequency of tumour formation but that the tumours showed reduced malignancy and an increased level of apoptosis (98).

The second association of IGFs with malignant disease comes from analysis of the effects of the tumour suppressor gene *WT1* which is frequently mutated in Wilms' tumour, a paediatric tumour of the kidney (see Chapter 10). *WT1* encodes a zinc-finger DNA-binding protein that functions as a transcriptional repressor. IGFII is overexpressed in Wilms' tumours in which the *WT1* gene is inactivated and this seems to be due to relief of transcriptional repression of the *IGFII* gene by *WT1* (99). In addition the *IGFII* gene is normally subject to genetic imprinting in that transcription of the gene is predominantly from the paternal allele. Beckwith–Wiedemann syndrome is manifest as growth abnormalities resulting from tissue hypertrophy and is associated with a predisposition to Wilms' tumours. In many Beckwith–Weidemann patients the maternal *IGFII* gene is lost and the paternal gene duplicated resulting in enhanced *IGFII* production (100).

2.8 Chemokines

Chemokines are small (typically 6 to 10 kDa) peptides which were initially identified as mediators of inflammatory responses by induction of chemotaxis and activation of inflammatory target cells such as neutrophils and macrophages (reviewed in ref. 101). Over 20 distinct chemokines have been identified which show approximately 20% overall identity at the sequence level. The chemokine family can be further sub-divided into two classes, designated C–C and C–X–C, based upon the sequence of the first two cysteine residues. The C–C and C–X–C families are clustered together in distinct chromosomal locations suggesting that the family as a whole has undergone rapid evolution by gene duplication and divergence. The two families also appear to exhibit distinct preferences for different target cell types: C–C chemokines are potent activators of neutrophils and C–X–C chemokines act primarily on macrophages. The three-dimensional structures of two chemokines, IL-8 (102) and RANTES (103) show considerable overall similarity in terms of their peptide fold (Fig. 2) and have been classified as belonging to a new structural superfamily of 'alpha + beta cytokines' denoted by the presence of a single region of alpha helix and a beta sheet motif (reviewed in ref. 104).

Many chemokines have been identified as genes whose expression is induced by the action of other growth factors and cytokines (e.g. KC; ref. 105) and are actively expressed in solid tumours associated with inflammatory involvement and macrophage or neutrophil invasion. Inflammatory cells themselves release growth factors such as PDGF and TGFβ1 following activation by chemokines. This class of molecules therefore plays an important role in mediating tumour cell/stromal interactions. It has recently become apparent that C–X–C chemokines may play a more direct, if complex, role in tumour growth. Chemokines of the C–X–C class which contain the amino acid sequence motif ELR have been demonstrated to have angiogenic activity (e.g. PF4) which can be inhibited by C–X–C chemokines (e.g. gro-beta) which lack the ELR motif (106–108). These findings indicate that chemokine expression by either tumour cells themselves, or elicited from stromal cells by the action of tumour-derived growth factors, have the potential to regulate tumour growth by modulation of angiogenesis. It further seems clear that the exact cocktail of chemokines expressed in the tumour microenvironment (in turn determined by the extent of inflammatory invasion) is likely to have a strong influence on the tumour growth. The chemokines also clearly illustrate a situation in which indirect expression of specific growth factors via regulatory cascades can have a significant input into the biological behaviour of tumour cells *in vivo*.

2.9 Cytokines

The term cytokine has become a generic name for growth factors but more strictly represents a large family of growth factors with diverse biological functions which share a diagnostic three-dimensional structure comprising four alpha helical domains linked by polypeptide loops (the helix bundle, Fig. 2). The prototypic member of the cytokine family is growth hormone (109). Within the helical bundle family, three subgroups can be defined; long chain (such as growth hormone) and short chain (such as interleukin-2), based upon the length and disposition of the regions of alpha helix, and dimeric (such as interferon gamma and interleukin-5) which have eight alpha helices in the form of a duplicated four helix bundle structure (110).

Many members of the cytokine family were originally isolated as 'interleukins' or factors that mediate signalling between cells of the haemopoetic system. It has now become clear that this distinction is somewhat artificial since many interleukins (such as interleukin-6) have widespread functions outside the immune system (reviewed in ref. 111). These include not only induction of cell multiplication and suppression of apoptosis but also induction of differentiation and cell death. 'Polyfunctional' cytokines such as IL-6 therefore exemplify the multifactorial actions of growth factors. It is little wonder, therefore, that such cytokines have been implicated in promotion of tumour cell growth in many different systems via autocrine activation as well as suppression of tumour cell growth via induction of differentiation and cell death.

Some members of the cytokine family, by contrast, have highly specific cellular targets *in vivo*. These include G-CSF which is a specific growth factor for granulocyte precursors, and IL-2 which is a specific growth factor for T cells. In the last few years, these highly specific cytokines have proved to be valuable agents for the treatment of naturally occurring tumours since they are able to specifically amplify or modulate a defined and restricted set of target cell types. The clinical applications of specific cytokines can range from amplification of specific haemopoetic subpopulations following radiotherapy, chemotherapy, or bone marrow transplantation (112), to the activation of anti-tumour immune functions (113), and to direct and indirect effects on tumour cell multiplication *in vivo*. The emerging lesson from these studies is that the objective of controlling the signalling environment of tumour cells is wholly realistic provided that the relevant growth factors are highly specific in action or that their action is restricted by some means to the tumour microenvironment.

3. Conclusions

Growth factors, taken as a whole, are a large and highly diverse group of molecules. They exhibit a wide variety of different biological effects on different target cell types. Within this complexity some common principles can be put forward. First, growth factors can be placed into a relatively small number of families which has great value in understanding and manipulating ligand / receptor specificity. Secondly, most if not all growth factors are essentially locally acting intercellular mediators with a variety of different mechanisms for restricting dissemination *in vivo*. Thirdly, growth factors are linked into regulatory circuits involving other growth factors. Finally, the same agent may exhibit quite distinct effects on different types of cells. The value of these principles in terms of oncogenesis is that whilst growth factor activation undoubtedly plays a significant role in the induction of some types of tumour, perhaps their broader biological functions in tumour biology are equally important.

References

1. Sporn, M. and Roberts, A. (1988) Growth factors are multifunctional. *Nature*, **332**, 217.
2. Folkman, J. (1995) Angiogenesis in cancer, vascular, rheumatoid and other disease. *Nature Med.*, **1**, 27.
3. Klagsbrun, M. and D'Amore, P. A. (1991) Regulators of angiogenesis. *Annu. Rev. Physiol.*, **53**, 217.
4. Radinsky, R. (1991) Growth factors and their receptors in metastasis. *Semin. Cancer Biol.*, **2**, 169.
5. Sporn, M. B. and Roberts, A. B. (1992) Autocrine secretion—10 years later. *Ann. Intern. Med.*, **117**, 408.

6. Wilkie, A. O. M., Morriss-Kay, G., Jones, E. Y., and Heath, J. K. (1995) Functions of fibroblast growth factors and their receptors: evidence from mouse and human genetics. *Curr. Biol.*, **5**, 500.

7. Armelin, H. A. (1973) Pituitary extracts and steroid hormones in the control of 3T3 cell growth. *Proc. Natl. Acad. Sci. USA*, **70**, 2702.

8. Thomas, K. A., Riley, M. C., Lemmon, S. K., Baglan, N. C., and Bradshaw, R. A. (1980) Brain fibroblast growth factor: nonidentity with myelin basic protein fragments. *J. Biol. Chem.*, **255**, 5517.

9. Zhu, X., Komiya, H., Chirino, A., Faham, S., Fox, G. M., Arakawa, T., *et al.* (1991) Three-dimensional structures of acidic and basic fibroblast growth factors. *Science*, **251**, 90.

10. Dickson, C., Smith, R., Brookes, S., and Peters, G. (1984) Tumorigenesis by mouse mammary tumor virus: proviral activation of a cellular gene in the common integration region *int-2*. *Cell*, **37**, 529.

11. Dickson, C. and Peters, G. (1987) Potential oncogene product related to growth factors. *Nature*, **326**, 833.

12. Delli Bovi, P., Curatola, A. M., Kern, F. G., Greco, A., Ittmann, M., and Basilico, C. (1987) An oncogene isolated by transfection of Kaposi's sarcoma DNA encodes a growth factor that is a member of the FGF family. *Cell*, **50**, 729.

13. Sakamoto, H., Mori, M., Taira, M., Yoshida, T., Matsukawa, S., Shimizu, K., *et al.* (1986) Transforming gene from human stomach cancers and a noncancerous portion of stomach mucosa. *Proc. Natl. Acad. Sci. USA*, **83**, 3997.

14. Zhan, X., Bates, B., Hu, X., and Goldfarb, M. (1988) The human FGF-5 oncogene encodes a novel protein related to fibroblast growth factors. *Mol. Cell. Biol.*, **8**, 3487.

15. Marics, I., Adelaide, J., Raybaud, F., Mattei, M.-G., Coulier, F., Planche, J., *et al.* (1989) Characterization of the *HST*-related *FGF6* gene, a new member of the fibroblast growth factor gene family. *Oncogene*, **4**, 335.

16. Finch, P. W., Rubin, J. S., Miki, T., Ron, D., and Aaronson, S. A. (1989) Human KGF is FGF-related with properties of a paracrine effector of epithelial cell growth. *Science*, **245**, 752.

17. Tanaka, A., Miyamoto, K., Minamino, N., Takeda, M., Sato, M., Matsuo, H., *et al.* (1992) Cloning and characterization of an androgen-induced growth factor essential for the androgen-dependent growth of mouse mammary carcinoma cells. *Proc. Natl. Acad. Sci. USA*, **89**, 8928.

18. Miyamoto, M., Naruo, K., Seko, C., Matsumoto, S., Kondo, T., and Kurokawa, T. (1993) Molecular cloning of a novel cytokine cDNA encoding the ninth member of the fibroblast growth factor family, which has a unique secretion property. *Mol. Cell. Biol.*, **13**, 4251.

19. Yayon, A., Klagsbrun, M., Esko, J. D., Leder, P., and Ornitz, D. M. (1991) Cell surface, heparin-like molecules are required for binding of basic fibroblast growth factor to its high affinity receptor. *Cell*, **64**, 841.

20. Ornitz, D. M., Yayon, A., Flanagan, J. G., Svahn, C. M., Levi, E., and Leder, P. (1992) Heparin is required for cell-free binding of basic fibroblast growth factor to a soluble receptor and for mitogenesis in whole cells. *Mol. Cell. Biol.*, **12**, 240.

21. Spivak Kroizman, T., Lemmon, M. A., Dikic, I., Ladbury, J. E., Pinchasi, D., Huang, J., *et al.* (1994) Heparin-induced oligomerization of FGF molecules is responsible for FGF receptor dimerization, activation, and cell proliferation. *Cell*, **79**, 1015.

22. Turnbull, J. E., Fernig, D. G., Ke, Y., Wilkinson, M. C., and Gallagher, J. T. (1992) Identification of the basic fibroblast growth factor binding sequence in fibroblast heparin sulfate. *J. Biol. Chem.*, **267**, 10337.

23. Ishihara, M. (1994) Structural requirements in heparin for binding and activation of FGF-1 and FGF-4 are different from that for FGF-2. *Glycobiology*, **4**, 817.

24. Aviezer, D., Hecht, D., Safran, M., Eisinger, M., David, G., and Yayon, A. (1994) Perlecan, basal lamina proteoglycan, promotes basic fibroblast growth factor-receptor binding, mitogenesis and angiogenesis. *Cell*, **79**, 1005.

25. Bennett, K. L., Jackson, D. G., Simon, J. C., Tanczos, E., Peach, R., Modrell, B., *et al.* (1995) CD44 isoforms containing exon V3 are responsible for the presentation of heparin-binding growth factor. *J. Cell Biol.*, **128**, 687.

26. Nurcombe, V., Ford, M. D., Wildschut, J. A., and Bartlett, P. F. (1993) Developmental regulation of neural response to FGF-1 and FGF-2 by heparan sulfate proteoglycan. *Science*, **260**, 103.

27. Kandel, J., Bossy-Wetzel, E., Radvanyi, F., Klagsbrun, M., Folkman, J., and Hanahan, D. (1991) Neovascularization is associated with a switch to the export of bFGF in the multistep development of fibrosarcoma. *Cell*, **66**, 1095.

28. Savage, C., Inagami, T., and Cohen, S. (1972) The primary structure of epidermal growth factor. *J. Biol. Chem.*, **247**, 7612.

29. Carpenter, G. and Cohen, S. (1979) Epidermal growth factor. *Annu. Rev. Biochem.*, **48**, 193.

30. Carpenter, G., Stoscheck, C. M., Preston, Y. A., and DeLarco, J. E. (1981) Antibodies to the epidermal growth factor receptor block the biological activities of sarcoma growth factor. *Proc. Natl. Acad. Sci. USA*, **80**, 5627.

31. Derynck, R. (1980) Transforming growth factor alpha. *Cell*, **54**, 593.

32. Gray, A., Dull, T., and Ullrich, A. (1983) Nucleotide sequence of epidermal growth factor cDNA predicts a 128,000 molecular weight precursor. *Nature*, **303**, 722.

33. Derynck, R., Roberts, A. B., Winkler, M. E., Chen, E. Y., and Goeddel, D. V. (1984) Human transforming growth factor-alpha: precursor structure and expression in *E. coli*. *Cell*, **38**, 287.

34. Campbell, I., Cooke, R., Baron, M., Harvey, T., and Tappin, M. (1989) The solution structures of EGF and TGF alpha. *Prog. Growth Factor Res.*, **1**, 13.

35. Plowman, G. D., Green, J. M., McDonald, V. L., Neubauer, M. G., Disteche, C. M., Todaro, G. J., *et al.* (1990) The amphiregulin gene encodes a novel epidermal growth factor-related protein with tumor-inhibitory activity. *Mol. Cell. Biol.*, **10**, 1969.

36. Johnson, G. R. and Wong, L. (1994) Heparan sulfate is essential to amphiregulin induced mitogenic signaling by the epidermal growth factor receptor. *J. Biol. Chem.*, **269**, 27149.

37. Thorne, B. A. and Plowman, G. D. (1994) The heparin-binding domain of amphiregulin necessitates the precursor pro-region for growth factor secretion. *Mol. Cell. Biol.*, **14**, 1635.

38. Prigent, S. A. and Lemoine, N. R. (1992) The type 1 (EGFR-related) family of growth factor receptors and their ligands. *Prog. Growth Factor Res.*, **4**, 1.

39. Shing, Y., Christofori, G., Hanahan, D., Ono, Y., Sasada, R., Igarashi, K., *et al.* (1993) Betacellulin: a mitogen from pancreatic beta cell tumors. *Science*, **259**, 1604.

40. Higashiyama, S., Abraham, J. A., and Klagsbrun, M. (1993) Heparin-binding EGF-like growth factor stimulation of smooth muscle cell migration: dependence on interactions with cell surface heparan sulfate. *J. Cell Biol.*, **122**, 933.

41. No, M., Raab, G., Lau, K., Abraham, J. A., and Klagsbrun, M. (1994) Purification and characterization of transmembrane forms of heparin-binding EGF-like growth factor. *J. Biol. Chem.*, **269**, 31315.

42. Thompson, S. A., Higashiyama, S., Wood, K., Pollitt, N. S., Damm, D., McEnroe, G., *et al.* (1994) Characterization of sequences within heparin-binding EGF-like growth factor that mediate interaction with heparin. *J. Biol. Chem.*, **269**, 2541.

43. Wen, D., Peles, E., Cupples, R., Suggs, S. V., Bacus, S. S., Luo, Y., *et al.* (1992) Neu differentiation factor: a transmembrane glycoprotein containing an EGF domain and an immunoglobulin homology unit. *Cell*, **69**, 559.

44. Peles, E. and Yarden, Y. (1993) Neu and its ligands: from an oncogene to neural factors. *Bioessays*, **15**, 815.

45. Falls, D. L., Rosen, K. M., Corfas, G., Lane, W. S., and Fischbach, G. D. (1993) ARIA, a protein that stimulates acetylcholine receptor synthesis, is a member of the neu ligand family. *Cell*, **72**, 801.

46. Jhappan, C., Stahle, C., Harkins, R. N., Fausto, N., Smith, G. H., and Merlino, G. T. (1990) TGFalpha overexpression in transgenic mice induces liver neoplasia and abnormal development of the mammary gland and pancreas. *Cell*, **61**, 1137.

47. Sandgren, E. P., Luetteke, N. C., Palmiter, R. D., Brinster, R. L., and Lee, D. C. (1990) Overexpression of TGFalpha in transgenic mice: Induction of epithelial hyperplasia, pancreatic metaplasia, and carcinoma of the breast. *Cell*, **61**, 1121.

48. Vassar, R., Hutton, M. E., and Fuchs, E. (1991) Transgenic overexpression of transforming growth factor alpha bypasses the need for Ha-Ras mutations in mouse skin tumorigenesis. *Mol. Cell. Biol.*, **12**, 4643.

49. Heldin, C.-H., Westermark, B., and Wasteson, A. (1979) Platelet derived growth factor: purification and partial characterisation. *Proc. Natl. Acad. Sci. USA*, **76**, 3722.

50. Betsholtz, C., Johnsson, A., Heldin, C., Westermark, B., Lind, P., Urdea, M., *et al.* (1986) cDNA sequence and chromosomal localisation of human platelet derived growth factor A chain and its expression in tumour cells. *Nature*, **320**, 695.

51. Johnsson, A., Heldin, C.-H., Wasteson, A., Westermark, B., Deuel, T., Huang, J., *et al.* (1984) The c-sis gene encodes a precursor of the B chain of platelet-derived growth factor. *EMBO J.*, **3**, 921.

52. Oefner, C., D'Arcy, A., Winkler, F., Eggimann, B., and Hosang, M. (1992) Crystal structure of platelet derived growth factor. *EMBO J.*, **11**, 3921.

53. Murray Rust, J., McDonald, N. Q., Blundell, T. L., Hosang, M., Oefner, C., Winkler, F., *et al.* (1993) Topological similarities in TGF-beta 2, PDGF-BB and NGF define a superfamily of polypeptide growth factors. *Structure*, **1**, 153.

54. Andersson, M., Ostman, A., Westermark, B., and Heldin, C.-H. (1994) Characterization of the retention motif in the C-terminal part of the long splice form of platelet-derived growth factor A-chain. *J. Biol. Chem.*, **269**, 926.

55. Orr-Urtreger, A. and Lonai, P. (1992) Platelet-derived growth factor A and its receptor are expressed in separate but adjacent cell layers of the mouse embryo. *Development*, **115**, 289.

56. Vassbotn, F. S., Andersson, M., Westermark, B., Heldin, C. H., and Ostman, A. (1993) Reversion of autocrine transformation by a dominant negative platelet-derived growth factor mutant. *Mol. Cell. Biol.*, **13**, 4066.

57. Conn, G., Bayne, M. L., Soderman, D. D., Kwok, P. W., Sullivan, K. A., Palisi, T. M., *et al.* (1990) Amino acid and cDNA sequences of a vascular endothelial cell mitogen

that is homologous to platelet-derived growth factor. *Proc. Natl. Acad. Sci. USA*, **87**, 2628.

58. Park, J. E., Keller, G. A., and Ferrara, N. (1993) The vascular endothelial growth factor (VEGF) isoforms: differential deposition into the subepithelial extracellular matrix and bioactivity of extracellular matrix-bound VEGF. *Mol. Biol. Cell*, **4**, 1317.

59. Mustonen, T. and Alitalo, K. (1995) Endothelial receptor tyrosine kinases involved in angiogenesis. *J. Cell Biol.*, **129**, 895.

60. Kim, K. J., Li, B., Winer, J., Armanini, M., Gillett, N., Phillips, H. S., *et al.* (1993) Inhibition of vascular endothelial growth factor-induced angiogenesis suppresses tumour growth *in vivo*. *Nature*, **362**, 841.

61. Millauer, B., Shawver, L. K., Plate, K. H., Risau, W., and Ullrich, A. (1994) Glioblastoma growth inhibited *in vivo* by a dominant-negative Flk-1 mutant. *Nature*, **367**, 576.

62. Goldberg, M. A. and Schneider, T. J. (1994) Similarities between the oxygen sensing mechanisms regulating the expression of vascular endothelial growth factor and erythropoietin. *J. Biol. Chem.*, **269**, 4355.

63. Nusse, R. and Varmus, H. E. (1982) Many tumours induced by the mouse mammary tumour virus contain a provirus integrated in the same region of the host genome. *Cell*, **31**, 99.

64. Nusse, R. and Varmus, H. E. (1992) Wnt genes. *Cell*, **69**, 1073.

65. MacArthur, C. A., Shankar, D. B., and Shackleford, G. M. (1995) Fgf-8, activated by proviral insertion, cooperates with the Wnt-1 transgene in murine mammary tumorigenesis. *J. Virol.*, **69**, 2501.

66. Lee, F. S., Lane, T. F., Kuo, A., Shackleford, G. M., and Leder, P. (1995) Insertional mutagenesis identifies a member of the Wnt gene family as a candidate oncogene in the mammary epithelium of int-2/Fgf-3 transgenic mice. *Proc. Natl. Acad. Sci. USA*, **92**, 2268.

67. Bradley, R. S. and Brown, A. M. (1995) A soluble form of Wnt-1 protein with mitogenic activity on mammary epithelial cells. *Mol. Cell. Biol.*, **15**, 4606.

68. Karnovsky, A. and Klymkowsky, M. W. (1995) Anterior axis duplication in Xenopus induced by the over-expression of the cadherin-binding protein plakoglobin. *Proc. Natl. Acad. Sci. USA*, **92**, 4522.

69. Hinck, L., Nelson, W. J., and Papkoff, J. (1994) Wnt-1 modulates cell-cell adhesion in mammalian cells by stabilizing beta-catenin binding to the cell adhesion protein cadherin. *J. Cell. Biol.*, **124**, 729.

70. Kingsley, D. M. (1994) The TGF-beta superfamily: new members, new receptors, and new genetic tests of function in different organisms. *Genes Dev.*, **8**, 133.

71. Ciccodicola, A., Dono, R., Obici, S., Simeone, A., Zollo, M., Persico, M. G., *et al.* (1978) Sarcoma growth factor from conditioned medium of virally transformed cells is composed of both type alpha and type beta transforming growth factors. *EMBO J.*, **8**, 1987.

72. Flaumenhaft, R., Abe, M., Sato, Y., Miyazono, K., Harpel, J., Heldin, C. H., *et al.* (1993) Role of the latent TGF-beta binding protein in the activation of latent TGF-beta by co-cultures of endothelial and smooth muscle cells. *J. Cell Biol.*, **120**, 995.

73. Harpel, J. G., Metz, C. N., Kojima, S., and Rifkin, D. B. (1992) Control of transforming growth factor-beta activity: latency vs. activation. *Prog. Growth Factor Res.*, **4**, 321.

74. Taipale, J., Miyazono, K., Heldin, C. H., and Keski Oja, J. (1994) Latent transforming growth factor-beta 1 associates to fibroblast extracellular matrix via latent TGF-beta binding protein. *J. Cell Biol.*, **124**, 171.

75. Lopez Casillas, F., Payne, H. M., Andres, J. L., and Massague, J. (1994) Betaglycan can act as a dual modulator of TGF-beta access to signaling receptors: mapping of ligand binding and GAG attachment sites. *J. Cell Biol.*, **124**, 557.

76. Daopin, S., Li, M., and Davies, D. R. (1993) Crystal structure of TGF-beta 2 refined at 1.8 Å resolution. *Proteins*, **17**, 176.

77. Sporn, M. B. and Roberts, A. B. (1992) Transforming growth factor-beta: recent progress and new challenges. *J. Cell Biol.*, **119**, 1017.

78. Pierce, D. F., Jr., Gorska, A. E., Chytil, A., Meise, K. S., Page, D. L., Coffey, R. J., Jr., *et al.* (1995) Mammary tumor suppression by transforming growth factor beta 1 transgene expression. *Proc. Natl. Acad. Sci. USA*, **92**, 4254.

79. Fynan, T. M. and Reiss, M. (1993) Resistance to inhibition of cell growth by transforming growth factor-beta and its role in oncogenesis. *Crit. Rev. Oncol.*, **4**, 493.

80. Wright, J. A., Turley, E. A., and Greenberg, A. H. (1993) Transforming growth factor beta and fibroblast growth factor as promoters of tumor progression to malignancy. *Crit. Rev. Oncol.*, **4**, 473.

81. Markowitz, S., Wang, J., Myeroff, L., Parsons, R., Sun, L., Lutterbaugh, J., *et al.* (1995) Inactivation of the type II TGF-beta receptor in colon cancer cells with microsatellite instability. *Science*, **268**, 1336.

82. Park, K., Kim, S. J., Bang, Y. J., Park, J. G., Kim, N. K., Roberts, A. B., *et al.* (1994) Genetic changes in the transforming growth factor beta (TGF-beta) type II receptor gene in human gastric cancer cells: correlation with sensitivity to growth inhibition by TGF-beta. *Proc. Natl. Acad. Sci. USA*, **91**, 8772.

83. Glick, A. B., Lee, M. M., Darwiche, N., Kulkarni, A. B., Karlsson, S., and Yuspa, S. H. (1994) Targeted deletion of the TGF-beta 1 gene causes rapid progression to squamous cell carcinoma. *Genes Dev.*, **8**, 2429.

84. Hahn, S. A., Schutte, M., Hoque, A. T., Moskaluk, C. A., da Costa, L. T., Rozenblum, E., *et al.* (1996) DPC4, a candidate tumor suppressor gene at human chromosome 18q21.1. *Science*, **271**, 350.

85. Noble, N. A., Harper, J. R., and Border, W. A. (1992) *In vivo* interactions of TGF beta and extracellular matrix. *Prog. Growth Factor Res.*, **4**, 369.

86. Roberts, A. B., McCune, B. K., and Sporn, M. B. (1992) TGF-beta: regulation of extracellular matrix. *Kidney Int.*, **41**, 557.

87. Naldini, L., Weidner, K. M., Vigna, E., Gaudino, G., Bardelli, A., Ponzetto, C., *et al.* (1991) Scatter factor and hepatocyte growth factor are indistinguishable ligands for the MET receptor. *EMBO J.*, **10**, 2867.

88. Gaudino, G., Follenzi, A., Naldini, L., Collesi, C., Santoro, M., Gallo, K. A., *et al.* (1994) RON is a heterodimeric tyrosine kinase receptor activated by the HGF homologue MSP. *EMBO J.*, **13**, 3524.

89. Naldini, L., Tamagnone, L., Vigna, E., Sachs, M., Hartmann, G., Birchmeier, W., *et al.* (1992) Extracellular proteolytic cleavage by urokinase is required for activation of hepatocyte growth factor/scatter factor. *EMBO J.*, **11**, 4825.

90. Lyon, M., Deakin, J. A., Mizuno, K., Nakamura, T., and Gallagher, J. T. (1994) Interaction of hepatocyte growth factor with heparan sulfate. Elucidation of the major heparan sulfate structural determinants. *J. Biol. Chem.*, **269**, 11216.

91. Sonnenberg, E., Meyer, D., Weidner, K. M., and Birchmeier, C. (1993) Scatter factor/hepatocyte growth factor and its receptor, the c-met tyrosine kinase, can mediate a

signal exchange between mesenchyme and epithelia during mouse development. *J. Cell Biol.*, **123**, 223.

92. Bellusci, S., Moens, G., Gaudino, G., Comoglio, P., Nakamura, T., Thiery, J. P., *et al.* (1994) Creation of an hepatocyte growth factor/scatter factor autocrine loop in carcinoma cells induces invasive properties associated with increased tumorigenicity. *Oncogene*, **9**, 1091.

93. Brinkmann, V., Foroutan, H., Sachs, M., Weidner, K. M., and Birchemier, W. (1995) Hepatocyte growth factor/scatter factor induces a variety of tissue-specific morphogenic programs in epithelial cells. *J. Cell Biol.*, **131**, 573.

94. DeChiara, T., Efstradiatis, A., and Robertson, E. (1990) A growth-deficiency phenotype in heterozygous mice carrying an insulin-like growth factor II gene disrupted by gene targeting. *Nature*, **345**, 78.

95. Dull, T., Gray, A., Hayflick, J., and Ullrich, A. (1984) Insulin-like growth factor gene organisation in relation to insulin gene family. *Nature*, **310**, 777.

96. Jones, J. I., Gockerman, A., Busby, W. H., Jr., Camacho-Hubner, C., and Clemmons, D. R. (1993) Extracellular matrix contains insulin-like growth factor binding protein-5: potentiation of the effects of IGF-I. *J. Cell Biol..*, **121**, 679.

97. Harrington, E. A., Bennett, M. R., Fanidi, A., and Evan, G. I. (1994) c-Myc induced apoptosis in fibroblasts is inhibited by specific cytokines. *EMBO J.*, **13**, 3286.

98. Christofori, G., Naik, P., and Hanahan, D. (1994) A second signal supplied by insulin-like growth factor II in oncogene-induced tumorigenesis. *Nature*, **369**, 414.

99. Drummond, I. A., Madden, S. L., Rohwer-Nutter, P., Bell, G. I., Sukhatme, V. P., and Rauscher, F. J. (1992) Repression of the insulin-like growth factor II gene by the Wilms tumor suppressor WT1. *Science*, **257**, 674.

100. Kubota, T., Saitoh, S., Matsumoto, T., Narahara, K., Fukushima, Y., Jinno, Y., *et al.* (1994) Excess functional copy of allele at chromosomal region 11p15 may cause Wiedemann-Beckwith (EMG) syndrome. *Am. J. Med. Genet.*, **49**, 378.

101. Schall, T. J., Mak, J. Y., DiGregorio, D., and Neote, K. (1993) Receptor/ligand interactions in the C-C chemokine family. *Adv. Exp. Med. Biol.*, **351**, 29.

102. Baldwin, E., Weber, R., Charles, R., Xuan, J., Appella, E., Yamada, M., *et al.* (1991) Crystal structure of interleukin 8: symbiosis of NMR and crystallography. *Proc. Natl. Acad. Sci. USA*, **88**, 502.

103. Skelton, N. J., Aspiras, F., Ogez, J., and Schall, T. J. (1995) Proton NMR assignments and solution conformation of RANTES, a chemokine of the C-C type. *Biochemistry*, **34**, 5329.

104. Clore, G. M. and Gronenborn, A. M. (1995) Three-dimensional structures of alpha and beta chemokines. *FASEB J.*, **9**, 57.

105. Bozic, C. R., Kolakowski, L. F., Jr., Gerard, N. P., Garcia Rodriguez, C., von Uexkull Guldenband, C., Conklyn, M. J., *et al.* (1995) Expression and biologic characterization of the murine chemokine KC. *J. Immunol.*, **154**, 6048.

106. Bussolino, F., Arese, M., Montrucchio, G., Barra, L., Primo, L., Benelli, R., *et al.* (1995) Platelet activating factor produced *in vitro* by Kaposi's sarcoma cells induces and sustains *in vivo* angiogenesis. *J. Clin. Invest.*, **96**, 940.

107. Cao, Y., Chen, C., Weatherbee, J. A., Tsang, M., and Folkman, J. (1995) gro-beta, a -C-X-C- chemokine, is an angiogenesis inhibitor that suppresses the growth of Lewis lung carcinoma in mice. *J. Exp. Med.*, **182**, 2069.

108. Strieter, R. M., Polverini, P. J., Kunkel, S. L., Arenberg, D. A., Burdick, M. D., Kasper, J.,

et al. (1995) The functional role of the ELR motif in CXC chemokine-mediated angiogenesis. *J. Biol. Chem.*, **270**, 27348.

109. De Vos, A. M., Ultsch, M., and Kossiakoff, A. A. (1992) Human growth hormone and the extracellular domain of its receptor: crystal structure of the complex. *Science*, **255**, 306.

110. Sprang, S. and Bazan, F. (1993) Cytokine structural taxonomy and mechanisms of receptor engagement. *Curr. Opin. Struct. Biol.*, **3**, 815.

111. Kishimoto, T., Akira, S., Narazaki, M., and Taga, T. (1995) Interleukin-6 family of cytokines and gp130. *Blood*, **86**, 1243.

112. Nemunaitis, J. (1994) Use of hematopoietic growth factors in marrow transplantation. *Curr. Opin. Oncol.*, **6**, 139.

113. Caron, P. C. and Scheinberg, D. A. (1994) Immunotherapy for acute leukemias. *Curr. Opin. Oncol.*, **6**, 14.

3 | Growth factor receptors in cell transformation

CARL-HENRIK HELDIN and LARS RÖNNSTRAND

1. Introduction

The growth of cells is regulated by polypeptide factors that stimulate or inhibit proliferation. More than 50 such growth regulatory factors are known (Chapter 2). They exert their effects on cells by binding to specific receptors at the cell surface. For factors that stimulate cell proliferation, activation of protein tyrosine kinases appears to be a common and maybe obligatory event. Several growth factors bind to receptors with intrinsic tyrosine kinase domains which are activated after ligand binding. Other growth factors bind receptors which after ligand binding form complexes that contain intracellular tyrosine kinases. In contrast, the well characterized growth inhibitory factors of the transforming growth factor β (TGFβ) family bind to receptors with intrinsic serine/threonine kinase domains.

There is ample evidence that constitutive activation of growth stimulatory pathways occurs in conjunction with cell transformation. Thus, subversion of mitogenic pathways may account for the loss of growth control that characterizes malignantly transformed cells (reviewed in ref. 1). There are examples of transformed cells that produce growth factors for which they carry the corresponding receptor, resulting in autocrine stimulation of growth. Growth factor receptors may also be present in too high amounts or may be mutated in a manner which results in constitutive activation in the absence of growth factor. Analogously, any of the intracellular components of the mitogenic pathway, which in the normal cell is controlled by growth factors, may be constitutively activated. It is also possible that loss of components in growth inhibitory pathways contribute to the uncontrolled growth of tumour cells.

This review focuses on perturbations at the growth factor receptor level in cell transformation.

2. Families of growth factor receptors

There are two main types of receptors for growth stimulatory factors, i.e. protein tyrosine kinase receptors and cytokine receptors. Based on their structural characteristics, these two types of receptors can be further divided into subfamilies.

The tyrosine kinase receptors contain a single transmembrane segment which

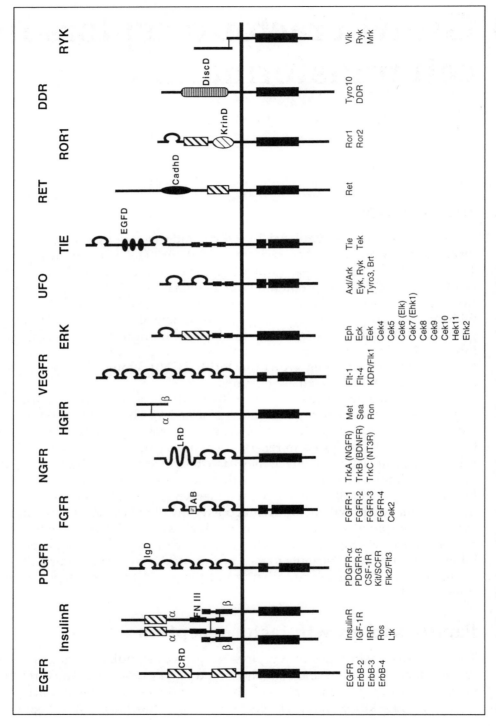

Fig. 1 Schematic illustration of protein tyrosine kinase receptor families. The prototype receptor for each family is indicated above the receptors, and the known members below. CRD, cysteine-rich domain; FN III, fibronectin type III-like domain; IgD, immunoglobulin-like domain; AB, acidic box; LRD, leucine-rich domain; EGFD, epidermal growth factor-like domain; CadhD, cadherin-like domain; KrinD, kringle-like domain; DiscD, discoidin-like domain.

divides the molecules into an amino terminal, extracellular, ligand-binding part and an intracellular part containing the kinase domain. Different structural motifs, such as immunoglobulin-like domains, fibronectin type III (FN III) domains, epidermal growth factor-like domains, and cysteine-rich domains, are often found in the extracellular parts of the receptors (Fig. 1). Another characteristic feature of certain subclasses of receptors is the presence of a stretch of amino acid residues which divides the kinase domain into two parts. About a dozen subfamilies can be distinguished with more than 50 currently known members (reviewed in ref. 2) (Fig. 1). There are several examples of orphan receptors, for which the ligands remain to be identified.

The cytokine receptors lack intrinsic enzymatic activities and after ligand binding they often form complexes with specific signal transducers which are also transmembrane molecules without intrinsic enzymatic activities (3, 4). The cytokine receptors are subdivided into two major families, i.e. class I and class II cytokine receptors. The class I cytokine receptors include receptors for many interleukins and colony stimulating factors and certain other factors and hormones. The extracellular portions of these proteins include one or two domains each containing two segments of FN III-like motifs, the W–S–X–W–S sequence, and four conserved cysteine residues (Fig. 2). The class I cytokine receptors can be further classified based on which signal transducer they associate with (see further below). The class II cytokine receptors, which include receptors for interferons and IL-10, are characterized by another motif of four cysteine residues, but lack the W–S–X–W–S motif.

3. Signal transduction via protein tyrosine kinase receptors

The available information supports the notion that a general mechanism for the activation of tyrosine kinase receptors involves ligand-induced receptor dimerization (reviewed in ref. 5). The dimerization brings the kinase domains of the two receptors close to each other and thereby promotes 'autophosphorylation' in *trans* between the two molecules. The autophosphorylation appears to serve two important functions: it locks the kinase in an active configuration and it provides binding sites in the receptors for downstream signal transduction molecules (see further below).

Certain growth factors, such as PDGF, SCF, and M-CSF, are dimeric molecules. In these cases, each molecule contains two identical receptor binding epitopes and forms stable dimers by simultaneously binding two receptors with high affinity. Other ligands are apparent monomers, like EGF. Interestingly, however, calorimetric studies have shown that a single EGF molecule can simultaneously bind two receptor molecules (6). FGF2 is also a monomeric molecule. Evidence has been presented that the ligand binds one receptor with high affinity and a second with lower affinity (7). Since signalling via FGF receptors is dependent on the presence of heparin or heparan sulfate (see Chapter 2) it is possible that the interaction between FGF and the second receptor is stabilized by heparin / heparan sulfate. An alternative mechanism has been

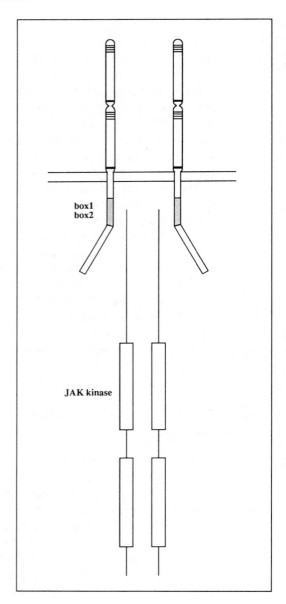

Fig. 2 Schematic illustration of a cytokine type I receptor, interacting with JAK kinases after ligand-induced homodimerization. Thin lines in the extra-cellular part of the receptors denote conserved cysteine residues, and thick lines the conserved W–S–X–W–S motif. The two kinase domains in each JAK kinase are illustrated by open rectangles.

suggested for FGF1, in which heparin stabilizes the formation of a dimeric ligand complex which thereby can induce receptor dimerization (8). Another variation on the dimerization theme is exemplified by ligands for the EPH-related tyrosine kinase receptors. These molecules are cell surface attached and do not activate their receptors in soluble form. The finding that antibody-mediated clustering leads to activation of receptors supports the notion that dimerization, in the normal case presumably facilitated by membrane attachment, is involved in the activation mechanism (9).

Autophosphorylation, which follows receptor dimerization, occurs on two different classes of sites. The first is the autophosphorylation of a tyrosine residue located inside the kinase domain which is conserved in almost all tyrosine kinases. In the insulin receptor (10) and the HGF receptor (11) phosphorylation at this and neighbouring positions has been shown to activate the kinases and allow the phosphorylation of other tyrosine residues in the receptors and in substrates. However, this model for activation of tyrosine kinase receptors does not explain how the reaction is initiated. It is possible that the receptor kinases have a low basal activity sufficient to accomplish activating phosphorylation of the other receptor in the dimer provided that the two receptors form a sufficiently stable dimer. Alternatively, the dimerization induces interactions between the kinase domains of the receptors which leads to alterations of their conformations and an increase in the V_{max} of the kinases. There are examples of receptors which are not regulated by phosphorylation in the kinase domain, such as EGF receptor in which the conserved tyrosine in the kinase domain does not appear to be autophosphorylated.

The other class of autophosphorylated tyrosine residues are normally located outside of the kinase domains. They serve the important function of providing docking sites for downstream signal transduction molecules containing SH2 domains (see Chapter 4 and ref. 12). The SH2 domain is a 100 amino acid motif which folds to form a surface which recognizes a phosphorylated tyrosine in a specific environment. One or two SH2 domains are present in a number of different signal transduction molecules; since they have different preferences regarding the amino acids surrounding the phosphorylated tyrosine, specificity in the interaction is achieved.

As an example, the PDGF receptor-β (PDGFRβ) contains at least nine autophosphorylation sites, Y857 in the kinase domain and at least eight additional tyrosines outside the kinase domain (Fig. 3) (reviewed in ref. 13). The SH2 domain molecules that interact with PDGFRβ fall into two categories, those which also have catalytic domains, such as phospholipase Cγ (PLCγ) protein tyrosine phosphatase 1D, GTPase activating protein for RAS (GAP), and SRC (Chapters 4 and 5), and those which do not have any intrinsic enzymatic activity but rather serve functions as adaptor molecules, such as GRB2, SHC, NCK and the regulatory p85 subunit of the phosphatidylinositol-3'-kinase (PI3K). The signal transduction molecules are activated either in conjunction with the binding to the receptor, or by subsequent phosphorylation by the receptors. Other signal transduction molecules may be constitutively active but translocated to the cell membrane by binding to an activated receptor, thus enabling them to interact with the next components in the signal transduction chain.

The tyrosine kinase receptors are activated by the homodimerization of two identical receptors, or by the heterodimerization of related receptors. As an example, the different isoforms of PDGF induce different dimeric complexes of α and β receptors. Whereas both α and β receptors mediate mitogenic signals, only the β receptor transduces a stimulatory signal for chemotaxis; in fact, the α receptor inhibits chemotaxis, at least in certain cell types (13). There is also a difference in the effects on the actin filament system; both receptors mediate stimulation of edge ruffling and loss of stress

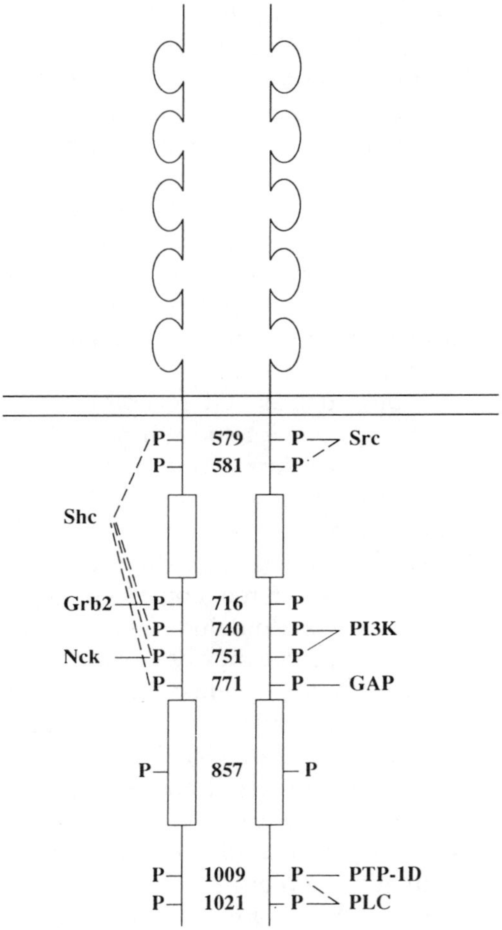

Fig. 3 Schematic illustration of the interaction between activated PDGF β receptors and downstream signal transduction molecules. Ligand binding induces dimerization and auto-phosphorylation of receptors. Auto-phosphorylated tyrosine residues in the juxtamembrane domain, the domain between the two parts of the kinase domain, and in the carboxy terminal tail of the receptor mediate interaction with SH2 domain containing molecules. Adaptor molecules are depicted on the left side and catalytically active signal transduction molecules to the right. Note that it is not known how many SH2 domain containing molecules can bind simultaneously to a receptor complex.

fibres, but only the β receptor mediates the formation of circular ruffles on the dorsal surface of the cell. These differences in the signalling via homodimeric receptor complexes of α or β receptors are likely to be due to differences in the autophosphorylation sites and in the substrate specificities of the two receptors. It is an interesting possibility that the heterodimeric αβ receptor complex has unique properties, for example through the presence of autophosphorylation sites in the heterodimer not found in homodimeric receptor complexes (14).

Members of the EGF receptor family also undergo heterodimerization after ligand binding. In addition to homodimers of EGF receptors, EGF induces the formation of a heterodimer of one EGF receptor and one ERBB2 molecule (15, 16). Moreover, signalling by NDF, a candidate ligand for ERBB2, is dependent on the formation of heterodimers between ERBB2 and ERBB3 or ERBB4 (17). Interestingly, the ERBB3 receptor lacks certain conserved amino acid residues in the kinase domain and has only a very low kinase activity (18). Its role in a heterodimer may be to be phosphorylated by the EGF receptor, ERBB2, or ERBB4, and to provide docking sites for downstream targets such as PI3K, since such sites are lacking in the other members of the EGF receptor family (15, 19–21).

4. Signal transduction via cytokine receptors

As with the tyrosine kinase receptors, the cytokine receptors undergo dimerization after ligand binding (Fig. 2). There are examples of cytokine receptors which undergo homodimerization, such as the receptors for erythropoietin, prolactin, growth hormone (GH) and granulocyte colony stimulating factor (G-CSF). The best characterized example is the GH receptor which has been crystallized together with its ligand (22–24). The monomeric GH molecule first binds with high affinity to one receptor molecule. Thereafter a second receptor is recruited to the complex; the binding of the second receptor is stabilized by interactions with the GH molecule as well as directly with the other receptor molecule in the dimer.

Other factors induce the formation of heteromeric complexes of receptors and signal transduction molecules that are structurally related to cytokine receptors. IL-3, GM-CSF, and IL-5 bind to specific α receptor subunits; each of the α receptors then interacts with a common β subunit which is required for high affinity binding and signal transduction (4).

The receptors for IL-6, LIF, oncostatin M, IL-11, and CNTF constitute another subfamily which all comprise heteromeric complexes between unique receptor molecules and the signal transducer gp130 (3). Signalling appears to be initiated by the formation of complexes containing homo- or heterodimers of gp130 and the ligand receptor.

Receptors for IL-2, IL-4, IL-7, and IL-9 form another subfamily, in which signalling is initiated by the formation of complexes between specific β subunits and a common γ subunit (25). In the case of IL-2, the binding is stabilized by an α subunit which is structurally unrelated to cytokine receptors.

The cytokine receptors and their signal transducers do not have intrinsic kinase activities, but some of them interact with cytoplasmic tyrosine kinases of the JAK family (26, 27) (Fig. 2). The activating event appears to be dimerization which brings two JAK kinases close to each other and possibly allows for their transphosphorylation and activation. The JAK family of tyrosine kinases has at least four members (JAK1, JAK2, JAK3, and TYK2) which interact in a specific manner with different cytokine receptors. The JAKs bind to regions in the juxtamembrane parts of the cytokine receptors, denoted box1 and box2. The different receptors interact with different JAKs. Thus, ligand binding induces homodimerization or heterodimerization of different members of the JAK family of tyrosine kinases.

Important substrates for the JAK family of kinases are members of the family of signal transducers and activators of transcription (STATs) (28). After phosphorylation, these molecules dimerize and translocate into the nucleus where they activate the transcription of specific genes. There are several members of the STAT family and it is likely that different JAKs phosphorylate STATs in differential manners.

5. Tyrosine kinase receptors in cell transformation

Insights into the possible importance of tyrosine kinase receptors in cell transformation have come from studies of acutely transforming retroviruses, transformation by chemical carcinogens, as well as 'spontaneous' human tumours (Chapter 1). The involvement of members of the major tyrosine kinase receptor families in carcinogenesis is summarized below.

5.1 The EGF receptor family

5.1.1 The EGF receptor (ERBB)

The EGF receptor is the prototype for a receptor family of four members, and is one of the most studied tyrosine kinase receptors. The discovery, in 1984, that the EGF receptor is the cellular counterpart of v-ERBB, the transforming protein of avian erythroblastosis virus (29), was the first finding that directly linked tyrosine kinase receptors to oncogene products. The oncogene v-ERBB codes for a mutated version of the chicken EGF receptor, with a very short extracellular part and the whole intracellular domain of the EGF receptor, apart from the most carboxy terminal region (30). The lack of the carboxy terminal sequences is of major importance for the transforming activity of v-ERBB, since this region contains regulatory sequences, including two serine phosphorylation sites (31, 32) and tyrosine autophosphorylation sites (33). Point mutations in the kinase domain also contribute to the transforming activity of v-ERBB (34).

The c-ERBB locus has also been found to be activated by the integration of avian leukosis virus DNA, leading to the production of amino terminally truncated variants of the EGF receptor (35). Interestingly, the amino terminally truncated EGF receptors induce predominantly erythroleukaemias, but acquire the ability to also induce fibrosarcomas after point mutation of a residue in the ATP-binding pocket of the kinase domain (36). This mutated receptor shows increased autophosphorylation and phosphorylation of certain substrates, providing a possible explanation for the increased tumorigenicity (37).

A role for the EGF receptor in human tumorigenesis is suggested by the fact that it is frequently found to be overexpressed or mutated in several different human tumour types. For instance, the EGF receptor gene is amplified in approximately 20–40% of human glioblastomas (38–40). In conjunction with amplification in glioblastomas, deletions in the extracellular domain (41, 42), as well as in the cytoplasmic part of the EGF receptor (43), are commonly seen. Such mutations can lead to a constitutively activated receptor kinase (44). Amplification of the EGF receptor also occurs in a variety of epithelial tumours, albeit with lower frequencies (10–15%), including head and neck squamous cell carcinomas, breast tumours (45, 46), oesophageal tumours (47), and urogenital tumours (48). Amplification was found to be accompanied by overexpression of the EGF receptor (for review see ref. 49). Consistent with a role of EGF receptor overactivity in cell transformation, Moroni *et al.* (50) were able to reverse the transformed phenotype of a human epidermoid carcinoma cell line by expression of EGF receptor antisense RNA. Whereas amplified EGF receptors often contain structural alterations, overexpression of the normal human EGF receptor was also found to lead to transformation of fibroblasts in culture, and to the induction of tumours in animals (51).

The expression of ligands for the EGF receptor and other members of the EGF receptor family, such as TGFα, amphiregulin, and cripto, has been described in colorectal tumours (52) and in a variety of other tumour cells (53). The co-expression of both receptor and ligand suggests an autocrine or paracrine mode of growth stimulation, although it has been difficult to directly demonstrate such mechanisms. Using an antisense approach to inhibit expression of cripto, Ciardiello *et al.* (54) were able to reverse the tumorigenicity of a colon carcinoma cell line.

5.1.2 ERBB2/NEU

The oncogene *NEU* was first identified in chemically induced neuroblastomas in rat (55) and subsequently shown to encode a protein of the same family as the EGF receptor. The transforming protein in these tumours was found to differ from its normal counterpart by only a single base substitution, changing valine at position 664 in the transmembrane region to a glutamic acid residue (56). This single amino acid substitution, V664E, has been proposed to lead to a constitutively dimerized and activated receptor (57). Consistent with this notion, a pentapeptide comprising amino acid residues 661–665 of wild-type NEU was found to inhibit the growth of NEU-expressing cells, presumably by interaction with the transmembrane part of the receptor leading to inhibition of receptor dimerization (58).

The human counterpart of NEU was subsequently isolated and termed ERBB2 (or HER2) (59, 60), due to its similarity with the EGF receptor (ERBB). The activating point mutation found in chemically-induced rat neuroblastomas has not been found in human tumours. A possible explanation is that, because of differences in the DNA sequence between rat and human, a replacement of V with E in humans would require two bases to be mutated, rather than one, thus making it less likely to occur. High expression of normal human ERBB2 also results in transformation of NIH/3T3 cells (61, 62).

Amplification and overexpression of *ERBB2* has been found in a variety of human tumours, including carcinomas of the breast, ovaries, colon, lung, liver, stomach, kidney, oesophagus, salivary gland, and bladder (reviewed in 63, 64). Amplification of *ERBB2* occurs in approximately 20% of invasive breast carcinomas. Particularly in lymph node-positive patients, *ERBB2* amplification and protein overexpression seem to be associated with poor prognosis (65, 66). No or very weak correlation with poor prognosis was found in node-negative patients (66), and overexpression did not correlate with the presence of lymph node metastases. Thus, it is possible that *ERBB2* amplification increases the growth rate but not the metastatic potential of tumour cells. More than 50% of all ductal carcinoma *in situ* (DCIS) express *ERBB2*. In most cases of DCIS, consisting of large cells, overexpression of *ERBB2* is found, while over-expression is rare in DCIS of the small cell type (67, 68). Since DCIS is believed to be a precursor lesion of metastatic breast cancer, these data suggest that *ERBB2* has a role in the early stages of breast tumorigenesis.

Transgenic mice carrying either an activated form of *NEU* or the wild-type proto-oncogene under the transcriptional control of the mouse mammary tumour virus promoter, frequently develop mammary carcinomas (69–71). Induction of mammary tumours in transgenic mice expressing wild-type *NEU* occurs through in-frame deletions of 7–12 amino acids in the extracellular region proximal to the transmembrane domain; the introduction of these mutations into the wild-type *NEU* cDNA has been shown to increase its transforming ability (72).

5.1.3   ERBB3

The third member of the EGF receptor family, *ERBB3*, was cloned by low stringency hybridization using *v-ERBB* to probe a normal genomic DNA library (73). Increased levels of *ERBB3* mRNA have been demonstrated in certain human mammary tumour cell lines (73) and in human breast cancers (74). High expression of ERBB3 correlated with the presence of lymph node metastases. No amplification of the *ERBB3* gene was seen in these tumours. Overexpression of *ERBB3* has also been observed in epidermoid carcinoma of the larynx and oesophageal carcinoma (75).

5.1.4   ERBB4

ERBB4, the fourth member of the EGF receptor family, was recently cloned (76). ERBB4 has been shown to be overexpressed in a human mammary tumour cell line, but its role in human tumours remains to be elucidated.

5.2   The PDGF receptor family

5.2.1   PDGF α and β receptors

PDGF α and β receptors are structurally related tyrosine kinase receptors that bind the PDGF isoforms with different specificities. The finding that the *SIS* oncogene is related to the gene for the B-chain of PDGF, and that *SIS*-transformation of cells occurs by autocrine stimulation involving a PDGF-like molecule (reviewed in ref. 77 and Chapter 2), prompted investigations to explore whether PDGF receptor pathways are overactive in human malignancies. Unlike the situation for members of the EGF receptor family, amplification of the PDGF receptors is uncommon. There are, however, reports that the α receptor is amplified in about 5% of glioblastomas (78, 79).

The α receptor is expressed in normal glial cells (80), as well as in benign and malignant glioma (81–83). It is possible that overactivity of the PDGF α receptor contributes to the uncontrolled growth of glioma tumour cells, since PDGF A- and B-chains are expressed at higher amounts in malignant glioblastomas than in benign tumours (82). Interestingly, the PDGF β receptor is not expressed at any appreciable amounts in glioma cells, but is expressed in a malignancy-dependent manner in the supporting stromal cells (82, 84, 85). These observations suggest that the two PDGF receptors are involved in two separate autocrine and paracrine mechanisms in human glioma, one involving the α receptor in the tumour cell compartment, and the other involving the β receptor in the stromal compartment. This may be of importance for the balanced growth of different cell types in glioblastomas. The notion that activation of PDGF receptors is of importance for glioma cell growth is further supported by the findings that a dominant negative form of PDGF (86), or a truncated PDGF receptor acting in a dominant negative manner (87), inhibit glioma cell growth. Also, fibromas and fibrosarcomas express PDGF and PDGF receptors in a malignancy-dependent manner, suggesting that the activation of PDGF receptors contributes to the uncontrolled growth of these tumour types (88–91).

Direct confirmation of the oncogenic potential of the PDGF β receptor came from the recent demonstration that the common translocation between chromosomes 5 and 12 in chronic myelomonocytic leukaemia, involves the fusion of gene sequences coding for the kinase domain of the β receptor with the gene for an ETS-like transcription factor, TEL (ref. 92; and Chapter 1). It is possible, but remains to be shown, that the fusion with TEL causes a constitutive activation of the PDGF receptor kinase by induction of dimerization.

The PDGF receptors have also been implicated in transformation by bovine papilloma virus type 1. The E5 transforming protein of this virus is a small hydrophobic protein of 44 amino acid residues which occurs as a disulfide-bonded dimer. E5 has been shown to interact with the transmembrane part of the PDGF β receptor and promote ligand-independent dimerization (93, 94; Chapter 1). It is possible that E5 of human and bovine papilloma virus may also activate other growth factor receptors, such as the EGF receptor (95).

5.2.2 Stem cell factor receptor (KIT)

The *KIT* oncogene was originally isolated from a feline sarcoma virus (96). The transforming protein was found to consist of the kinase domain of a tyrosine kinase receptor, later identified as the SCF receptor (97, 98), and viral *gag*-encoded sequences. The *c-KIT* gene has been shown to be the target of the spontaneous dominant white spotting (W) mutation in mice (99). Analyses of mice homozygous for W mutations have revealed defects in the development of haematopoietic, melanogenic, and gametogenic lineages (reviewed in ref. 100). The SCF receptor is expressed in cells of these lineages, as well as in benign tumours originating therefrom. Interestingly, however, no expression was found in malignant melanoma, breast cancers, and certain other malignant tumours (101–104). Thus, there are indications that a deregulated SCF receptor kinase in certain situations, such as fibrosarcomas of cats infected with the feline sarcoma virus, acts as a dominant oncoprotein, whereas the SCF receptor in other contexts, such as in melanomas, may have the properties of a tumour suppressor gene product.

5.2.3 Colony stimulating factor-1 receptor (FMS)

The CSF1 receptor gene was transduced by feline leukaemia virus as the *v-FMS* oncogene (105; and Chapter 1). The v-FMS product differs structurally from the natural CSF1 receptor; the 40 carboxy terminal amino acid residues in the CSF1 receptor, containing an important regulatory tyrosine residue, have been replaced with 11 other amino acid residues in v-FMS (106). Moreover, v-FMS contains a mutation in the extracellular domain, replacing leucine 301 with a serine residue (107). Both these structural alterations contribute to ligand-independent activation of the receptor kinase, and to the transforming activity.

The CSF1 receptor is also implicated in the development of myelomonocytic leukaemia in mice, where it is activated at high frequency by proviral insertion (108). In humans, *FMS* mutations have been described in patients with myelodysplastic syndrome (109).

5.3 The insulin-like growth factor I receptor

The IGFI receptor belongs to the same family of tyrosine kinase receptors as the insulin receptor (110), with which it bears about 70% sequence similarity. Primary breast tumours generally express high levels of IGFI receptor (111–113), and amplification of the *IGFI* receptor gene has been observed (114). Some cell lines have also been shown to produce IGFI, suggesting a possible role for IGFI in autocrine stimulation of breast cancer cell growth (Chapter 2).

Interestingly, even though IGFI is a growth factor for most normal cells, it cannot sustain cell growth on its own; other growth factors, such as PDGF, are also required to induce an efficient proliferative response (115, 116). These early findings were recently extended by *in vivo* studies on animals with the gene for IGFI receptor knocked-out by homologous recombination. These mice were born with a size of only 30% of their wild-type littermates (117, 118). Interestingly, in contrast to cells from wild-type mice, cells derived from such knock-out mice could not be transformed by the SV40 T antigen, by an activated and overexpressed *H-RAS* gene, or by a combination of both (119, 120). This resistance to transformation could be reversed by stably transfecting the IGFI receptor negative cells with a plasmid expressing the wild-type IGFI receptor (119, 121). Furthermore, the transformed phenotype, measured as colony formation in soft agar, could be reversed by expressing antisense RNA to the IGFI receptor or by incubating cells with antisense oligonucleotides (119, 120, 122–125). Antisense RNA to the IGFI receptor was furthermore shown to inhibit growth of human melanoma and glioma cells in nude mice (123, 124).

The observations described above suggest that the IGFI receptor has an important role in cell growth which is qualitatively different from that of most other growth factor receptors. A clue to the nature of such a function is the recent observation that IGFI inhibits the apoptosis induced by the topoisomerase inhibitor etoposide (126) or by overexpression of c-*MYC* (127). Thus, in the absence of the IGFI receptor, a large fraction of cells may die through apoptosis, thereby preventing efficient tumour growth. The central role of the IGFI receptor in growth of tumour cells, makes it an interesting target for therapeutic interventions (128).

5.4 The neurotrophin receptor family

The *TRKA* oncogene, originally isolated from a colon carcinoma biopsy, was found to consist of a fusion of genes encoding a tyrosine kinase and non-muscular tropomyosin (129). More recently normal *TRKA* has been shown to code for the receptor for nerve growth factor (NGF). The related TRKB and TRKC have subsequently been shown to be receptors for brain-derived neurotrophic factor (BDNF) and neurotrophin-3 (NT3), respectively (130). A clue to the mechanism of activation of the *TRKA* oncogene was unravelled when it was shown that the fusion with tropomyosin caused dimerization of the TRKA protein, leading to constitutive activation of its tyrosine kinase activity (131). Since then, a number of examples have been described where the *TRKA* sequence has been fused to genes coding for proteins that normally form dimers in cells, leading to the synthesis of a constitutively dimerized and active tyrosine kinase. Examples include the *TRK2ʰ* oncogene, isolated from a breast carcinoma cell line, which consists of the *TRKA* proto-oncogene fused to the gene for the ribosomal large subunit protein L7a (132), and *TRK* T1, isolated from a human papillary thyroid carcinoma, which consists of *TRKA* fused to the gene for TPR, a transcription factor with two leucine zipper motifs (133, 134). Also other cases of rearrangement of *TRKA* have been described in papillary thyroid carcinomas (135, 136).

Whereas the fusion of TRKA with different proteins leads to a constitutively activated receptor and to a growth signal in several cell types, there are also examples where TRKA may have a tumour suppressor effect. In non-advanced stages of neuroblastoma, a high frequency of expression of TRK was observed which correlated inversely with *N-MYC* gene amplification (137). Co-expression of mRNA for TRKA and the low affinity NGF receptor in neuroblastoma correlated with a favourable prognosis (138–140). The tumours expressing TRKA and the low affinity NGF receptor also regressed spontaneously or responded to conventional therapy. These observations are consistent with the notion that loss of NGF receptors is an important step in the genesis of neuroblastomas.

5.5 Angiogenic receptors

The growth of solid tumours is absolutely dependent on their ability to stimulate ingrowth of blood vessels (141). One mechanism involves the release of angiogenic factors from the tumour cells, but angiogenic factors may also be derived from, for example, macrophages recruited by the tumour cells. Two well characterized families of angiogenic factors act by binding to tyrosine kinase receptors, i.e. members of the FGF family which bind to a family of receptors with two or three immunoglobulin-like extracellular domains, and VEGF which binds to two related receptors with seven immunoglobulin-like extracellular domains (Fig. 1).

There are several observations that support the notion that VEGF has an important role in the vascularization of brain tumours. Thus, VEGF mRNA has been found to be increased in glioma cells (85, 142) and its presence correlated with the vascularity of the tumours (143). The VEGF receptor FLT is not expressed in normal brain endothelium but is induced in the endothelium of brain tumours, suggesting a paracrine effect of VEGF (144). The importance of VEGF for angiogenesis of gliomas and other tumours is also supported by *in vivo* studies. Expression of a dominant-negative VEGF receptor was shown to slow down glioma growth in nude mice (145), as was the administration of antibodies against VEGF (146). VEGF may also be important for the angiogenesis of other types of tumours, including meningiomas (143), and kidney and bladder carcinomas (147). There is also evidence that VEGF acts as a regulator of neovascularization and cyst formation in von Hippel–Lindau disease-associated and sporadic haemangioblastomas (148).

FGFs may also be important for the vascularization of certain types of tumours. The expression of FGF1 has been shown to be associated with a switch to an angiogenic phase during the development of dermal fibrosarcoma in a transgenic mouse model (149). Moreover, neutralizing antibodies against FGF1 have been shown to inhibit angiogenesis in an *in vitro* model system (150) as well as *in vivo* (151). It should be pointed out that overexpression of FGF receptors by certain tumour cells may also contribute to their growth, for example, melanomas (152). Moreover, FGF receptor genes have been found to be amplified in some breast cancers (153). Similarly, there is an example of an orphan receptor, TIE (Fig. 1), which is overexpressed in the vascular endothelium of metastatic melanomas (154).

Angiogenesis is crucial for the metastatic spread of tumours to distant sites, and the numbers of microvessels in different human cancers correlate with their ability to invade and produce metastases (reviewed in ref. 155). The observation that removal of the primary tumour often leads to a rapid growth of metastases was the basis for the identification of an anti-angiogenic factor; angiostatin is a 38 kDa fragment of plasminogen, which is produced by certain tumours and inhibits angiogenesis (156). Other angiogenesis inhibitors, such as thrombospondin (157) and a still unidentified factor (158), are under the control of the tumour suppressor p53 (see Chapter 9). Inactivation of p53 may thus lead to a decreased secretion of these inhibitors and increased angiogenesis.

5.6 The hepatocyte growth factor receptor

The *MET* oncogene was identified in human osteosarcoma cells treated with the carcinogen methyl-nitro-nitroso-guanidine (159) and subsequently shown to code for a mutated version of the receptor for HGF (160, 161). The transforming protein is a fusion of the kinase domain of the HGF receptor and TPR, a transcription factor containing leucine zippers. The transforming effect is mediated by dimerization induced by the leucine zipper of TPR followed by activation of the HGF receptor kinase (161a).

Overexpression of *c-MET* has been reported in a number of tumours of epithelial origin, including carcinomas of the colorectum (162), thyroid (163), ovaries (164), stomach (165), pancreas (166), and in hepatocellular carcinomas (167). An aberrant and overexpressed transcript has been found in certain gastric carcinomas (168), and amplification of the *c-MET* proto-oncogene has also been observed in a gastric carcinoma cell line (169). The *MET* gene has also been shown to undergo spontaneous amplification in NIH/3T3 cells grown *in vitro* (170). A correlation between expression of *c-MET* and progression of malignant melanoma has been observed (171).

Co-expression of *c-MET* and its ligand, HGF, has been found to be associated with increased tumorigenicity in a model system (172). The observation that HGF and its receptor are co-expressed in certain pancreatic cancers (173), suggests that autocrine growth stimulation may occur also in human tumours.

5.7 Orphan receptors

5.7.1 RET

The *RET* oncogene was originally identified as a recombination of two sequences of human DNA which most likely occurred during transfection of NIH/3T3 cells (174). The *c-RET* gene encodes a tyrosine kinase receptor containing a cadherin-like structure (Fig. 1), and is expressed in the peripheral nervous system (reviewed in ref. 175). The ligand for the RET protein remains to be identified.

The RET tyrosine kinase has been found to be activated in thyroid tumours (see Chapter 1). The activation mechanism involves the fusion of the kinase domain of RET with other sequences including the regulatory subunit of the cAMP-dependent protein kinase (176). Since in the latter case the fusion partner normally occurs as a dimer, it is possible that it causes dimerization and thereby activation of the RET kinase.

Recent studies have revealed that mutations in the c-*RET* gene are associated with the development of multiple endocrine neoplasia (MEN) 2A and 2B, familial medullary thyroid carcinoma, and Hirschsprung disease (Chapter 1 and 177–182). Since mice with the *c-RET* gene disrupted showed phenotypes similar to Hirschsprung disease (183), it is likely that the abnormalities seen in this disease are due to inactivation of c-RET. In contrast, the mutations seen in MEN2A, MEN2B, and familial medullary thyroid carcinoma may represent gain-of-function mutations. Consistent with this possibility, MEN2A mutations in the extracellular domain of c-RET, converting a cysteine residue to other residues, were found to induce ligand-independent dimerization and activation of the receptor (184, 185). Apparently, the loss of the cysteine residue left another cysteine residue unpaired and thus available to form a disulfide bond with the corresponding residue in another receptor molecule. In contrast, a MEN2B mutation inside the kinase domain, M918T, led to quantitatively and qualitatively altered catalytic properties of the RET kinase (185).

5.7.2 ROS

The *v-ROS* oncogene was originally identified as the transforming sequence of avian sarcoma virus UR2 (186). The corresponding normal gene encodes a large tyrosine kinase receptor, the ligand for which remains to be found. The loss of regulatory extracellular sequences is important for the constitutive activation of the ROS kinase and its transforming properties (187).

6. Cytokine receptors

6.1 Erythropoietin receptor

The erythropoietin receptor has the structure of a typical cytokine receptor and is activated by ligand-induced homodimerization, leading to the activation of the JAK2 tyrosine kinase which is widely expressed in different haematopoietic progenitor cells (188). The erythropoietin receptor has been shown to acquire transforming properties by an arginine to cysteine mutation in the extracellular domain. The mechanism for activation involves ligand-independent formation of homodimeric receptor molecules stabilized by a disulfide bond between the introduced cysteine residues in the extracellular parts of the receptors (189, 190).

The erythropoietin receptor has also been implicated in the transforming mechanisms of Friend spleen focus-forming virus which causes erythroleukaemia in mice (191). The gp55 glycoprotein of the virus envelope interacts directly with the erythropoietin receptor and thereby activates it (192–194). The interaction is highly specific and a dominant negative erythropoietin receptor inhibits gp55-dependent transformation (195). The critical interaction between the erythropoietin receptor and gp55 occurs in the transmembrane regions, but a site of interaction is also present in the extracellular domain (191).

6.2 Thrombopoietin receptor (MPL)

Although most of the receptor genes that have been transduced by oncogenic retroviruses code for tyrosine kinases, there is one example of a cytokine receptor which was identified as the product of a viral oncogene, i.e. MPL (196, 197). Recently, c-MPL was shown to be the receptor for thrombopoietin (198).

Analysis of the expression of MPL in human haematopoietic malignancies revealed that the expression was increased in 26 of 51 patients with acute myeloblastic leukaemia and in 5 of 16 patients with myelodysplastic syndrome (199). Moreover, amplification of *MPL* was observed in one patient with acute myeloblastic leukaemia.

7. Mechanisms of oncogenic activation of growth factor receptors

Protein tyrosine kinase receptors as well as cytokine receptors are activated by homo- or heterodimerization induced by ligand binding (5). Dimerization appears to be sufficient for receptor activation and, consequently, mutations in the receptors which induce dimerization will induce a proliferative signal even in the absence of ligand.

As has been exemplified above, mutations which promote dimerization of growth factor receptors are often seen in transformed cells. There are, however, several different mechanisms by which growth factor receptors become constitutively activated by dimerization and thereby contribute to the loss of growth control that characterizes transformed cells.

One mechanism to achieve an increased amount of dimeric receptors is to express an increased number of receptors per cell. Overexpression of a normal receptor, even in the absence of ligand, will shift the equilibrium from monomeric, inactive receptors to dimeric or oligomeric, active receptors. A concomitant expression of the corresponding ligand will of course reinforce the signal. Increased numbers of receptors can occur after increased transcriptional activation of a normal gene or after amplification of a gene. Amplification of growth factor receptors is most common for members of the EGF receptor family (200).

Another mechanism for receptor activation is a mutation in the receptor that promotes ligand-independent dimerization. One example is the erythropoietin receptor in which an R to C mutation in the extracellular domain has been found to lead to the formation of a disulfide bond between two receptors (190). Analogously, the loss of a cysteine residue in the extracellular domain of the orphan receptor RET in MEN2A allows the formation of a disulfide bond between the unpaired cysteine residues in two receptors (184, 185). Experimental introduction of an extra cysteine residue in the extracellular domain of the EGF receptor likewise causes the formation of dimeric, disulfide-bonded and activated receptors (201). It is possible that the activating L to S mutation in codon 301 of the CSF1 receptor (107) promotes receptor–receptor interactions. Another example is the replacement of valine in the transmembrane part of ERBB2 with a glutamic acid residue, which has been proposed to lead to a constitutively dimerized and activated receptor (57). Amplification of the EGF receptor is often accompanied by structural alterations which lead to increased dimerization of the product (43, 44).

A third type of mechanism to dimerize tyrosine kinases is via the formation of fusion proteins between a tyrosine kinase domain and a protein which is a functional dimer. Examples include the TRK, RET, and MET receptors, which have been found as fusion proteins together with, for example, tropomyosin, TPR, or the regulatory subunit of the cAMP-dependent protein kinase (134). Each of these fusion partners is able to form homodimers; therefore in the fusion proteins they will bring together the kinase domains, which may allow their autophosphorylation and activation.

Finally, there are examples of viral proteins which interact with growth factor receptors in a manner which may promote receptor dimerization. For instance, the E5 protein of papilloma virus can bind to the PDGF β receptor (93, 94) and possibly also the EGF receptor (95). Since the E5 protein is a small membrane protein which occurs as a disulfide-bonded dimer, it may interact in a symmetric manner with two receptors and thus promote receptor dimerization. It is also possible that gp55 of Friend spleen focus-forming virus activates the erythropoietin receptor through the formation of receptor dimers, although this has not been shown directly (191).

There are, however, other principally different mechanisms whereby tyrosine kinase receptors can acquire transforming properties, such as by mutations in the kinase domain of the receptor leading to an increased catalytic activity of the kinase or to an altered substrate specificity. Examples include mutations in the EGF receptor in cells transformed by avian leukosis virus (37), and mutations in the RET protein tyrosine kinase receptor seen in MEN2B (185). Such mutations could expand quantitatively and qualitatively the repertoire of substrates in the target cells, and thereby shift the balance in cells towards growth stimulation and transformation.

In addition to mutations in receptors that alter the substrate specificity, increase the catalytic activity, or promote dimerization and activation, mutations that perturb regions involved in negative regulation of receptor function may also contribute to the transforming properties. Examples include loss of a regulatory tyrosine residue in the carboxy terminus of the CSF1 receptor (106), and loss of regulatory regions in the carboxy terminus of the EGF receptor containing regulatory serine phosphorylation sites (31, 32) as well as autophosphorylation sites (33). Loss of such negative regulatory sites may contribute to excessive receptor activity and transformation. A negative regulatory region has recently been identified in the erythropoietin receptor (202) and may occur in other cytokine receptors. However, whether mutations in such regions of cytokine receptors contribute to cell transformation remains to be elucidated.

In conclusion, several different types of mutations that affect the activation of growth factor receptors have been identified. Often, a combination of different mutations in a given receptor is necessary to achieve full transforming activity.

8. Concluding remarks

Mutated versions of receptors for growth stimulating factors have been identified as dominantly acting oncogenes of acutely transforming retroviruses, in tumours induced by chemical carcinogens, as well as in human tumours. Overexpression of normal receptors has also been associated with the development of tumours. However, in particular types of tumours the expression of certain growth factor receptors has been shown to correlate with good prognosis, for example the receptors for NGF and SCF in neuroblastoma and melanoma, respectively (103, 104, 139). Presumably, the activity of these receptors is correlated with the maintenance of differentiation of these cell types. However, it remains to be determined whether the expression of these receptors is the cause or the effect of the differentiated phenotype of the tumour cells.

The increasing knowledge about growth factor receptors in cell transformation has opened up certain possibilities of using receptors as targets in anti-tumour therapy. The overexpression of specific receptors in certain tumour types, such as EGF receptor in glioblastoma, provides an opportunity for therapeutic intervention. Toxic EGF conjugates or receptor antibodies could be targeted directly to the tumour cells and leave normal cells less affected. Given the central and ubiquitous role of the IGFI receptor in cell growth and transformation, it is possible that the growth of many different tumour types could be slowed down by inhibition of IGFI receptor activation. Moreover, angiogenesis factors or their receptors could be targets for therapeutic interventions; inhibition of tumour angiogenesis may provide a general method to slow down the growth of solid tumours.

Acknowledgements

We thank Ingegärd Schiller for valuable help in the preparation of this manuscript, and Peter Blume-Jensen for drawing Fig. 1.

References

1. Aaronson, S. A. (1991) Growth factors and cancer. *Science*, **254**, 1146.
2. Fantl, W. J., Johnson, D. E., and Williams, L. T. (1993) Signalling by receptor tyrosine kinases. *Annu. Rev. Biochem.*, **62**, 453.
3. Kishimoto, T., Taga, T., and Akira, S. (1994) Cytokine signal transduction. *Cell*, **76**, 253.
4. Mui, A. L.-F. and Miyajima, A. (1994) Cytokine receptors and signal transduction. *Prog. Growth Factor Res.*, **5**, 15.
5. Heldin, C.-H. (1995) Dimerization of cell surface receptors in signal transduction. *Cell*, **80**, 213.
6. Lemmon, M. A. and Schlessinger, J. (1994) Regulation of signal transduction and signal diversity by receptor oligomerization. *Trends Biochem. Sci.*, **19**, 459.
7. Springer, B. A., Pantoliano, M. W., Barbera, F. A., Gunyuzlu, P. L., Thompson, L. D., Herblin, W. F., *et al.* (1994) Identification and concerted function of two receptor binding surfaces on basic fibroblast growth factor required for mitogenesis. *J. Biol. Chem.*, **269**, 26879.
8. Spivak-Kroizman, T., Lemmon, M. A., Dikic, I., Ladbury, J. E., Pinchasi, D., Huang, J., *et al.* (1994) Heparin-induced oligomerization of FGF molecules is responsible for FGF receptor dimerization, activation, and cell proliferation. *Cell*, **79**, 1015.
9. Davis, S., Gale, N. W., Aldrich, T. H., Maisonpierre, P. C., Lhotak, V., Pawson, T., *et al.* (1994) Ligands for EPH-related receptor tyrosine kinases that require membrane attachment or clustering for activity. *Science*, **266**, 816.
10. White, M. F., Shoelson, S. E., Keutmann, H., and Kahn, C. R. (1988) A cascade of tyrosine autophosphorylation in the β-subunit activates the phosphotransferase of the insulin receptor. *J. Biol. Chem.*, **263**, 2969.
11. Naldini, L., Vigna, E., Ferracini, R., Longati, P., Gandino, L., Prat, M., *et al.* (1991) The tyrosine kinase encoded by the *MET* proto-oncogene is activated by autophosphorylation. *Mol. Cell. Biol.*, **11**, 1793.
12. Pawson, T. (1995) Protein modules and signalling networks. *Nature*, **373**, 573.
13. Claesson-Welsh, L. (1994) Platelet-derived growth factor receptor signals. *J. Biol. Chem.*, **269**, 32023.
14. Rupp, E., Siegbahn, A., Rönnstrand, L., Wernstedt, C., Claesson-Welsh, L., and Heldin, C.-H. (1994) A unique autophosphorylation site in the platelet-derived growth factor α receptor from a heterodimeric receptor complex. *Eur. J. Biochem.*, **225**, 29.
15. Soltoff, S. P., Carraway III, K. L., Prigent, S. A., Gullick, W. G., and Cantley, L. C. (1994) ErbB3 is involved in activation of phosphatidylinositol 3-kinase by epidermal growth factor. *Mol. Cell. Biol.*, **14**, 3550.

16. Wada, T., Qian, X., and Greene, M. I. (1990) Intermolecular association of the p185[neu] protein and EGF receptor modulates EGF receptor function. *Cell*, **61**, 1339.

17. Carraway, K. L., III and Cantley, L. C. (1994) A Neu acquaintance for erbB3 and erbB4: A role for receptor heterodimerization in growth signaling. *Cell*, **78**, 5.

18. Prigent, S. A. and Gullick, W. J. (1994) Identification of c-erbB-3 binding sites for phosphatidylinositol 3'-kinase and SHC using an EGF receptor/c-erbB-3 chimera. *EMBO J.*, **13**, 2831.

19. Fedi, P., Pierce, J. H., Di Fiore, P. P., and Kraus, M. H. (1994) Efficient coupling with phosphatidylinositol 3-kinase, but not phospholipase Cγ or GTPase-activating protein, distinguishes ErbB-3 signaling from that of other ErbB/EGFR family members. *Mol. Cell. Biol.*, **14**, 492.

20. Kita, Y. A., Barff, J., Luo, Y., Wen, D., Brankow, D., Hu, S., *et al.* (1994) NDF/heregulin stimulates the phosphorylation of Her3/erbB3. *FEBS Lett.*, **349**, 139.

21. Sliwkowski, M. X., Schaefer, G., Akita, R. W., Lofgren, J. A., Fitzpatrick, V. D., Nuijens, A., *et al.* (1994) Coexpression of *erb*B2 and *erb*B3 proteins reconstitutes a high affinity receptor for heregulin. *J. Biol. Chem.*, **269**, 14661.

22. Cunningham, B. C., Ultsch, M., De Vos, A. M., Mulkerrin, M. G., Clausner, K. R., and Wells, J. A. (1991) Dimerization of the extracellular domain of the human growth hormone receptor by a single hormone molecule. *Science*, **254**, 821.

23. De Vos, A. M., Ultsch, M., and Kossiakoff, A. A. (1992) Human growth hormone and extracellular domain of its receptor: Crystal structure of the complex. *Science*, **255**, 306.

24. Ultsch, M., De Vos, A. M., and Kossiakoff, A. A. (1991) Crystals of the complex between human growth hormone and the extracellular domain of its receptor. *J. Mol. Biol.*, **22**, 865.

25. Kawahara, A., Minami, Y., and Taniguchi, T. (1994) Evidence for a critical role for the cytoplasmic region of the interleukin 2 (IL-2) receptor γ chain in IL-2, IL-4, and IL-7 signalling. *Mol. Cell. Biol.*, **14**, 5433.

26. Ihle, J. N., Witthuhn, B. A., Quelle, F. W., Yamamoto, K., Thierfelder, W. E., Kreider, B., *et al.* (1994) Signaling by the cytokine receptor superfamily: JAKs and STATs. *Trends Biochem. Sci.*, **19**, 222.

27. Ziemiecki, A., Harpur, A. G., and Wilks, A. F. (1994) JAK protein tyrosine kinases: their role in cytokine signalling. *Trends Cell Biol.*, **4**, 207.

28. Darnell, J. E., Jr., Kerr, I. M., and Stark, G. R. (1994) Jak-STAT pathways and transcriptional activation in response to IFNs and other extracellular signaling proteins. *Science*, **264**, 1415.

29. Downward, J., Yarden, Y., Mayes, E., Scrace, G., Totty, N., Stockwell, P., *et al.* (1984) Close similarity of epidermal growth factor receptor and v-*erb*-B oncogene protein sequences. *Nature*, **307**, 521.

30. Ullrich, A., Coussens, L., Hayflick, J. S., Dull, T. J., Gray, A., Tam, A. W., *et al.* (1984) Human epidermal growth factor receptor cDNA sequence and aberrant expression of the amplified gene in A431 epidermoid carcinoma cells. *Nature*, **309**, 418.

31. Countaway, J. L., Nairn, A. C., and Davis, R. J. (1992) Mechanism of desensitization of the epidermal growth factor receptor protein-tyrosine kinase. *J. Biol. Chem.*, **267**, 1129.

32. Theroux, S. J., Taglienti-Sian, C., Nair, N., Countaway, J. L., Robinson, H. L., and Davis, R J. (1992) Increased oncogenic potential of ErbB is associated with the loss of a COOH-terminal domain serine phosphorylation site. *J. Biol. Chem.*, **267**, 7967.

33. Downward, J., Parker, P., and Waterfield, M. D. (1984) Autophosphorylation sites on the epidermal growth factor receptor. *Nature*, **311**, 483.

34. Massoglia, S., Gray, A., Dull, T. J., Munemitsu, S., Kung, H.-J., Schlessinger, J., *et al.* (1990) Epidermal growth factor receptor cytoplasmic domain mutations trigger ligand-independent transformation. *Mol. Cell. Biol.*, **10**, 3048.

35. Nilsen, T. W., Maroney, P. A., Goodwin, R. G., Rottman, F. M., Crittenden, L. B., Raines, M. A., *et al.* (1985) c-*erb*B activation in ALV-induced erythroblastosis: novel RNA processing and promoter-insertion result in the expression of an amino-truncated EGF receptor. *Cell*, **41**, 719.

36. Shu, H.-K. G., Pelley, R. J., and Kung, H.-J. (1990) Tissue-specific transformation by epidermal growth factor receptor: A single point mutation within the ATP-binding pocket of the *erbB* product increases its intrinsic kinase activity and activates its sarcomagenic potential. *Proc. Natl. Acad. Sci. USA*, **87**, 9103.

37. Shu, H.-K. G., Chang, C.-M., Ravi, L., Ling, L., Castellano, C. M., Walter, E., *et al.* (1994) Modulation of erbB kinase activity and oncogenic potential by single point mutations in the glycine loop of the catalytic domain. *Mol. Cell. Biol.*, **14**, 6868.

38. Bigner, S. H., Mark, J., Burger, P. C., Mahaley Jr., S., Bullard, D. E., Muhlbaier, L. H., *et al.* (1988) Specific chromosomal abnormalities in malignant human gliomas. *Cancer Res.*, **88**, 405.

39. Ekstrand, A. J., James, C. D., Cavenee, W. K., Seliger, B., Pettersson, R. F., and Collins, V. P. (1991) Genes for epidermal growth factor receptor, transforming growth factor alpha, and epidermal growth factor and their expression in human gliomas *in vivo*. *Cancer Res.*, **51**, 2164.

40. Libermann, T. A., Nusbaum, H. R., Razon, N., Kris, R., Lax, I., Soreq, H., *et al.* (1985) Amplification, enhanced expression and possible rearrangement of EGF-receptor gene in primary human brain tumours of glial origin. *Nature*, **313**, 144.

41. Sugawa, N., Ekstrand, A. J., James, C. D., and Collins, V. P. (1990) Identical splicing of aberrant epidermal growth factor receptor transcripts from amplified rearranged genes in human glioblastomas. *Proc. Natl. Acad. Sci. USA*, **87**, 8602.

42. Yamazaki, H., Fukui, Y., Ueyama, Y., Tamaoki, N., Kawamoto, T., Taniguchi, S., *et al.* (1988) Amplification of the structurally and functionally altered epidermal growth factor receptor gene (c-*erbB*) in human brain tumors. *Mol. Cell. Biol.*, **8**, 1816.

43. Ekstrand, A. J., Sugawa, N. D., James, C. D., and Collins, V. P. (1992) Amplified and rearranged epidermal growth factor receptor genes in human glioblastomas reveal deletions of sequences encoding portions of the N- and/or C-terminal tails. *Proc. Natl. Acad. Sci. USA*, **89**, 4309.

44. Nishikawa, R., Ji, X.-D., Harmon, R. C., Lazar, C. S., Gill, G. N., Cavenee, W. K., *et al.* (1994) A mutant epidermal growth factor receptor common in human glioma confers enhanced tumorigenicity. *Proc. Natl. Acad. Sci. USA*, **91**, 7727.

45. Filmus, J., Pollak, M. N., Cailleau, R., and Buick, R. N. (1985) MDA-468, a human breast cancer cell line with a high number of epidermal growth factor (EGF) receptors, has an amplified EGF receptor gene and is growth inhibited by EGF. *Biochem. Biophys. Res. Commun.*, **128**, 898.

46. Ro, J., North, S. M., Gallick, G. E., Hortobagyi, G. N., Gutterman, J. U., and Blick, M. (1988) Amplified and overexpressed epidermal growth factor receptor gene in uncultured primary human breast carcinoma. *Cancer Res.*, **48**, 161.

47. Hollstein, M. C., Smits, A. M., Galiana, C., Yamasaki, H., Bos, J. L., Mandard, A., *et al.* (1988) Amplification of epidermal growth factor receptor gene but no evidence of *ras* mutations in primary human esophageal cancers. *Cancer Res.*, **48**, 5119.

48. Berger, M. S., Greenfield, C., Gullick, W. J., Haley, J., Downward, J., Neal, D. E., *et al.* (1987) Evaluation of epidermal growth factor receptors in bladder tumours. *Br. J. Cancer*, **56**, 533.

49. Gullick, W. J. (1991) Prevalence of aberrant expression of the epidermal growth factor receptor in human cancers. *Br. Med. Bull.*, **47**, 87.

50. Moroni, M. C., Willingham, M. C., and Beguinot, L. (1992) EGF-R antisense RNA blocks expression of the epidermal growth factor receptor and suppresses the transforming phenotype of a human carcinoma cell line. *J. Biol. Chem.*, **267**, 2714.

51. Velu, T. J., Beguinot, L., Vass, W. C., Willingham, M. C., Merlino, G. T., Pastan, I., *et al.* (1987) Epidermal growth factor-dependent transformation by a human EGF receptor proto-oncogene. *Science*, **238**, 1408.

52. Ciardiello, F., Kim, N., Saeki, T., Dono, R., Persico, M. G., Plowman, G. D., *et al.* (1991) Differential expression of epidermal growth factor-related proteins in human colorectal tumors. *Proc. Natl. Acad. Sci. USA*, **88**, 7792.

53. Nistér, M., Libermann, T. A., Betsholtz, C., Pettersson, M., Claesson-Welsh, L., Heldin, C.-H., *et al.* (1988) Expression of messenger RNAs for platelet-derived growth factor and transforming growth factor-α and their receptors in human malignant glioma cell lines. *Cancer Res.*, **48**, 3910.

54. Ciardiello, F., Tortora, G., Bianco, C., Selvam, M. P., Basolo, F., Fontanini, G., *et al.* (1994) Inhibition of CRIPTO expression and tumorigenicity in human colon cancer cells by antisense RNA and oligodeoxynucleotides. *Oncogene*, **9**, 291.

55. Shih, C., Padhy, L. C., Murray, M., and Weinberg, R. A. (1981) Transforming genes of carcinomas and neuroblastomas introduced into mouse fibroblasts. *Nature*, **290**, 261.

56. Bargmann, C. I., Hung, M.-C., and Weinberg, R. A. (1986) Multiple independent activations of the *neu* oncogene by a point mutation altering the transmembrane domain of p185. *Cell*, **45**, 649.

57. Weiner, D. B., Liu, J., Cohen, J. A., Williams, W. V., and Greene, M. I. (1989) A point mutation in the *neu* oncogene mimics ligand induction of receptor aggregation. *Nature*, **339**, 230.

58. Lofts, F. J., Hurst, H. C., Sternberg, M. J. E., and Gullick, W. J. (1993) Specific short transmembrane sequences can inhibit transformation by the mutant *neu* growth factor receptor *in vitro* and *in vivo*. *Oncogene*, **8**, 2813.

59. Coussens, L., Yang-Feng, T. L., Liao, Y.-C., Chen, E., Gray, A., McGrath, J., *et al.* (1985) Tyrosine kinase receptor with extensive homology to EGF receptor shares chromosomal location with *neu* oncogene. *Science*, **230**, 1132.

60. King, C. R., Kraus, M. H., and Aaronson, S. A. (1985) Amplification of a novel v-*erb*B-related gene in a human mammary carcinoma. *Science*, **229**, 974.

61. Di Fiore, P. P., Pierce, J. H., Kraus, M. H., Segatto, O., King, C. R., and Aaronson, S. A. (1987) *erb*B-2 is a potent oncogene when overexpressed in NIH/3T3 cells. *Science*, **237**, 178.

62. Hudziak, R. M., Schlessinger, J., and Ullrich, A. (1987) Increased expression of the putative growth factor receptor p185[HER2] causes transformation and tumorigenesis of NIH 3T3 cells. *Proc. Natl. Acad. Sci. USA*, **84**, 7159.

63. Brandt-Rauf, P. W., Pincus, M. R., and Carney, W. P. (1994) The c-*erb*B-2 protein in oncogenesis: Molecular structure to molecular epidemiology. *Crit. Rev. Oncogenesis*, **5**, 313.

64. Hynes, N. E. and Stern, D. F. (1994) The biology of erbB-2/neu/HER-2 and its role in cancer. *Biochim. Biophys. Acta*, **1198**, 165.

65. Lovekin, C., Ellis, I. O., Locker, A., Robertson, J. F. R., Bell, J., Nicholson, R., *et al.* (1991) c-erbB-2 oncoprotein expression in primary and advanced breast cancer. *Br. J. Cancer,* **63**, 439.

66. Slamon, D. J., Godolphin, W., Jones, L. A., Holt, J. A., Wong, S. G., Keith, D. E., *et al.* (1989) Studies of the HER-2/*neu* proto-oncogene in human breast and ovarian cancer. *Science,* **224**, 707.

67. Ramachandra, S., Machin, L., Ashley, S., Monaghan, P., and Gusterson, B. A. (1990) Immunohistochemical distribution of c-erbB-2 in *in situ* breast carcinoma—A detailed morphological analysis. *J. Pathol.,* **161**, 7.

68. Van de Vijver, M. J., Peterse, J. L., Mooi, W. J., Wisman, P., Lomans, J., Dalesio, O., *et al.* (1988) *Neu*-protein overexpression in breast cancer. Association with comedo-type ductal carcinoma *in situ* and limited prognostic value in stage II breast cancer. *N. Engl. J. Med.,* **319**, 1239.

69. Bouchard, L., Lamarre, L., Tremblay, P. J., and Jolicoeur, P. (1989) Stochastic appearance of mammary tumors in transgenic mice carrying the MMTV/c-*neu* oncogene. *Cell,* **57**, 931.

70. Guy, C. T., Webster, M. A., Schaller, M., Parsons, T. J., Cardiff, R. D., and Muller, W. J. (1992) Expression of the *neu* protooncogene in the mammary epithelium of transgenic mice induces metastatic disease. *Proc. Natl. Acad. Sci. USA,* **89**, 10578.

71. Muller, W. J., Sinn, E., Pattengale, P. K., Wallace, R., and Leder, P. (1988) Single-step induction of mammary adenocarcinoma in transgenic mice bearing the activated c-*neu* oncogene. *Cell,* **54**, 105.

72. Siegel, P. M., Dankort, D. L., Hardy, W. R., and Muller, W. J. (1994) Novel activating mutations in the *neu* proto-oncogene involved in induction of mammary tumors. *Mol. Cell. Biol.,* **14**, 7068.

73. Kraus, M. H., Issing, W., Miki, T., Popescu, N. C., and Aaronson, S. A. (1989) Isolation and characterization of ERBB3, a third member of the ERBB/epidermal growth factor receptor family: Evidence for overexpression in a subset of human mammary tumors. *Proc. Natl. Acad. Sci. USA,* **86**, 9193.

74. Lemoine, N. R., Barnes, D. M., Hollywood, D. P., Hughes, C. M., Smith, P., Dublin, E., *et al.* (1992) Expression of the *ERBB3* gene product in breast cancer. *Br. J. Cancer,* **66**, 1116.

75. Issing, W. J., Heppt, W. J., and Kastenbauer, E. R. (1993) *erb*B-3, a third member of the *erb*B/epidermal growth factor receptor gene family: its expression in head and neck cancer cell lines. *Eur. Arch. Otorhinolaryngol.,* **250**, 392.

76. Plowman, G. D., Culouscou, J. M., Whitney, G. S., Green, J. M., Carlton, G. W., Foy, L., *et al.* (1993) Ligand-specific activation of HER4/p180erbB4, a fourth member of the epidermal growth factor receptor family. *Proc. Natl. Acad. Sci. USA,* **90**, 1746.

77. Westermark, B., Betsholtz, C., Johnsson, A., and Heldin, C.-H. (1987) Acute transformation by simian sarcoma virus is mediated by an externalized PDGF-like growth factor. In *Viral carcinogenesis* (ed. N. O. Kjeldgaard and J. Forchhammer), pp. 445–57. Munksgaard, Copenhagen.

78. Fleming, T. P., Saxena, A., Clark, W. C., Robertson, J. T., Oldfield, E. H., Aaronson, S. A., *et al.* (1992) Amplification and/or overexpression of platelet-derived growth factor receptors and epidermal growth factor receptor in human glial tumors. *Cancer Res.,* **52**, 4550.

79. Kumabe, T., Sohma, Y., Kayama, T., Yoshimoto, T., and Yamamoto, T. (1992) Amplifi-

cation of α-platelet-derived growth factor receptor gene lacking an exon coding for a portion of the extracellular region in a primary brain tumor of glial origin. *Oncogene*, **7**, 627.

80. Hart, I. K., Richardson, W. D., Heldin, C.-H., Westermark, B., and Raff, M. C. (1989) PDGF receptors on cells of the oligodendrocyte-type-2 astrocyte (O-2A) cell lineage. *Development*, **105**, 595.

81. Guha, A., Dashner, K., Black, P. M., Wagner, J. A., and Stiles, C. D. (1995) Expression of PDGF and PDGF receptors in human astrocytoma operation specimens supports the existence of an autocrine loop. *Int. J. Cancer*, **60**, 168.

82. Hermanson, M., Funa, K., Hartman, M., Claesson-Welsh, L., Heldin, C.-H., Westermark, B., *et al.* (1992) Platelet-derived growth factor and its receptors in human glioma tissue: Expression of messenger RNA and protein suggests the presence of autocrine and paracrine loops. *Cancer Res.*, **52**, 3213.

83. Maxwell, M., Naber, S. P., Wolfe, H. J., Galanopoulos, T., Hedley-Whyte, E. T., Black, P. M., and Antoniades, H. N. (1990) Coexpression of platelet-derived growth factor (PDGF) and PDGF-receptor genes by primary human astrocytomas may contribute to their development and maintenance. *J. Clin. Invest.*, **86**, 131.

84. Hermanson, M., Nistér, M., Betsholtz, C., Heldin, C.-H., Westermark, B., and Funa, K. (1988) Endothelial cell hyperplasia in human glioblastoma: Coexpression of mRNA for platelet-derived growth factor (PDGF) B chain and PDGF receptor suggests autocrine growth stimulation. *Proc. Natl. Acad. Sci. USA*, **85**, 7748.

85. Plate, K. H., Breier, G., Weich, H. A., and Risau, W. (1992) Vascular endothelial growth factor is a potential tumour angiogenesis factor in human gliomas *in vivo*. *Nature*, **359**, 845.

86. Shamah, S. M., Stiles, C. D., and Guha, A. (1993) Dominant-negative mutants of platelet-derived growth factor revert the transformed phenotype of human astrocytoma cells. *Mol. Cell. Biol.*, **13**, 7203.

87. Strawn, L. M., Mann, E., Elliger, S. S., Chu, L. M., Germain, L. L., Niederfellner, G., *et al.* (1994) Inhibition of glioma cell growth by a truncated platelet-derived growth factor-β receptor. *J. Biol. Chem.*, **269**, 21215.

88. Alman, B. A., Goldberg, M. J., Naber, S. P., Galanopoulous, T., Antoniades, H. N., and Wolfe, H. J. (1992) Aggressive fibromatosis. *J. Pediatr. Orthop.*, **12**, 1.

89. Palman, C., Bowen-Pope, D. F., and Brooks, J. J. (1992) Platelet-derived growth factor receptor (beta-subunit) immunoreactivity in soft tissue tumors. *Lab. Invest.*, **66**, 108.

90. Smits, A., Funa, K., Vassbotn, F. S., Beausang-Linder, M., af Ekenstam, F., Heldin, C.-H., *et al.* (1992) Expression of platelet-derived growth factor and its receptors in proliferative disorders of fibroblastic origin. *Am. J. Pathol.*, **140**, 639.

91. Wang, J., Coltrera, M. D., and Gown, A. M. (1994) Cell proliferation in human soft tissue tumors correlates with platelet-derived growth factor B chain expression: An immunohistochemical and *in situ* hybridization study. *Cancer Res.*, **54**, 560.

92. Golub, T. R., Barker, G. F., Lovett, M., and Gilliland, D. G. (1994) Fusion of PDGF receptor β to a novel *ets*-like gene, *tel*, in chronic myelomonocytic leukemia with t(5;12) chromosomal translocation. *Cell*, **77**, 307.

93. Nilson, L. A. and DiMaio, D. (1993) Platelet-derived growth factor receptor can mediate tumorigenic transformation by the bovine papillomavirus E5 protein. *Mol. Cell. Biol.*, **13**, 4137.

94. Petti, L. and DiMaso, D. (1994) Specific interaction between the bovine papillomavirus

E5 transforming protein and the β receptor for platelet-derived growth factor in stably transformed and acutely transfected cells. *J. Virol.*, **68**, 3582.

95. Cohen, B. D., Goldstein, D. J., Rutledge, L., Vass, W. C., Lowy, D. R., Schlegel, R., *et al.* (1993) Transformation-specific interaction of the bovine papillomavirus E5 oncoprotein with the platelet-derived growth factor receptor transmembrane domain and the epidermal growth factor receptor cytoplasmic domain. *J. Virol.*, **67**, 5303.

96. Besmer, P., Murphy, J. E., George, P. C., Qiu, F., Bergold, P. J., Lederman, L., *et al.* (1986) A new acute transforming feline retrovirus and relationship of its oncogene v-*kit* with the protein kinase gene family. *Nature*, **320**, 415.

97. Yarden, Y., Kuang, W.-J., Yang-Feng, T., Coussens, L., Munemitsu, S., Dull, T. J., *et al.* (1987) Human proto-oncogene c-*kit*: a new cell surface receptor tyrosine kinase for an unidentified ligand. *EMBO J.*, **6**, 3341.

98. Zsebo, K. M., Williams, D. A., Geissler, E. N., Broudy, V. C., Martin, F. H., Atkins, H. L., *et al.* (1990) Stem cell factor is encoded at the *SI* locus of the mouse and is the ligand for the c-*kit* tyrosine kinase receptor. *Cell*, **63**, 213.

99. Chabot, B., Stephenson, D. A., Chapman, V. M., Besmer, P., and Bernstein, A. (1988) The proto-oncogene c-*kit* encoding a transmembrane tyrosine kinase receptor maps to the mouse W locus. *Nature*, **335**, 88.

100. Lev, S., Blechman, J. M., Givol, D., and Yarden, Y. (1994) Steel factor and c-kit protooncogene: Genetic lessons in signal transduction. *Crit. Rev. Oncogenesis*, **5**, 141.

101. Funasaka, Y., Boulton, T., Cobb, M., Yarden, Y., Fan, B., Lyman, S. D., *et al.* (1992) c-Kit-kinase induces a cascade of protein tyrosine phosphorylation in normal human melanocytes in response to mast cell growth factor and stimulates mitogen-activated protein kinase but is down-regulated in melanomas. *Mol. Biol. Cell*, **3**, 197.

102. Lassam, N. and Bickford, S. (1992) Loss of c-kit expression in cultured melanoma cells. *Oncogene*, **7**, 51.

103. Natali, P. G., Nicotra, M. R., Sures, I., Mottolese, M., Botti, C., and Ullrich, A. (1992) Breast cancer is associated with loss of the c-kit oncogene product. *Int. J. Cancer*, **52**, 713.

104. Natali, P. G., Nicotra, M. R., Sures, I., Santoro, E., Bigotti, A., and Ullrich, A. (1992) Expression of c-kit receptor in normal and transformed human nonlymphoid tissues. *Cancer Res.*, **52**, 6139.

105. Sherr, C. J., Rettenmier, C. W., Sacca, R., Roussel, M. F., Look, A. T., and Stanley, E. R. (1985) The c-*fms* proto-oncogene product is related to the receptor for the mononuclear phagocyte growth factor, CSF-1. *Cell*, **41**, 665.

106. Coussens, L., Van Beveren, C., Smith, D., Chen, E., Mitchell, R. L., Isacke, C., *et al.* (1986) Structural alteration of viral homologue of receptor proto-oncogene *fms* at carboxyl terminus. *Nature*, **320**, 277.

107. Roussel, M. F., Downing, J. R., Rettenmier, C. W., and Sherr, C. J. (1988) A point mutation in the extracellular domain of the human CSF-1 receptor (c-*fms* proto-oncogene product) activates its transforming potential. *Cell*, **55**, 979.

108. Gisselbrecht, S., Fichelson, S., Sola, B., Bordereaux, D., Hampe, A., Andre, C., *et al.* (1987) Frequent c-fms activation by proviral insertion in mouse myeloblastic leukaemias. *Nature*, **329**, 259.

109. Jacobs, A. (1992) Gene mutations in myelodysplasia. *Leuk. Res.*, **16**, 47.

110. Ullrich, A., Gray, A., Tam, A. W., Yang-Feng, T., Tsubokawa, M., Collins, C., *et al.* (1986) Insulin-like growth factor I receptor primary structure: comparison with insulin receptor suggests structural determinants that define functional specificity. *EMBO J.*, **5**, 2503.

111. Foekens, J. A., Portengen, H., van Putten, W. L. J., Trapman, A. M. A. C., Reubi, J.-C., Alexieva-Figusch, J., *et al.* (1989) Prognostic value of receptors for insulin-like growth factor 1, somatostatin, and epidermal growth factor in human breast cancer. *Cancer Res.*, **49**, 7002.

112. Pekonen, F., Partanen, S., Mäkinen, T., and Rutanen, E.-M. (1988) Receptors for epidermal growth factor and insulin-like growth factor I and their relation to steroid receptors in human breast cancer. *Cancer Res.*, **48**, 1343.

113. Peyrat, J.-P., Bonneterre, J., Beuscart, R., Djiane, J., and Demaille, A. (1988) Insulin-like growth factor 1 receptors in human breast cancer and their relation to estradiol and progesterone receptors. *Cancer Res.*, **48**, 6429.

114. Berns, E. M., Klijn, J. G., van Staveren, I. L., Portengen, H., and Foekens, J. A. (1992) Sporadic amplification of the insulin-like growth factor 1 receptor gene in human breast tumors. *Cancer Res.*, **52**, 1036.

115. Scher, C. D., Shepard, R. C., Antoniades, H. N., and Stiles, C. D. (1979) Platelet-derived growth factor and the regulation of the mammalian fibroblast cell cycle. *Biochim. Biophys. Acta*, **560**, 217.

116. Stiles, C. D., Capone, G. T., Scher, C. D., Antoniades, H. N., Van Wyk, J. J., and Pledger, W. J. (1979) Dual control of cell growth by somatomedins and platelet-derived growth factor. *Proc. Natl. Acad. Sci. USA*, **76**, 1279.

117. Baker, J., Liu, J.-P., Robertson, E. J., and Efstratiadis, A. (1993) Role of insulin-like growth factors in embryonic and postnatal growth. *Cell*, **75**, 73.

118. Liu, J.-P., Baker, J., Perkins, A. S., Robertson, E. J., and Efstratiadis, A. (1993) Mice carrying null mutations of the genes encoding insulin-like growth factor I (*Igf-1*) and type 1 IGF receptor (*Igf1r*). *Cell*, **75**, 59.

119. Sell, C., Rubini, M., Rubin, R., Liu, J.-P., Efstratiadis, A., and Baserga, R. (1993) Simian virus 40 large tumor antigen is unable to transform mouse embryonic fibroblasts lacking type 1 insulin-like growth factor receptor. *Proc. Natl. Acad. Sci. USA*, **90**, 11217.

120. Sell, C., Dumenil, G., Deveaud, C., Miura, M., Coppola, D., DeAngelis, T., *et al.* (1994) Effect of a null mutation of the insulin-like growth factor I receptor gene on growth and transformation of mouse embryo fibroblasts. *Mol. Cell. Biol.*, **14**, 3604.

121. Coppola, D., Ferber, A., Miura, M., Sell, C., D'Ambrosio, C., Rubin, R., *et al.* (1994) A functional insulin-like growth factor I receptor is required for the mitogenic and transforming activities of the epidermal growth factor receptor. *Mol. Cell. Biol.*, **14**, 4588.

122. Baserga, R., Sell, C., Porcu, P., and Rubini, M. (1994) The role of the IGFI receptor in the growth and transformation of mammalian cells. *Cell Prolif.*, **27**, 63.

123. Resnicoff, M., Coppola, D., Sell, C., Rubin, R., Ferrone, S., and Baserga, R. (1994) Growth inhibition of human melanoma cells in nude mice by antisense strategies to the type 1 insulin-like growth factor receptor. *Cancer Res.*, **54**, 4848.

124. Resnicoff, M., Sell, C., Rubini, M., Coppola, D., Ambrose, D., Baserga, R., *et al.* (1994) Rat glioblastoma cells expressing an antisense RNA to the insulin-like growth factor-1 (IGF1) receptor are nontumorigenic and induce regression of wild-type tumors. *Cancer Res.*, **54**, 2218.

125. Valentinis, B., Porcu, P. L., Quinn, K., and Baserga, R. (1994) The role of the insulin-like growth factor I receptor in the transformation by simian virus 40 T antigen. *Oncogene*, **9**, 825.

126. Sell, C., Baserga, R., and Rubin, R. (1995) Insulin-like growth factor I (IGFI) and the IGFI receptor prevent etoposide-induced apoptosis. *Cancer Res.*, **55**, 303.

127. Harrington, E. A., Bennett, M. R., Fanidi, A., and Evan, G. I. (1994) c-*myc* induced apoptosis in fibroblasts is inhibited by specific cytokines. *EMBO J.*, **13**, 3286.

128. Baserga, R. (1995) The insulin-like growth factor I receptor: A key to tumor growth? *Cancer Res.*, **55**, 249.

129. Martin-Zanca, D., Hughes, S. H., and Barcacid, M. (1986) A human oncogene formed by the fusion of truncated tropomyosin and protein tyrosine kinase sequences. *Nature*, **319**, 743.

130. Barbacid, M., Lamballe, F., Pulido, D., and Klein, R. (1991) The *trk* family of tyrosine protein kinase receptors. *Biochim. Biophys. Acta*, **1072**, 115.

131. Coulier, F., Martin-Zanca, D., Ernst, M., and Barbacid, M. (1989) Mechanism of activation of the human *trk* oncogene. *Mol. Cell. Biol.*, **9**, 15.

132. Ziemiecki, A., Müller, R. G., Xiao-Chang, F., Hynes, N. E., and Kozma, S. (1990) Oncogenic activation of the human *trk* proto-oncogene by recombination with the ribosomal large subunit protein L7a. *EMBO J.*, **9**, 191.

133. Greco, A., Pierotti, M. A., Bongarzone, I., Pagliardini, S., Lanzi, C., and Della Porta, G. (1992) Trk-t1 is a novel oncogene formed by the fusion of tpr and trk genes in a human papillary thyroid carcinoma. *Oncogene*, **7**, 237.

134. Rodrigues, G. A. and Park, M. (1994) Oncogenic activation of tyrosine kinases. *Curr. Opin. Genet. Dev.*, **4**, 15.

135. Bongarzone, I., Pierotti, M. A., Monzini, N., Mondellini, P., Manenti, G., Donghi, R., *et al.* (1989) High frequency of activation of tyrosine kinase oncogenes in human papillary thyroid carcinoma. *Oncogene*, **4**, 1457.

136. Sozzi, G., Bongarzone, I., Miozzo, M., Cariani, C. T., Mondellini, P., Calderone, C., *et al.* (1992) Cytogenetic and molecular genetic characterization of papillary thyroid carcinomas. *Genes Chrom. Cancer*, **5**, 212.

137. Borrello, M. G., Bongarzone, I., Pierotti, M. A., Luksch, R., Gasparini, M., Collini, P., *et al.* (1993) *trk* and *ret* proto-oncogene expression in human neuroblastoma specimens: high frequency of *trk* expression in non-advanced stages. *Int. J. Cancer*, **54**, 540.

138. Kogner, P., Barbany, G., Dominici, C., Castello, M. A., Raschellá, G., and Persson, H. (1993) Coexpression of messenger RNA for *TRK* protooncogene and low affinity nerve growth factor receptor in neuroblastoma with favorable prognosis. *Cancer Res.*, **53**, 2044.

139. Nakagawara, A., Arima-Nakagawara, M., Scavarda, N. J., Azar, C. G., Cantor, A. B., and Brodeur, G. M. (1993) Association between high levels of expression of the TRK gene and favorable outcome in human neuroblastoma. *N. Engl. J. Med.*, **328**, 847.

140. Suzuki, T., Bogenmann, E., Shimada, H., Stram, D., and Seeger, R. C. (1993) Lack of high-affinity nerve growth factor receptors in aggressive neuroblastomas. *J. Natl. Cancer Inst.*, **85**, 377.

141. Folkman, J. and Shing, Y. (1992) Angiogenesis. *J. Biol. Chem.*, **267**, 10931.

142. Shweiki, D., Itin, A., Soffer, D., and Keshet, E. (1992) Vascular endothelial growth factor induced by hypoxia may mediate hypoxia-initiated angiogenesis. *Nature*, **359**, 843.

143. Samoto, K., Ikezaki, K., Ono, M., Shono, T., Kohno, K., Kuwano, M., *et al.* (1995) Expression of vascular endothelial growth factor and its possible relation with neovascularization in human brain tumors. *Cancer Res.*, **55**, 1189.

144. Plate, K. H., Breier, G., Millauer, B., Ullrich, A., and Risau, W. (1993) Up-regulation of vascular endothelial growth factor and its cognate receptors in a rat glioma model of tumor angiogenesis. *Cancer Res.*, **53**, 5822.

145. Millauer, B., Shawver, L. K., Plate, K. H., Risau, W., and Ullrich, A. (1994) Glioblastoma growth inhibited *in vivo* by a dominant-negative Flk-1 mutant. *Nature*, **367**, 576.

146. Kim, K. J., Li, B., Winer, J., Armanini, M., Gillett, N., Phillips, H. S., *et al.* (1993) Inhibition of vascular endothelial growth factor-induced angiogenesis suppresses tumour growth *in vivo*. *Nature*, **362**, 841.

147. Brown, L. F., Berse, B., Jackman, R. W., Tognazzi, K., Manseau, E. J., Dvorak, H. F., *et al.* (1993) Increased expression of vascular permeability factor (vascular endothelial growth factor) and its receptors in kidney and bladder carcinomas. *Am. J. Pathol.*, **143**, 1255.

148. Wizigmann-Voos, S., Breier, G., Risau, W., and Plate, K. H. (1995) Up-regulation of vascular endothelial growth factor and its receptors in von Hippel–Lindau disease-associated and sporadic hemangioblastomas. *Cancer Res.*, **55**, 1358.

149. Kandel, J., Bossy, W. E., Radvanyi, F., Klagsbrun, M., Folkman, J., and Hanahan, D. (1991) Neovascularization is associated with a switch to the export of bFGF in the multistep development of fibrosarcoma. *Cell*, **66**, 1095.

150. Abe, T., Okamura, K., Ono, M., Kohno, K., Mori, T., Hori, S., and Kuwano, M. (1993) Induction of vascular endothelial tubular morphogenesis by human glioma cells. A model system for tumor angiogenesis. *J. Clin. Invest.*, **92**, 54.

151. Hori, A., Sasada, R., Matsutani, E., Naito, K., Sakura, Y., Fujita, T., *et al.* (1991) Suppression of solid tumor growth by immunoneutralizing monoclonal antibody against human basic fibroblast growth factor. *Cancer Res.*, **51**, 6180.

152. Halaban, R., Funasaka, Y., Lee, J., Rubin, J., Ron, D., and Birnbaum, D. (1991) Fibroblast growth factors in normal and malignant melanocytes. In *Fibroblast growth factors in normal and malignant melanocytes*. The New York Academy of Sciences, New York.

153. Adnane, J., Gaudray, P., Dionne, C. A., Crumley, G., Jaye, M., Schlessinger, J., Jeanteur, P., *et al.* (1991) BEK and FLG, two receptors to members of the FGF family, are amplified in subsets of human breast cancers. *Oncogene*, **6**, 659.

154. Kaipainen, A., Vlaykova, T., Hatva, E., Böhling, T., Jekunen, A., Pyrhönen, S., *et al.* (1994) Enhanced expression of the Tie receptor tyrosine kinase messenger RNA in the vascular endothelium of metastatic melanomas. *Cancer Res.*, **54**, 6571.

155. Fidler, I. J. and Ellis, L. M. (1994) The implications of angiogenesis for the biology and therapy of cancer metastasis. *Cell*, **79**, 185.

156. O'Reilly, M. S., Holmgren, L., Shing, Y., Chen, C., Rosenthal, R. A., Moses, M., *et al.* (1994) Angiostatin: A novel angiogenesis inhibitor that mediates the suppression of metastases by a lewis lung carcinoma. *Cell*, **79**, 315.

157. Dameron, K. M., Volpert, O. V., Tainsky, M. A., and Bouck, N. (1994) Control of angiogenesis in fibroblasts by p53 regulation of thrombospondin-1. *Science*, **265**, 1582.

158. Van Meir, E. G., Polverini, P. J., Chazin, V. R., Su Huang, H.-J., de Tribolet, N., and Cavenee, W. K. (1994) Release of an inhibitor of angiogenesis upon induction of wild type *p53* expression in glioblastoma cells. *Nat. Genet.*, **8**, 171.

159. Cooper, C. S., Park, M., Blair, D. G., Tainsky, M. A., Huebner, K., Croce, C. M., *et al.* (1984) Molecular cloning of a new transforming gene from a chemically transformed human cell line. *Nature*, **311**, 29.

160. Bottaro, D. P., Rubin, J. S., Faletto, D. L., Chan, A. M.-L., Kmiecik, T. E., Vande Woude, G. F., *et al.* (1991) Identification of the hepatocyte growth factor receptor as the c-*met* proto-oncogene product. *Science*, **251**, 802.

161. Park, M., Dean, M., Kaul, K., Braun, M. J., Gonda, M. A., and Vande Woude, G. (1987)

Sequence of *MET* protooncogene cDNA has features characteristic of the tyrosine kinase family of growth-factor receptors. *Proc. Natl. Acad. Sci. USA*, **84**, 6379.

161a. Rodrigues, G. A. and Park, M. (1993) Dimerization mediated through a leucine zipper activates the oncogenic potential of the *met* receptor tyrosine kinase. *Mol. Cell. Biol.*, **13**, 6711.

162. Liu, C., Park, M., and Tsao, M.-S. (1992) Overexpression of c-*met* proto-oncogene but not epidermal growth factor receptor or c-*erb*B-2 in primary human colorectal carcinomas. *Oncogene*, **7**, 181.

163. Di Renzo, M. F., Olivero, M., Ferro, S., Prat, M., Bongarzone, I., Pilotti, S., *et al.* (1992) Overexpression of the c-*MET*/HGF receptor gene in human thyroid carcinomas. *Oncogene*, **7**, 2549.

164. Di Renzo, M. F., Olivero, M., Katsaros, D., Crepaldi, T., Gaglia, P., Zola, P., *et al.* (1994) Overexpression of the *MET*/HGF receptor in ovarian cancer. *Int. J. Cancer*, **58**, 658.

165. Kuniyasu, H., Yasui, W., Kitadai, Y., Yokozaki, H., Ito, H., and Tahara, E. (1992) Frequent amplification of the c-*met* gene in scirrhous type stomach cancer. *Biochem. Biophys. Res. Commun.*, **189**, 227.

166. Di Renzo, M. F., Poulsom, R., Olivero, M., Comoglio, P. M., and Lemoine, N. R. (1995) Expression of the *Met*/hepatocyte growth factor receptor in human pancreatic cancer. *Cancer Res.*, **55**, 1129.

167. Boix, L., Rosa, J. L., Ventura, F., Castells, A., Bruix, J., Rodés, J., *et al.* (1994) c-*met* mRNA overexpression in human hepatocellular carcinoma. *Hepatology*, **19**, 88.

168. Kuniyasu, H., Yasui, W., Yokozaki, H., Kitadai, Y., and Tahara, E. (1993) Aberrant expression of c-*met* mRNA in human gastric carcinomas. *Int. J. Cancer*, **55**, 72.

169. Ponzetto, C., Giordano, S., Peverali, F., Della Valle, G., Abate, M. L., Vaula, G., *et al.* (1991) c-*met* is amplified but not mutated in a cell line with an activated *met* tyrosine kinase. *Oncogene*, **6**, 553.

170. Cooper, C. S., Tempest, P. R., Beckman, M. P., Heldin, C.-H., and Brookes, P. (1986) Amplification and overexpression of the *met* gene in spontaneously transformed NIH3T3 mouse fibroblasts. *EMBO J.*, **5**, 2623.

171. Natali, P. G., Nicotra, M. R., Di Renzo, M. F., Prat, M., Bigotti, A., Cavaliere, R., *et al.* (1993) Expression of the c-Met/HGF receptor in human melanocytic neoplasms: demonstration of the relationship to malignant melanoma tumour progression. *Br. J. Cancer*, **68**, 746.

172. Rong, S., Bodescot, M., Blair, D., Dunn, J., Nakamura, T., Mizuno, K., *et al.* (1992) Tumorigenicity of the *met* proto-oncogene and the gene for hepatocyte growth factor. *Mol. Cell. Biol.*, **12**, 5152.

173. Ebert, M., Yokoyama, M., Friess, H., Büchler, M. W., and Korc, M. (1994) Coexpression of the c-*met* proto-oncogene and hepatocyte growth factor in human pancreatic cancer. *Cancer Res.*, **54**, 5775.

174. Takahashi, M. and Cooper, G. M. (1987) *ret* transforming gene encodes a fusion protein homologous to tyrosine kinases. *Mol. Cell. Biol.*, **7**, 1378.

175. Schneider, R. (1992) The human protooncogene *ret*: a communicative cadherin? *Trends Biochem. Sci.*, **17**, 468.

176. Bongarzone, I., Monzini, N., Borrello, M. G., Carcano, C., Ferraresi, G., Aroghi, E., *et al.* (1993) Molecular characterization of a thyroid tumor-specific transforming sequence formed by the fusion of *ret* tyrosine kinase and the regulatory subunit RIα of cyclic AMP-dependent protein kinase. *Mol. Cell. Biol.*, **13**, 358.

177. Carlson, K. M., Dou, S., Chi, D., Scavarda, N., Toshima, K., Jackson, C. E., et al. (1994) Single missense mutation in the tyrosine kinase catalytic domain of the RET protooncogene is associated with multiple endocrine neoplasia type 2B. Proc. Natl. Acad. Sci. USA, **91**, 1579.

178. Donis-Keller, H., Dou, S., Chi, D., Carlson, K. M., Toshima, K., Lairmore, T. C., et al. (1993) Mutations in the RET proto-oncogene are associated with MEN 2A and FMTC. Hum. Mol. Genet., **2**, 851.

179. Edery, P., Lyonnet, S., Mulligan, L. M., Pelet, A., Dow, E., Abel, L., et al. (1994) Mutations of the RET proto-oncogene in Hirschsprung's disease. Nature, **367**, 378.

180. Hofstra, R. M. W., Landsvater, R. M., Ceccherini, I., Stulp, R. P., Stelwagen, T., Luo, Y., et al. (1994) A mutation in the RET proto-oncogene associated with multiple endocrine neoplasia type 2B and sporadic medullary thyroid carcinoma. Nature, **367**, 375.

181. Mulligan, L. M., Kwok, J. B. J., Healey, C. S., Elsdon, M. J., Eng, C., Gardner, E., et al. (1993) Germ-line mutations of the RET proto-oncogene in multiple endocrine neoplasia type 2A. Nature, **363**, 458.

182. Romeo, G., Ronchetto, P., Luo, Y., Barone, V., Seri, M., Ceccherini, I., et al. (1994) Point mutations affecting the tyrosine kinase domain of the REF proto-oncogene in Hirschsprung's disease. Nature, **367**, 377.

183. Schuchardt, A., D'Agati, V., Larsson-Blomberg, L., Costantini, F., and Pachnis, V. (1994) Defects in the kidney and enteric nervous system of mice lacking the tyrosine kinase receptor Ret. Nature, **367**, 380.

184. Asai, N., Iwashita, T., Matsuyama, M., and Takahashi, M. (1995) Mechanism of activation of the ret proto-oncogene by multiple endocrine neoplasia 2A mutations. Mol. Cell. Biol., **15**, 1613.

185. Santoro, M., Carlomagno, F., Romano, A., Bottaro, D. P., Dathan, N. A., Grieco, M., et al. (1995) Activation of RET as a dominant transforming gene by germline mutations of MEN2A and MEN2B. Science, **267**, 381.

186. Balduzzi, P. C., Notter, M. F. D., Morgan, H. R., and Shibuya, M. (1981) Some biological properties of two new avian sarcoma viruses. J. Virol., **40**, 268.

187. Zong, C. S., Poon, B., Chen, J., and Wang, L. H. (1993) Molecular and biochemical bases for activation of the transforming potential of the proto-oncogene c-ros. J. Virol., **67**, 6453.

188. Witthuhn, B. A., Quelle, F. W., Silvennoinen, O., Yi, T., Tang, B., Miura, O., et al. (1993) Jak2 associates with the erythropoietin receptor and is tyrosine phosphorylated and activated following stimulation with erythropoietin. Cell, **74**, 227.

189. Longmore, G. D., Watowich, S. S., Hilton, D. J., and Lodish, H. F. (1993) The erythropoietin receptor: Its role in hematopoiesis and myeloproliferative diseases. J. Cell Biol., **123**, 1305.

190. Yoshimura, A., Longmore, G., and Lodish, H. F. (1990) Point mutation in the exoplasmic domain of the erythropoietin receptor resulting in hormone-independent activation and tumorigenicity. Nature, **348**, 647.

191. D'Andrea, A. D., Moreau, J. F., and Showers, M. O. (1992) Molecular mimicry of erythropoietin by the spleen focus-forming virus gp55 glycoprotein: the first stage of Friend virus-induced erythroleukemia. Biochim. Biophys. Acta, **1114**, 31.

192. Hoatlin, M. E., Kazak, S. L., Lilly, F., Chakraborti, A., Kozak, C. A., and Kabat, D. (1990) Activation of erythropoietin receptors by Friend viral gp55 and by erythropoietin and down-modulation by the murine $Fv-2^r$ resistance gene. Proc. Natl. Acad. Sci. USA, **87**, 9985.

193. Li, J.-P., D'Andrea, A. D., Lodish, H. F., and Baltimore, D. (1990) Activation of cell growth by binding of Friend spleen focus-forming virus gp55 glycoprotein to the erythropoietin receptor. *Nature*, **343**, 762.

194. Zon, L. I., Moreau, J.-F., Koo, J.-W., Mathey-Prevot, B., and D'Andrea, A. D. (1992) The erythropoietin receptor transmembrane region is necessary for activation by the friend spleen focus-forming virus gp55 glycoprotein. *Mol. Cell. Biol.*, **12**, 2949.

195. Barber, D. L., DeMartino, J. C., Showers, M. O., and D'Andrea, A. D. (1994) A dominant negative erythropoietin (EPO) receptor inhibits EPO-dependent growth and blocks F-gp55-dependent transformation. *Mol. Cell. Biol.*, **14**, 2257.

196. Souyri, M., Vigon, I., Penciolelli, J. F., Heard, J. M., Tambourin, P., and Wendling, F. (1990) A putative truncated cytokine receptor gene transduced by the myeloproliferative leukemia virus immortalizes hematopoietic progenitors. *Cell*, **63**, 1137.

197. Vigon, I., Mornon, J. P., Cocault, L., Mitjavila, M. T., Tambourin, P., Gisselbrecht, S., *et al.* (1992) Molecular cloning and characterization of MPL, the human homolog of the v-mpl oncogene: identification of a member of the hematopoietic growth factor receptor superfamily. *Proc. Natl. Acad. Sci. USA*, **89**, 5640.

198. Metcalf, D. (1994) Blood. Thrombopoietin—at last. *Nature*, **369**, 519.

199. Vigon, I., Dreyfus, F., Melle, J., Viguie, F., Ribrag, V., Cocault, L., *et al.* (1993) Expression of the c-mpl proto-oncogene in human hematologic malignancies. *Blood*, **82**, 877.

200. Brison, O. (1993) Gene amplification and tumor progression. *Biochim. Biophys. Acta*, **1155**, 25.

201. Sorokin, A., Lemmon, M. A., Ullrich, A., and Schlessinger, J. (1994) Stabilization of an active dimeric form of the epidermal growth factor receptor by introduction of an inter-receptor disulfide bond. *J. Biol. Chem.*, **269**, 9752.

202. Klingmüller, U., Lorenz, U., Cantley, L. C., Neel, B. G., and Lodish, H. F. (1995) Specific recruitment of SH-PTP1 to the erythropoietin receptor causes inactivation of JAK2 and termination of proliferative signals. *Cell*, **80**, 729.

4 | Oncogenic cytoplasmic protein tyrosine kinases

SERGE ROCHE and SARA A. COURTNEIDGE

1. Introduction

Phosphorylation on tyrosine residues accounts for only 0.05% of total protein phosphorylation in mammalian cells, yet protein tyrosine kinases play important roles in the intracellular transduction of extracellular signals. They are involved in various biological responses including cell growth and differentiation, cell motility, and cell secretion. Protein tyrosine kinases can be divided into two groups: receptor and non-receptor tyrosine kinases. The receptor class comprises a family of cell surface proteins, which act as receptors for a variety of ligands. They are composed of an extracellular domain which contains the ligand binding site, a transmembrane domain, and a cytoplasmic domain that contains catalytic activity. This class of kinase is detailed in Chapter 3. Members of the second class of tyrosine kinases do not have extracellular sequences and do not span the plasma membrane. They can be located in the cytoplasm, on the inner part of the plasma membrane, or in the nucleus. The cytoplasmic tyrosine kinases have been subclassified into a number of families based upon their structural homology. To date there are at least seven subgroups of non-receptor tyrosine kinases, consisting of the SRC, FPS, ABL, CSK, SYK, JAK, BTK, and FAK families. The different members of each family are listed in Table 1. They are quite diverse in tissue expression, structure, or function (for reviews see refs 1 and 2). Generally the sequences of the subgroups diverge significantly except for the presence of the catalytic domain and some additional sequences involved in protein–protein interactions. Many are involved in cell growth and several have been found as oncogenes: this includes *v-SRC, v-YES*, and *v-FGR* as members of the SRC family, *v-FPS/FES* in the FPS family, and *v-ABL* and BCR–ABL in the ABL family. They have been frequently transduced by animal RNA tumour viruses except for the cellular fusion BCR–ABL protein found in human chronic myelogenous leukaemia (Chapter 1). In this chapter we will concentrate on the oncogenic properties of cytoplasmic tyrosine kinases with particular attention to the interaction of these oncogenes with intracellular signalling networks.

Table 1 Cytoplasmic protein tyrosine kinases

	Cellular form	Oncogenic form
SRC family	c-SRC (pp60$^{c\text{-SRC}}$)	v-SRC (pp60$^{v\text{-SRC}}$)
	c-YES (p62$^{c\text{-YES}}$)	v-YES (pp90$^{gag\text{-v-YES}}$, pp80$^{gag\text{-v-YES}}$)
	FYN (p59^{FYN})	
	YRK (p60^{YRK})	
	c-FGR (p55$^{c\text{-FGR}}$)	v-FGR (p70$^{gag\text{-actin-v-FGR}}$)
	LCK (p56^{LCK})	
	HCK (P50^{HCK})	
	LYN (p56^{LYN})	
	BLK (p57^{BLK})	
FPS family	c-FPS/FES (p98$^{c\text{-FPS}}$, p92$^{c\text{-FES}}$)	v-FPS/FES (p130$^{gag\text{-v-FPS}}$, p110$^{gag\text{-v-FES}}$)
	FER	
	FLK	
ABL family	ABL (p145$^{c\text{-ABL}}$)	v-ABL (p160$^{gag\text{-v-ABL}}$, p95$^{gag\text{-fv-ABL}}$)
		BCR–ABL (p185$^{BCR\text{-ABL}}$, p210$^{BCR\text{-ABL}}$)
	ARG	
CSK family	CSK	
	MTK, HYL, ISK, CTK, HTK	
SYK family	SYK (p72^{SYK})	
	ZAP-70	
JAK family	JAK1	
	JAK2	
	JAK3	
	TYK2	
BTK family	BTK, ATK, BPK	
	TEK	
	ITK	
FAK family	FAK (pp125^{FAK})	

2. Description

2.1 SRC family

The SRC family of tyrosine kinases is composed of nine members in higher eukaryotes of which three, SRC, YES, and FGR, have viral counterparts. The first viral form identified was pp60$^{v\text{-SRC}}$, the transforming product of the chicken retrovirus Rous sarcoma virus (RSV) (for review see ref. 3). Later the cellular homologue of v-SRC was identified as c-SRC. Both have protein tyrosine kinase activity. Like v-SRC, viral YES and FGR transforming products were found in the genomes of animal transforming retroviruses: for example the avian Yamaguchi-73 and Esh sarcoma viruses, encode pp90$^{gag\text{-v-YES}}$ and pp80$^{gag\text{-v-YES}}$ respectively (4, 5) and the Gardner Rasheed feline sarcoma virus (GR-FeSV) encodes p70$^{gag\text{-actin-v-FGR}}$ (6). Cellular SRC and YES are widely expressed and are generally co-expressed in the same cell types, in contrast to FGR whose expression is restricted to myeloid cells (7, 8). SRC and YES are highly expressed in brain, platelets, and epithelial cells (reviewed in ref. 9). However, they can be preferentially expressed in some tissue such as chromaffin cells, osteoclasts, or differentiated keratinocytes for SRC, and Purkinje cells, kidney tubules, and placenta for YES (9). SRC has three alternatively spliced forms, two known as neuronal SRC (or n-SRC) expressed in brain tissue (9). These alternative forms possess an insertion of six or eleven amino acids in the SH3 domain (see below). A third form has been detected in chicken skeletal muscle, in which the transcript lacks sequences within the kinase domain (9). c-FGR was first observed in Epstein–Barr virus (EBV)-transformed B cells but not in normal B cells (10). It is generally found in highly differentiated myeloid cells such as granulocytes and macrophages (7, 8). Like YES, no alternatively spliced forms have been detected.

The SRC family kinases may arise from the same ancestral gene, since the positions of intron/exon boundaries are highly conserved. In mammals SRC and HCK, another member of the SRC family, lie close to one another on the same chromosome suggesting recent gene duplication (11). SRC family members have been detected in simpler eukaryotic species such as the freshwater sponge (12); the fact that these primitive organisms express multiple SRC-like kinases suggests a specific role for individual kinases. However SRC-like kinases are not present in yeast, indicating that their function may be specific to multicellular organisms. Genetic analyses in mice have indicated a role for SRC family kinases during development. Generally, loss of a single function is not lethal to mice, but the strains show specific defects such as osteopetrosis in SRC null mutants (13), lymphoid defects in LCK (14) and FYN deficient mice (15, 16), and neural defects in FYN deficient mice (17). The combination of double null mutants severely increases lethality: for example mice that do not express YES are viable whereas mice mutants that express neither SRC nor YES die during embryogenesis (18). Similarly no defects have been observed in mice where *FGR* was knocked-out, whereas *FGR–HCK* double null mutants showed several defects in natural immunity (19). These genetic analyses indicate that several members of the SRC family have important functions during development and that as with SRC and YES, or FGR and HCK, these functions are partially overlapping.

2.2 FPS family

The oncogenic FPS/FES protein was originally found in several avian (v-FPS) and feline (v-FES) retroviruses (reviewed in ref. 20). Comparison of sequences revealed that both products arise from the same gene; the FPS/FES family will therefore be referred to as the FPS family in this chapter. Cellular FPS homologues have been identified (21), and are expressed in haematopoietic cells of the granulocytic and monocytic lineages (22, 23) and in endothelial cells (24). An alternative *FPS* transcript has been reported in human lymphoma and lymphoid leukaemia cell lines that encodes a predicted 17 kDa protein tyrosine kinase (25). The FPS family has two other members, called FER (26), identified by cDNA screening, and FLK (27), identified by screening a rat brain expression library with an anti-phosphotyrosine antibody. In contrast to FPS, FER is more widely expressed. Little is known about FPS function, but its specific expression during differentiation of macrophages indicates that it could have a role in the maturation of myeloid cells. This notion is further supported by the fact that overexpression of FPS in the human erythroleukaemia cell line K526 (that does not express the protein endogenously) induces cell differentiation (28). The function of FPS in endothelial cells has been unravelled recently by using transgenic mice expressing an activated allele of FPS: widespread hypervascularity progressing to haemangiomas was induced, suggesting an important role for FPS in endothelial cell growth and consequently in regulation of angiogenesis (24).

2.3 ABL family

The ABL family has two members, ABL and ARG. Three oncogenic forms of ABL have been described: two variants are the products of animal retroviruses, including the mouse Abelson leukaemia virus (AMuLV encoding v-ABL) and the Hardy Zuckerman-2 feline sarcoma virus (HZ2-FeSV encoding fv-ABL) (reviewed in refs 29 and 30). A third cellular oncogenic form has been detected in humans and is involved in chronic myelogenous leukaemia; the transforming product BCR–ABL consists of a fusion protein originating from the Philadelphia chromosome translocation in which the 5' sequences of the BCR gene become fused upstream of the second exon of the *ABL* sequence (29, 31; and Chapter 1). Alternative chimeric proteins, p210 and p185, which contain the amino terminal 927 or 426 amino acids of BCR respectively, are produced (29, 31). The *c-ABL* gene generates two alternative spliced products, called ABL-I and ABL-IV which differ in their amino terminal sequences (29, 30).

ABL is ubiquitously expressed in mammalian cells. *ABL* and *ARG* are highly related and are widely expressed during development (32, 33). Genetic analyses in *Drosophila* and in mice suggest that *ABL* is important for the viability of post-embryonic organisms. Mutations in *Drosophila ABL* cause death at the adult pupal stage of development (34). In contrast, the loss of *ABL* in mice does not impair the development of neonates. However, loss of *ABL* induces lymphopenia in 50% of mouse mutants, indicating that ABL may play an important role in lymphocyte proliferation (35, 36). The absence of a severe defect in *ABL* null mice could also result from ABL and ARG having partially redundant functions.

3. Oncogenic versus proto-oncogenic tyrosine kinases

Normal cytoplasmic tyrosine kinases differ from their transforming counterparts in several respects, including primary sequence, kinase activity, and cell localization. In particular, viral forms frequently lack regulatory sequences present in the cellular forms. Therefore a comparison between an oncogenic form and its normal counterpart allows a better understanding of how cytoplasmic tyrosine kinases can induce cell transformation and how the normal forms are regulated *in vivo*. Their comparative properties are summarized in Table 2.

Table 2 Viral versus cellular cytoplasmic tyrosine kinases

	Kinase activity	Cellular localization	Function
pp60^{c-SRC}	−/+	Plasma membrane, early endosomes	Cell growth activation
pp60^{v-SRC}	++	Plasma membrane, adhesion plaques, cytoskeleton	Cell transformation
p98^{c-FPS}	−/+	Cytoplasm	Cell differentiation
p130$^{gag-v-FPS}$	++	plasma membrane, cytoskeleton	Cell transformation
p145^{c-ABL}	−/+	Nucleus, cytoplasm, actin filament	Cell growth inhibition
p160$^{gag-v-ABL}$	++	Plasma membrane, adhesion plaque, actin filament	Cell transformation

3.1 Structure

Non-receptor tyrosine kinases frequently have homologous domains important for activity, regulation, and substrate recognition. These common domains are referred to as SRC homology, or SH domains. They are the SH1 domain (the kinase domain), SH2, and SH3 domains. A schematic representation of the different proto-oncogenic and oncogenic cytoplasmic tyrosine kinases is presented in Fig. 1.

3.1.1 Kinase domain

The kinase domain is about 250 amino acids long. This domain is common to receptor and non-receptor tyrosine kinases and is highly conserved during evolution. The catalytic unit contains an ATP-binding site which consists of a GXGXXGX(15–20)K motif (37). The lysine residue (K295 for SRC) is critical for activity since replacement of this amino acid abolishes catalytic activity (3, 37). All these kinases contain a major autophosphorylation site in the kinase domain (Y416 in SRC, Y713 in FPS, or Y412 in ABL) which can be important for the kinase activity: replacement of the conserved tyrosine with phenylalanine often reduces the activity *in vitro* as well as *in vivo* (38–42).

3.1.2 SH2 domain

The SH2 domain consists of approximately 100 amino acids. It was first described in v-FPS as a conserved entity that shows about 50% homology with the corresponding region in SRC (43). The SH2 domain is found in all three tyrosine kinase families under discussion here and is conserved in the viral forms. In addition to cytoplasmic tyrosine kinases, SH2 domains are also present in a large set of unrelated proteins.

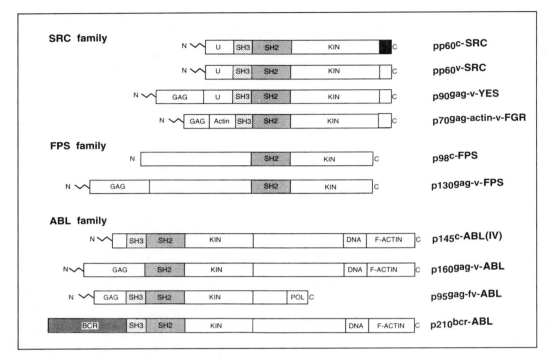

Fig. 1 Topography of the viral and cellular cytoplasmic tyrosine kinases. One representative member of the normal cellular forms and the known oncogenic forms of the cytoplasmic tyrosine kinases are shown. The presence of virally-encoded gag (GAG) and DNA polymerase (POL) sequences, the kinase region (KIN), the SH2, SH3, and unique (U) domains, as well as the DNA (DNA) and the F-actin (F-ACTIN) binding domains are indicated. (V\) indicates the presence of a myristyl group.

Most of these have roles in signal transduction networks, including enzymes such as phospholipase Cγ (PLCγ) and the tyrosine phosphatase SHP2, and adaptor molecules like SHC, GRB2, and the p85 subunit of the phosphatidylinositol-3-kinase (PI3K) (44). SH2 domains are involved in protein–protein interactions via the recognition of phosphorylated tyrosine residues (44, 45). The specific sequence surrounding the phosphotyrosine gives specificity to the association (46, 47). Crystallization and NMR studies have solved the SH2 structures of several proteins confirming such an interaction; these domains form compact, independently folded structures that are able to bind to specific phosphotyrosine containing peptides lying on a face of the domain (44, 46, 48).

3.1.3 SH3 domain

The SH3 domain consists of approximately 60 amino acids. It was first recognized in p47[gag–CRK], a transforming protein that has some homology with conserved regions in SRC and PLCγ (49, 50). An SH3 domain is included in most oncogenic cytoplasmic tyrosine kinases, except the FPS family and the feline form of v-ABL in HZ2-FeSV.

Like the SH2 sequences, a wide range of unrelated proteins contain SH3 domains. These include at least two families of proteins, the first of which are known to have functions in intracellular signalling networks, including enzymes (PLCγ, GAP) and adaptor proteins (p85 subunit of PI3K and the proteins NCK and GRB2) (51). The second family is composed of cytoskeleton-associated proteins such as α-spectrin and thermolysin I isoforms. SH3 domains are also detected in a number of unrelated proteins like the neutrophil/phagocyte oxidase factors p47 and p67 and some yeast proteins (46, 51). This domain is involved in protein–protein interaction through the recognition of small proline-rich regions where the surrounding amino acids in these sequences define the interaction specificity (46, 52, 53). The crystal structure of various SH3 entities has confirmed this interaction (54–56). A role has been proposed for this region in cellular localization and association with cytoskeletal components. Consistent with this idea, deletion of the SH3 domain redistributes the PLCγ and GRB2 proteins from membrane ruffles and actin stress fibres to the cytosol (57). Several proteins, including SRC and ABL kinases, PI3K and NCK possess a combination of SH2 and SH3 sequences which may allow them to complex with a large variety of proteins.

3.1.4 Specific sequences

In addition to the SH2, SH3, and kinase domains, cytoplasmic tyrosine kinases contain additional sequences which are specific to each family and may be important for cellular localization and/or for activity. Both viral and cellular SRC kinases are attached to the membrane via a myristylation site at the glycine at position 2 (58). In addition YES and FGR have palmitylation sites on cysteine residues within the first ten amino acids. Palmitylation increases the anchorage of these molecules to membranes (58). In contrast to YES, palmitylation of SRC has not been observed: instead the basic residues present in the amino terminal part of the molecule appear to contribute to the stabilization of the protein at the membrane (58). In both the v-YES and v-FGR oncoproteins, the amino terminal region of the kinase has been replaced by viral gag sequences (see Fig. 1) which locate the chimeric protein at the plasma membrane probably via myristylation. Lipid attachment sequences are followed by a sequence referred to as the unique domain. This region is about 70 amino acids long and is distinct from one member to another. However, the sequence is highly conserved during evolution, indicating that this region could be responsible for specific functions of each tyrosine kinase (1, 11), perhaps via protein–protein interactions. In favour of this idea, binding of LCK (a SRC family kinase) to CD4 in T lymphocytes involves the unique domain (59). Interestingly, the first 170 amino acids of c-FGR, including the unique domain, have been replaced in the viral form by a portion of gag fused to cellular actin sequences (6), suggesting that the unique domain is not absolutely required for cell transformation (Fig. 1). The last segment of the SRC family proteins is the carboxy terminal region, comprising amino acids 517–531 in avian c-SRC, often called the tail. This region diverges most between the cellular and viral proteins, but it is highly conserved among cellular members of the SRC family. Within the tail is a tyrosine that is highly phosphorylated *in vivo* (Y527 in c-SRC,

Y535 in c-YES, and Y511 in c-FGR). This residue is not present in any of the viral sequences, suggesting a crucial role for this tyrosine in regulation of the kinase activity (1, 3, 11).

In the FPS family, both viral and cellular forms of the protein contain an SH2 domain followed by the kinase domain (see Fig. 1). The SH2 domain is preceded by a long amino terminal domain which has been recently shown to have a role in protein interaction (60). In contrast to the SRC family, FPS proteins do not have SH3 domains or lipid modification sites. The viral p130$^{gag-FPS}$ and p110$^{gag-FES}$ proteins differ from the cellular counterparts by the replacement of the amino terminal region (the first 26 amino acids in the c-FPS product) with a portion of the viral structural protein gag, which contains a myristylation site (20).

Most ABL products contain an SH3 domain followed by an SH2 domain and the kinase domain (see Fig. 1). As seen in the SRC family, the ABL-IV form includes a myristylation site at the amino terminus which is not present in the alternatively spliced product, ABL-I (29). c-ABL contains a long carboxy terminal domain (474–1097 in mouse ABL) unique among the non-receptor tyrosine kinases (61). This region includes a DNA binding domain (836–935) followed by an F-actin binding region suggesting the existence of multiple functions for ABL. Although DNA binding activity has been shown *in vitro* (62), the responsible sequence does not share any homology with other known DNA-binding proteins. Specific interaction between ABL and the EP element of the human hepatitis B virus enhancer has been recently shown (63), but the exact sequence recognized by ABL has not been determined. The F-actin binding domain is involved in the association of ABL with actin filaments (64) and it shows a limited homology over 20–30 amino acids with actin-binding proteins like α-actinin and spectrin (61, 64). The kinase and the DNA binding domains are separated by a long sequence (about 360 amino acids) which might serve as a 'spacer'; interestingly this region contains a nuclear translocation sequence (61). The viral forms differ from the cellular ones in different regions of the molecule: in the A-MuLV oncoprotein the amino terminal region, including the SH3 domain, is replaced by a portion of the viral *gag* gene, whereas the HZ2-FeSV transforming product has the SH3 domain but lacks the carboxy terminal region (29) (see Fig. 1).

The cellular oncogene BCR–ABL comes from a genetic translocation observed in chronic myelogenous leukaemia where the *BCR* gene has been fused with *c-ABL* (Chapter 1). The resultant product comprises sequences from BCR fused to ABL sequences at the amino terminal region of the kinase. All the specific domains of ABL are present except for the myristylation site (29, 31). The *BCR* gene is widely expressed and encodes a 160 kDa protein that exhibits homologies with various other proteins: it has a serine/threonine kinase sequence in the amino terminal part of the molecule, a DBL homology domain, also known as a RAS guanine nucleotide exchange factor domain, and a GTPase-activating domain specific for the RAS-related proteins RAC1 and CDC42hs (31; and Chapter 5). In the context of the BCR–ABL fusion protein, only the serine/threonine kinase sequence has been retained.

3.2 Enzymatic activity

Transforming proteins show high activity *in vitro* as well as *in vivo* whereas proto-oncogenes are highly regulated *in vivo* and usually *in vitro*. A more detailed comparison of both cellular and viral products reveals additional characteristics about the mechanism of regulation. Except for the autophosphorylation site, the regulation of activity involves different mechanisms depending on the kinase family under consideration. SRC family kinases are negatively regulated by phosphorylation of a tyrosine residue present in the tail. Indeed, this tyrosine is stoichiometrically phosphorylated *in vivo* (65) and dephosphorylation or replacement by phenylalanine (Y527F in avian c-SRC) leads to a 10–20 fold increase in activity (40, 41, 66, 67). The absence of this tyrosine in the viral form explains in part the striking difference observed between the activities of viral and cellular kinases. Phosphorylation of Y527 is not due to SRC itself but to CSK (68) (i.e. carboxy terminal SRC kinase), a cytoplasmic tyrosine kinase distinct from the SRC family. This kinase phosphorylates other SRC family members *in vivo* including YES and FGR (1, 69). Mutagenesis studies in the SRC molecule point to a possible role of SH2 and SH3 domains in the regulation of its activity via an intramolecular mechanism. This model has been further confirmed by expressing SRC in yeast where neither SRC- nor CSK-like proteins are expressed; in this *in vivo* system, ectopically expressed SRC can be phosphorylated and regulated efficiently by co-expression of CSK (70–72). Using this system, it was shown that both the SH2 and the SH3 domains are required for regulation of SRC activity by CSK (see Fig. 2). The region with which the SH3 domain interacts is not known, but further mutagenesis studies suggest that the interaction involves the same residues in the SH3 domain as those required for intermolecular association with other proteins (73). *In vivo*, one would predict that activation of SRC family kinases could therefore occur either by dephosphorylation of the tail, or by association of either the SH2 or SH3 domain with high affinity ligands. In this case, the intramolecular interaction would be disrupted and kinase activity derepressed. In keeping with this, SRC, FYN, and YES have been shown to interact with the activated PDGF receptor via their SH2 domains (74, 75; and Chapter 3) and association induces activation of their intrinsic activity (Fig. 2C) (74, 76, 77). Another example of activation through dephosphorylation of the tail is the dephosphorylation of LCK by CD45, a transmembrane tyrosine phosphatase, which is required for T cell signalling (Fig. 2B) (78–80).

In addition to tyrosine phosphorylation, SRC kinases are subject to serine/threonine phosphorylation. SRC is phosphorylated at several serine and threonine residues in the amino terminal part of the molecule. SRC is constitutively phosphorylated on S17 by cAMP-dependent kinase, and on S12 by protein kinase C *in vivo* (3). The function of these phosphorylations is not known but mutation of these residues does not affect the kinase activity (3). SRC and possibly FYN and YES can also be phosphorylated in the unique domain on serine/threonine residues (T34, T46, and S72 in avian SRC) by cdc2 kinase during the M phase of the cell cycle (81). Their role in the *in vivo* activation of SRC observed during mitosis is not clear but *in vitro* (82) and

Fig. 2 Regulatory model of the SRC tyrosine kinase activity. (A) Repressed conformation of c-SRC involving an intramolecular interaction between the SH2 domain and the phosphotyrosine in the tail and between the SH3 domain and another part of the molecule which has yet to be identified. (B) Activated conformation of c-SRC involving the dephosphorylation of the tyrosine present in the tail. (C) Activated conformation of c-SRC showing the association of c-SRC with an SH2 binding protein. The presence of the SH2, SH3, unique (U), kinase (KIN) domains are shown.

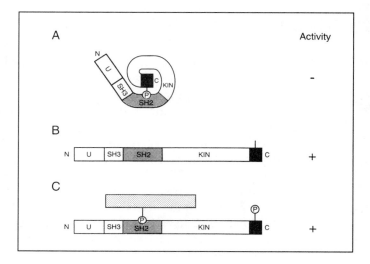

mutagenesis studies suggest that they are involved in activation of SRC during mitosis (83), perhaps by making SRC more susceptible to dephosphorylation of Y527 (81).

c-FPS activity is tightly regulated *in vivo* but in contrast to the SRC family, FPS does not contain any carboxy terminal inhibitory sequences, suggesting the existence of a distinct mechanism of regulation (20). An increase in activity generally correlates with tyrosine phosphorylation of the protein consistent with a positive regulation of FPS family by tyrosine phosphorylation (39, 42, 84–86). c-FPS autophosphorylates at two major sites including Y713 in the kinase domain (39, 87). Mutational analysis confirmed a role for both Y713 and the SH2 domain as positive regulators of the kinase activity, since deletion of either inhibited both $p92^{c\text{-}FES}$ and $p130^{gag\text{-}v\text{-}FPS}$ activities as well as the transforming capacity in the context of the viral oncoprotein (39, 88). Interestingly, an *in vitro* interaction has been observed between the SH2 domain and the autophosphorylation sites suggesting the existence of an intramolecular mechanism for kinase activation (39).

The main difference between the normal and oncogenic forms of FPS lies in the replacement of the first 26 amino acids of c-FPS by viral gag sequences. Overexpression of c-FPS using a retroviral expression vector does not induce cell transformation (89, 90) but addition of the gag sequence at the amino terminus does (24, 89, 91). Since the gag sequences endow FPS with a myristylation site, localization at the membrane is thought to be an important component in FPS-induced transformation. A role for the amino terminal sequence in the regulation of c-FPS activity has also been proposed, since this region is missing in the viral form (20). However, no important differences in the *in vitro* activity of cellular and viral kinases have been observed (89).

Regulation of ABL activity also occurs *in vivo*. Currently, two models are proposed for c-ABL inhibition both invoking an inhibitory function for the SH3 domain (Fig. 3). In keeping with this, several activated forms of ABL, including the product of A-

Fig. 3 Regulatory models of the ABL tyrosine kinase activity. (A) Repressed conformation of c-ABL involving the association of an inhibitor (I) that interacts with the SH3 domain of the kinase. (B) Repressed conformation of c-ABL involving an intramolecular interaction between the SH3 domain and the carboxy terminal region of the kinase. (C) Activated conformation of ABL in the context of BCR–ABL involving an intramolecular interaction between the SH2 domain of ABL and a region of BCR that is phosphorylated on both serine and threonine residues. The presence of SH2, SH3, and kinase (KIN) domains are shown.

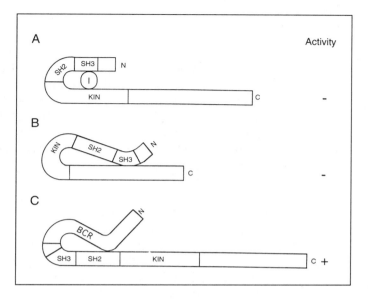

MuLV, lack an SH3 domain and deletion of this domain from c-ABL derepresses its activity *in vivo*. Furthermore, insertion of an SH3 domain into v-ABL inhibits its activity *in vitro* and its transforming ability *in vivo* (92). *In vitro* translation of *c-ABL* suggests that the kinase activity is regulated via a cellular inhibitor, so that the existence of an SH3 binding protein that would repress ABL activity has been postulated (93, and Fig. 3A). Several recent observations largely confirm this model: both wild-type and SH3-deleted c-ABL mutants show similar activity *in vitro* and *in vivo* when expressed in a neutral background such as in *Schizosaccharomyces pombe* (94). Therefore, the inhibitory effect of the SH3 domain may be mediated by a factor present in mammals and absent in fission yeast. Several SH3-binding proteins have been characterized (52, 53), including ABI1 and ABI2 (for ABL interactor 1 and 2) (95, 96). Both proteins are highly related and interact with ABL *in vitro* as well as *in vivo*. In addition, ABI proteins are substrates of ABL and modulate its transforming activity when overexpressed, suggesting that they could act as tumour suppressors (95, 96). However, whether ABI proteins are inhibitors of ABL kinase activity is not known and other ABI proteins that physiologically regulate ABL activity may exist. Interestingly, BCR–ABL and the HZ2-FeSV oncogenic products have retained the SH3 domain, indicating that in addition to an SH3-binding inhibitor, other factors could also affect the kinase activity (29, 31).

Although the data reported above largely confirm the first model, a second model has been proposed which involves an intramolecular interaction between the SH3 domain and the carboxy terminal region (Fig. 3B). In favour of the *cis*-inhibitory mechanism is the example of the HZ2-FeSV oncogene where the SH3 domain has been preserved but not the carboxy terminal region (29) and the existence of an oncogenic form of c-ABL where the exon encoding the last 644 amino acids has been deleted (97). An *in vitro* interaction between the SH3 domain and a specific sequence in the carboxy terminus has been observed, but the effect of this sequence on activity has not been reported (61). Another paradox is provided by BCR–ABL, where both SH3 and carboxy terminal regions are present (Fig. 3C). In this case, derepression of the activity may involve an interaction between the SH2 domain and the region encoded by the first exon of the BCR sequence. This model is supported by two observations: the ABL SH2 domain interacts specifically with the amino terminus of BCR *in vitro*, and deletion of either of these sequences inhibits cell transformation (98). In this particular case, SH2 domain association requires serine/threonine phosphorylation and not tyrosine phosphorylation as observed for most SH2 domains (98).

3.3 Subcellular localization

In addition to a change in kinase activity, oncogenic forms of cytoplasmic tyrosine kinases differ in subcellular localization, suggesting that this too may be important for cell transformation. This relocalization generally occurs to the plasma membrane or to the cytoskeletal matrix, but it can be different according to the kinase family. SRC tyrosine kinases are located at the plasma membrane, the perinuclear membrane, and in the endosomal compartments of the cell (99–101). In addition, while viral forms of SRC family kinases are abundant in focal adhesions, the cellular forms are poorly detected in this part of the cell (102, 103). A recent study has addressed the structural requirements for SRC to localize to the adhesion plaque. Both a derepressed conformation (where Y527 is not phosphorylated) and the SH3 domain are required (104).

c-FPS is largely cytosolic and recovered in detergent soluble fractions consistent with the absence of any lipid attachment site (20). In contrast to c-FPS, biochemical fractionation and immunofluorescence staining have shown that the v-FPS oncoprotein is largely present both in the plasma membrane and cellular matrix as observed for v-SRC and v-ABL oncoproteins (105–107).

In contrast to the SRC and FPS family kinases, c-ABL is largely nuclear: up to 20% of total ABL is present in the nucleus of liver cells (108). This localization correlates with the possible DNA binding function of c-ABL and its observed interaction with several nuclear proteins including the retinoblastoma protein (109, and Chapter 8) and RNA polymerase II (110). A structural study of the molecule suggests that both the SH3 domain and the nuclear translocation sequence are involved in nuclear localization (61). In contrast to the normal form, all activated forms of ABL are excluded from the nucleus, suggesting that DNA binding properties of c-ABL are dispensable for transformation, which has been confirmed by mutagenesis analysis (97). In addition, the exclusion of activated ABL from the nucleus might be involved in cell transformation: overexpression of c-ABL in fibroblasts does not induce cell transformation but inhibits the capacity of transfected cells to proliferate (111). Thus, exclusion of c-ABL from the nucleus by fusion with BCR may induce cell transformation partly by suppression of the inhibitory function related to nuclear localization of c-ABL.

In addition to its nuclear localization, c-ABL has also been detected in the cyto-plasm, including the cytosol and the actin filaments. In the case of BCR–ABL, the fused protein is exclusively associated with the actin bundles (64, 112) partly due to the amino terminal region of BCR: BCR–ABL forms multimers (113) and this homo-oligomerization requires the first 63 amino acids of BCR which increases the affinity of the F-actin binding domain for the actin filaments (64, 112, 113). Several explana-tions have been proposed for the varied localization of c-ABL, including the existence of two parallel functions of ABL in the cell, one in the nucleus and one at the cytoskeleton. On the other hand, a connection between the cytoskeleton and the nucleus has also been proposed (61), whereby ABL would participate in possible regulation of gene expression mediated by F-actin filaments.

4. Tyrosine kinases and cell transformation

Cell transformation can be induced by cytoplasmic tyrosine kinases in many ways, including overexpression of an activated form of the kinase, or activation of an endogenous kinase by DNA or RNA tumour virus products. In order to understand how cytoplasmic tyrosine kinases transform cells, extensive mutagenesis of various kinases has been performed and the transforming properties of the mutants analysed.

4.1 Change in activity

Cell transformation can be induced by a constitutive enzymatic activity as is the case with activated forms of c-SRC and FYN (40, 41, 66, 114) and SH3-deleted alleles of ABL (115). Cell transformation can also be achieved by high overexpression of the wild-type form where the level of expression is above a threshold so that cell factors cannot efficiently regulate it; 20-fold overexpression of c-SRC causes transformation (116), albeit less efficiently than v-SRC, possible because a proportion of the c-SRC is not regulated by CSK. Generally, viral tyrosine kinases show higher transforming activity compared to their cellular counterparts probably because of point mutations observed in the viral sequences (3).

4.2 Association with specific substrates

Changes in the activity and membrane localization of the kinase are not sufficient for cell transformation to occur: the activated kinase must also interact with specific sub-strates in order to induce full response. For example, truncation of the SH2 domain in v-SRC and in v-ABL severely affects their transforming abilities without affecting their kinase activities (117, 118), suggesting the existence of SH2-binding proteins important for oncogenic function. Similarly, the SRC SH3 domain can also be impor-tant for transforming activity: in the context of v-SRC an SH3 domain is not required for *in vivo* activity (117), whereas deletion of the similar sequence in activated c-SRC abrogates transformation of murine fibroblasts (73). Other specific regions of the tyrosine kinase can participate in the association of signalling proteins important for transforming effects. It has been recently shown that v-FPS forms complexes with the amino terminal sequence of the BCR protein (60). This association appears to be important for the biological activity of v-FPS, since deletion of the BCR-binding region impairs the capacity of the viral oncoprotein to induce cell transformation without affecting its kinase activity (119). When complexed, BCR becomes phosphorylated at residues that create a docking site for GRB2 (120), another signal molecule important for cell growth (60). In the context of BCR–ABL, the association involves the SH2 domain of GRB2 with the phosphotyrosine 177 of the BCR sequence (120, 121). GRB2 association appears to be required for cell transformation since mutation of Y177 in BCR–ABL inhibits cell transformation of Rat1 fibroblasts or primary bone marrow cultures (120).

4.3 Interaction with animal tumour viruses

Cytoplasmic tyrosine kinases can be involved in transformation by tumour viruses whose oncoproteins do not themselves have enzymatic activity. For example, SRC family tyrosine kinases have been implicated in cell transformation by the polyomavirus family of DNA tumour viruses (Chapter 1). c-SRC, c-YES, and FYN associate with the transforming product of the mouse polyomavirus, the middle T antigen (reviewed in ref. 122); complex formation with middle T antigen induces an increase in the kinase activity of SRC and YES mainly by prevention of phosphorylation of the tail by CSK (67). When complexed, middle T antigen becomes a substrate for the associated kinase, and tyrosine phosphorylation of different regions of the protein creates binding sites for SH2-containing proteins such as PI3K (123–126) and SHC (127, 128). Prevention of these associations by deletion of their binding sites impairs the ability of the middle T antigen to induce cell transformation (123, 127, 129).

Another example involves the retrovirally-encoded oncogene, *v-CRK* (49). Both v-CRK and c-CRK products encode proteins that comprise one SH2 and two SH3 domains, but lack kinase domains (52). Nevertheless, infection of fibroblasts with *v-CRK* induces tyrosine phosphorylation *in vivo*, indicating that a cellular tyrosine kinase has been activated during transformation. ABL may be the likely candidate, since it forms a stable complex with the v-CRK oncoprotein (130, 131) and CRK-associated kinase activity is drastically reduced in fibroblasts that do not express ABL (130). When complexed with CRK, ABL becomes largely depleted from the nucleus and relocated to the plasma membrane (130). Interaction with v-CRK involves a proline-rich region at the carboxy terminus of c-ABL and the first SH3 domain of CRK (52, 131). v-CRK may associate with important cellular proteins that can be phosphorylated by ABL, leading eventually to cell transformation.

5. Interaction with the intracellular signalling network

Oncogenic forms of cytoplasmic tyrosine kinases induce overt changes in cellular growth and dramatic alterations in cell morphology and adhesion. Both characteristics are due to activation of mitogenic signal pathways by phosphorylation and relocation of signalling molecules and possibly also to changes in structural protein assembly due to hyperphosphorylation.

5.1 Activation of the mitogenic signals

Many cytoplasmic tyrosine kinases are involved in cell growth pathways; for example, the cellular tyrosine kinases SRC, FYN, and YES can be activated by PDGF, CSF1, and EGF receptors (74, 76, 77, 132, 133) and FPS by GM-CSF, IL-3, and erythropoietin receptors (85, 86; and Chapter 3). The intracellular signals generated by the cellular kinases are generally necessary but not sufficient for cell growth (134, 135); oncogenic versions of these kinases activate in addition other signals which are sufficient to ensure cell growth. Consistent with this notion, signalling proteins stimulated or phosphorylated by oncogenic cytoplasmic tyrosine kinases are very similar to the ones induced by growth factor receptors (see Table 3; reviewed in ref. 45). These oncoproteins can activate the mitogenic signal at different levels of the intracellular signalling network: (a) at the receptor level by activation of the growth factor receptor (b) at the membrane with the use of docking proteins or (c) by direct interaction with signalling proteins. A constitutively active kinase stimulates mitogenic signals permanently so that cell proliferation is deregulated and the need for growth factors abrogated.

Oncogenic tyrosine kinases generally induce expression and secretion of growth factors that may account for cell proliferation observed in serum-free medium. For example, v-FPS induces the expression of TGFα, a ligand specific for EGF receptor (Chapter 3) in transformed rat embryo cells (136). Interestingly v-SRC can also interact directly with growth factor receptors. v-SRC phosphorylates the β subunit of the insulin-like growth factor I (IGF I) receptor, which triggers stimulation of the receptor kinase activity (137). Consistent with this activation, IRS1 (insulin receptor substrate

Table 3 Signalling proteins activated by the PDGF receptor and v-SRC

		Association	Phosphorylation	Activation
PDGF	c-SRC, FYN, c-YES	+	+	Yes
	PI3K	+	+	Yes
	ras GAP	+	+	No
	SHP2	+	+	Yes
	PLCγ1	+	+	Yes
	GRB2	+	−	
	SHC	+	+	
	NCK	+	+	
pp60^{v-SRC}	PI3K	+	+	Yes
	ras GAP	−	+	No
	SHP2	?	+	?
	PLCγ1	−	+	Yes
	GRB2	−	−	
	SHC	?	+	
	NCK	−	+	

1), an important substrate of the insulin receptor that is involved in signal transmission, becomes phosphorylated during v-SRC transformation (137).

Cytoplasmic tyrosine kinases can activate mitogenic signals by phosphorylating docking proteins, that then cause the relocation of SH2 domain-containing signalling proteins from the cytosol to the membrane. The best example is the middle T antigen mentioned earlier (122). A recently characterized cellular substrate of v-SRC has been proposed to have a similar function. This protein, called p130^{CAS}, stably associates with v-SRC *in vivo* (138). It contains one SH3 domain and 15 possible tyrosine phosphorylation sites that create potential binding sites for SH2 domain-containing proteins. In agreement with a possible docking function, the protein is largely located at the membrane in transformed cells (138); however, its possible role in signal transduction is rather elusive since associations with signalling molecules have not yet been reported.

Oncogenic cytoplasmic tyrosine kinases can interact with the mitogenic signalling network by direct association and phosphorylation of various second messenger proteins. Stimulation of RAS activity is known to be necessary and can be sufficient for cell proliferation (139, 140 and Chapter 5). Activation of this pathway is a common feature of all oncogenic cytoplasmic tyrosine kinases and plays an important role in transformation: neutralization of RAS protein *in vivo* reverts cell transformation induced by v-SRC or v-FPS (141). RAS activity can be regulated by SOS, a nucleotide exchange factor. In unstimulated cells, SOS is largely cytosolic and complexed with GRB2, an adaptor protein. Translocation of the GRB2/SOS complex to the membrane is sufficient to fully stimulate RAS activity (reviewed in Chapter 5, see also refs 45, 46). Oncogenic cytoplasmic tyrosine kinases activate RAS either indirectly, by tyrosine phosphorylation of BCR or SHC proteins (60, 121, 142, 143) that associate with the GRB2 SH2 domain (60, 121, 143, 144), or by direct association with the GRB2 SH2 domain (120, 121, 143); both lead to membrane translocation of GRB2/SOS. v-SRC might also activate the pathway downstream of RAS by direct activation of the serine/threonine kinase RAF, an effector of RAS (Chapter 5 and ref. 140): oncogenic forms of SRC can stimulate RAF activity *in vivo* (145–147) and strongly potentiate RAS-induced RAF activation through tyrosine phosphorylation of the kinase (146). RAF activation may be an important step for the oncogenic effect since inhibition of its activity reverts v-SRC-induced cell transformation (148).

Oncogenic cytoplasmic tyrosine kinases also activate RAS-independent signalling pathways necessary for efficient proliferation. For example, the SH2 domain-deleted version of BCR–ABL still associates with GRB2 but fails to induce cell transformation, suggesting that in the context of BCR–ABL, RAS activation is not sufficient to induce cell transformation. Consistent with this notion, expression of MYC is able to rescue the transforming phenotype, probably in a RAS-independent manner (149). A link between MYC expression and cytoplasmic tyrosine kinases has also been established for the SRC family. MYC expression appears to be a downstream event of the mitogenic signal generated by SRC, FYN, and YES in fibroblasts, since MYC can restore the biological response induced by various growth factors in cells where SRC family kinases are inhibited (150). Again, as suggested in the case of BCR–ABL, MYC rescue appears to occur in a RAS-independent fashion.

PI3K is another important component of the oncogenic signal induced by cytoplasmic tyrosine kinases; this enzyme phosphorylates phosphoinositides leading to the generation of PI3P, PI(3,4)P$_2$, and PIP$_3$. The function of these lipids is currently unknown but they are proposed to play second messenger roles (151, 152). This lipid kinase activity is associated with most tyrosine kinases (129). This association with oncoproteins recruits the enzyme to the membrane where its substrates are localized (151, 152). This translocation is absolutely required for *in vivo* activation: BCR–ABL associates with PI3K in fibroblasts but fails to induce PI(3,4)P$_2$ and PIP$_3$ generation *in vivo* when it is not associated with the membrane (153). The lipid kinase interacts with cytoplasmic tyrosine kinases in at least two ways; in the case of v-ABL by association with its SH2 domain, and in the case of SRC family tyrosine kinases by association with their SH3 domains (151, 152). Association of PI3K with other proteins increases its enzymatic activity by an allosteric mechanism (154–156), which is important for the generation of the signal (157). Complex formation with tyrosine kinases frequently also induces tyrosine phosphorylation of PI3K, but the role of this phosphorylation is currently unknown (151, 152, 158). Consistent with an important function for this enzyme in cell proliferation and cell transformation, inhibition of the PI3K activity blocks the capacity of various mitogens to induce DNA synthesis (157), and prevention of its association with tyrosine kinases generally correlates with an impairment of biological functions (129, 152). Recent data have proposed a link between PI3K activity and p70 S6 serine/threonine kinase (159, 160), an enzyme involved in increasing the rate of protein synthesis (161). Activation of S6 kinase is an important event of the mitogenic signal (162) which occurs in a RAS-independent way (163). While these reports suggest a role of PI3K in stimulation of S6 kinase activity, mutagenesis studies suggest the existence of another signal molecule involved in this process (163). Whether PI3K is related to this pathway needs to be clarified.

Activated cytoplasmic tyrosine kinases activate and phosphorylate a number of additional signalling proteins that are also activated by growth factor receptors (see Table 3 and Chapter 3). For example, high phospholipase C and D activities have been found in *v-SRC* and *v-FES* transformed cells (164, 165). A number of other proteins have been characterized by their ability to interact with the SH2 or SH3 domains of cytoplasmic tyrosine kinases *in vitro* (52, 53, 166), but their role in cell transformation is currently unknown. One of these binding proteins is SAM68 (SRC associated in mitosis), a 68kDa protein that can interact with the SH3 and SH2 domain of SRC family kinases *in vitro* as well as *in vivo*, and becomes an *in vivo* substrate of SRC during mitosis (167–169). SAM68 is largely nuclear (S. Fumagalli and S. A. Courtneidge, unpublished observation) and can associate with RNA *in vitro* (169), consistent with a possible function in RNA maturation. SAM68 can also complex with several signal molecules including GRB2 and PLCγ *in vitro* and in overexpression systems *in vivo* (170). The function of this SRC substrate is not known, but its intriguing properties suggest the existence of a link between the signal transduction network and RNA processing.

In addition to growth factor stimulation, SRC, FYN, and YES are also activated during mitosis (81, 171). Their activity appears to be required for fibroblast cell division (171) indicating that in addition to S phase entry, SRC kinases generate signals that are important for the G2/M transition (see Chapter 7). Consequently, these data suggest that oncogenic forms of the SRC family may affect cell growth at several phases of the cell cycle.

5.2 Interaction with cytoskeletal proteins

Cell transformation is accompanied by a dramatic cytoskeletal rearrangement that requires the tyrosine kinase activity of the oncoprotein. In transformed cells, actin fibres are dissolved and aggregates of F-actin form rosette-like structures called podosomes (172). Changes in cytoskeletal architecture are attributed to tyrosine phosphorylation of various cytoskeletal proteins including annexin, tensin, ezrin, and vinculin (3). The transforming activity of various SRC mutants correlates with the degree of their association with detergent insoluble cytoskeleton elements (102). Several associated proteins have now been characterized; for example AFAP-110 (for actin filament-associated protein of 110kDa), an actin associated protein is phosphorylated and stably complexed with v-SRC in chick embryo fibroblasts (173). This association requires the SH3 domain of the enzyme. Once phosphorylated, AFAP-110 stably interacts with the SH2 domain of SRC (173). Another example is the p80/p85 actin-binding protein referred to as cortactin. P80/85 contains an SH3 domain and associates with SRC in transformed cells (174, 175). This protein is found to be tyrosine phosphorylated during cell transformation and also after stimulation with growth factors such as FGF (176).

Cell adhesion plays an important role in the proliferation of untransformed cells and inhibition of this process blocks the capacity of cells to proliferate (177). Activation of cell adhesion receptors triggers several intracellular signals including activation of PI(4)P-5 kinase (responsible for PI4,5P$_2$ synthesis) and RAS activity (178, 179). In transformed cells, the adhesion requirement is overcome and the cells grow in an anchorage independent manner. One explanation is that transforming tyrosine kinases constitutively activate the cell signalling machinery induced by integrin engagement, which then provides the signals necessary for cell growth. Recently, the molecular understanding of integrin signalling has been advanced by the characterization of a cytoplasmic tyrosine kinase called focal adhesion kinase (FAK) (180). This enzyme comprises a putative integrin binding site, a catalytic domain, and focal adhesion targeting sequences, but it lacks SH2 or SH3 domains. FAK can be activated by fibronectin, but also by several mitogens, including PDGF, lysophosphatidic acid, and bombesin (181). Stimulation of FAK triggers its activation and association with several proteins, including SRC, FYN (182), and GRB2 (183). c-SRC activation occurs via association of its SH2 domain (184); when complexed, SRC phosphorylates FAK at novel tyrosine residues (185) and thus appears to fully stimulate FAK activity. GRB2 association involves Y925 of FAK and the SH2 domain of GRB2, and leads to RAS activation (183). In *v-SRC* transformed cells, activation of FAK and its association with GRB2 is constitutive, so that integrin-mediated RAS activation is deregulated

(183). This constant activation may largely explain the ability of transformed cells to grow in soft agar.

In parallel with RAS activation, FAK is able to complex PI3K (186). The role of this association is unclear but a possible role in the formation of membrane ruffles has been proposed. In favour of this idea, PI3K mediates membrane ruffling induced by some growth factors, such as the insulin and the PDGF receptors (187, 188). Also, a v-SRC mutant that cannot associate with PI3K induces only a partially transformed phenotype where the cells show a fusiform morphology (189). Finally, another component of the integrin signalling machinery involves paxillin, a cytoskeletal protein which is able to bind to the SH3 domain of SRC tyrosine kinases *in vitro* (190) and to the carboxy terminus of FAK (181). Its function is not known but paxillin can be phosphorylated by SRC *in vivo*, which could also create binding sites for other signalling molecules (181).

6. Implication in human tumours

6.1 The SRC family tyrosine kinases

SRC family tyrosine kinases have been well defined as oncoproteins in animals, but their involvement in human tumours is not clearly established. Activated mutants of LCK have been observed in humans (see below), and although no other cases of mutant SRC family kinases have been reported, some changes in activity have been observed. For example, overexpression and high kinase activity of SRC and YES have been observed in primary colon cancers (191) and in various human melanomas (192) suggesting a role of these kinases in tumour development. Another example involves breast cancers where a major proportion of primary tumours (> 80%) exhibits high SRC activity (193). Evidence supporting a role for SRC in mammary tumorigenesis *in vivo* comes from transgenic mice expressing the polyoma middle T antigen. Expression of middle T under the control of the mouse mammary tumour virus promoter leads to the development of mammary tumours (194), and high SRC kinase activity was observed in the transformed tissues. In contrast, development of mammary tumours was highly reduced when middle T antigen was expressed in the mammary epithelium of mice lacking SRC (195). The mechanism of activation of SRC in tumours is not yet fully established, but correlative evidence suggests that it could occur via its interaction with receptor tyrosine kinases. For example, in 30% of human breast cancers the genes encoding the EGF receptor and the highly related ERBB2/HER2 are amplified and the proteins overexpressed (see Chapters 1 and 3) and this expression generally correlates with elevated SRC activity (196). A link between SRC and EGF receptor has been established: overexpression of SRC can potentiate the EGF mitogenic response in cell culture (197) and SRC family kinases are required for the EGF mitogenic response in rodent fibroblasts (134). *In vivo*, SRC potentiates tumour formation in nude mice by cells expressing high levels of the EGF receptor (198). Taken together, these observations strongly suggest that SRC is an integral compo-

nent of the intracellular signal induced by EGF family receptors and raises the possibility that both kinases co-operate in mammary tumour development *in vivo*.

An oncogenic form of LCK, another member of the SRC family, has been recently
characterized in two transformed human T cell lines, suggesting a role for this tyrosine kinase in development of some T cell leukaemias. LCK is known to play an
important role in T cell receptor signalling (1). In these transformed cells, the *LCK*
gene has been translocated downstream of the *TCRβ* gene (Chapter 1), leading to
deregulated expression of LCK (199). In addition the LCK protein expressed in these
cells has three point mutations in the unique domain and kinase domain, plus an
insertion of three amino acids between the SH2 domain and the kinase domain (199).
The oncogenic activity of this mutant form of LCK has been further confirmed by its
ability to transform rodent fibroblasts *in vitro* (199). This suggests that LCK can be
oncogenically activated in T cells via both deregulated expression due to chromosomal translocation, and an increase of its activity by mutation.

6.2 The BCR–ABL tyrosine kinase

Oncogenic activation of c-ABL is a major component of chronic myelogenous
leukaemia (CML) and some acute lymphoblastic leukaemia (ALL) (for review see
29–31, 200). CML is a clonal cancer arising from neoplastic transformation of a
haematopoietic stem cell. Activation of c-ABL occurs via a reciprocal chromosomal
translocation, t(9;22)(q34;q11), that gives rise to the Philadelphia chromsome (Ph^1
Chapter 1). This cytogenetic aberration occurs in more than 90% of patients with
CML. The translocation results in the transposition of *c-ABL* on chromosome 9 to
chromosome 22, in close apposition to the *BCR* gene. The rearranged gene encodes
the fusion proteins p210$^{BCR–ABL}$ and p185$^{BCR–ABL}$ (29, 31, 200). As detailed earlier, these
chimeric proteins show deregulated kinase activity *in vitro* and transform rat fibroblasts and pre-B cells. The oncoproteins are clearly involved in tumour development
in vivo since, when introduced into bone marrow, BCR–ABL is able to induce a
myelogenous-like leukaemia in mice (201, 202). This has been further confirmed by
generation of transgenic mice expressing BCR–ABL (203).

CML is characterized by two distinct states: a chronic phase where the myeloid
progenitors rapidly proliferate but still differentiate, and a state where immature pre-
B cells rapidly proliferate but no longer differentiate (blast crisis) (29, 31, 200).
BCR–ABL is found in both phases with no obvious alteration in expression during
progression to acute leukaemia, suggesting that it has a role in myeloid growth but
is not sufficient to induce the blast crisis. In favour of this hypothesis, murine progenitor B cells overexpressing ectopic BCR–ABL proliferate in culture but retain the
ability to differentiate to mature immunoglobulin-secreting B cells (204). Similarly,
multipotent haematopoietic cells infected with a BCR–ABL expressing retrovirus
show a reduced requirement for growth factors to proliferate but are still able to
differentiate and do not form tumours in mice (205). Therefore, BCR–ABL must be an
important component for the chronic phase, but development of the terminal phase
may be due to a secondary, unknown event. Since there are a wide array of cytoge-

netic abnormalities observed in the blast crisis phase, it is possible that many different molecular events are capable of mediating this transition. However there is no consistent evidence of enhanced BCR–ABL transcription or of secondary activating mutations in the BCR–ABL protein during this development. One possibility is that MYC overexpression would co-operate with BCR–ABL; consistent with this idea, most tumours that develop in mice expressing v-ABL contain a translocation of the c-MYC gene, resulting in its overexpression (206). Furthermore, both genes can co-operate in vivo as shown by the shorter latency of tumours observed in double ABL–MYC transgenic mice (206). However, the possible involvement of MYC in CML needs to be further established.

7. Concluding remarks and perspectives

Characterization of viral forms of cytoplasmic tyrosine kinases has permitted unravelling of the molecular mechanisms of cell proliferation and cell transformation induced by tyrosine phosphorylation. Comparison of viral versus cellular tyrosine kinases has led to an understanding of the mechanisms by which the cellular counterparts are regulated. Importantly they have also permitted the definition of homology domains such as SH2 and SH3, known to play crucial roles in protein–protein interaction, and involved in the generation of various intracellular signals. Although the actions of oncogenic cytoplasmic tyrosine kinases are now broadly defined, the functions of the cellular counterparts are for the most part still obscure. One main reason is the difference in cell function, enzymatic activity, and substrate specificity: while v-ABL induces transformation in various cell types, overexpression of c-ABL inhibits cell growth (111). Similarly, the viral oncoproteins activate several signal pathways common to receptor tyrosine kinases whereas the cellular forms may activate specific pathways whose components are still largely unknown. Another important aspect of cellular tyrosine kinases involves substrate specificity. This question may not be best studied with viral transforming products because their high constitutive activity may mask specificity. For the future, it will be important to characterize in more detail how cellular cytoplasmic tyrosine kinases act in cell signalling networks. Finally, in vitro studies and genetic analyses will reveal functional redundancies among members of the different kinase families. It will be important in the future to address the specific roles of individual family members.

Acknowledgements

S. R. is a scientist of the Institut National de la Santé Et de la Recherche Médicale (I.N.S.E.R.M.).

References

1. Courtneidge, S. A. (1994) Non-receptor protein tyrosine kinases. In *Frontiers in molecular biology: protein kinases* (ed. J. Woodgett), p. 212. Oxford University Press.

2. Superti-Furga, G. and Courtneidge, S. A. (1995) Structure-function relationship in Src family and related protein tyrosine kinases. *Bioessays*, **17**, 1.
3. Parsons, J. T. and Weber, M. J. (1989) Genetics of *src*: structure and functional organization of a protein tyrosine kinase. *Curr. Top. Microbiol. Immunol.*, **147**, 79.
4. Ghysdael, J., Neil, J. C., and Vogt, P. K. (1981) Esh avian sarcoma virus codes for a gag-linked transformation specific protein with an associated protein kinase activity. *Virology*, **111**, 386.
5. Kitamura, N., Kitamura, A., Toyoshima, Y., Hirayama, Y., and Yoshida, M. (1982) Avian sarcoma virus Y73 genome sequence and structural similarity to its transforming gene product to that of Rous sarcoma virus. *Nature*, **287**, 205.
6. Naharro, G., Robbins, K. C., and Reddy, E. P. (1984) Gene product of v-*fgr* onc: hybrid portion containing a portion of actin and a tyrosine-specific protein kinase. *Science*, **223**, 63.
7. Ley, T. J., Connolly, N. L., Katamine, S., Cheah, M. S., Senior, R. M., and Robbins, K. C. (1989) Tissue-specific expression and developmental regulation of the human *fgr* proto-oncogene. *Mol. Cell. Biol.*, **9**, 92.
8. Willman, C. L., Stewart, C. C., Griffith, J. K., Stewart, S. J., and Tomasi, T. B. (1987) Differential expression and regulation of the c-src and c-fgr protooncogenes in myelomonocytic cells. *Proc. Natl. Acad. Sci. USA*, **84**, 4480.
9. Twamley, G. M. and Courtneidge, S. A. (1996) Non receptor tyrosine kinases. In *Protein phosphorylation* (ed. P. Marks). Verlagchemie, Wheinheim.
10. Cheah, M. S. C., Ley, T. J., Tronick, S. R., and Robbins, K. C. (1986) Fgr proto-oncogene mRNA induced in B lymphocytes by Epstein–Barr virus infection. *Nature*, **319**, 238.
11. Cooper, J. A. (1990) The *src* family of protein-tyrosine kinases. In *Peptides and protein phosphorylation* (ed. B. E. Kemps), p. 104. CRC Press, Florida.
12. Ottilie, S., Raulf, F., Barnekow, A., Hannig, G., and Schartl, M. (1992) Multiple *src*-related kinase genes, *srk*1-4, in the fresh water sponge *Spongilla lacustris*. *Oncogene*, **7**, 1625.
13. Soriano, P., Montgomery, C., Geske, R., and Bradley, A. (1991) Targeted disruption of the c-*src* proto-oncogene leads to osteopetrosis in mice. *Cell*, **64**, 693.
14. Karnitz, L., Sutor, S. L., Torigoe, T., Reed, J. C., Bell, M. P., McKean, D. J., *et al.* (1992) Effects of p56^{lck} deficiency on the growth and cytolytic effector function of an interleukin-2-dependent cytotoxic T-cell line. *Mol. Cell. Biol.*, **12**, 4521.
15. Appleby, M. W., Gross, J. A., Cooke, M. P., Levin, S. D., Qian, X., and Perlmutter, R. M. (1992) Defective T cell receptor signaling in mice lacking the thymic isoform of p59^{fyn}. *Cell*, **70**, 751.
16. Stein, P. L., Lee, H.-M., Rich, S., and Soriano, P. (1992) pp59^{fyn} mutant mice display differential signaling in thymocytes and peripheral T cells. *Cell*, **70**, 741.
17. Yagi, T., Aizawa, S., Tokunaga, T., Shigetani, Y., Takeda, N., and Ikawa, Y. (1993) A role for Fyn tyrosine kinase in the suckling behaviour of neonatal mice. *Nature*, **366**, 742.
18. Stein, P. L., Vogel, H., and Soriano, P. (1994) Combined deficiencies of Src, Fyn, and Yes tyrosine kinases in mutant mice. *Genes Dev.*, **8**, 1999.
19. Lowell, C. A., Soriano, P., and Varmus, H. E. (1994) Functional overlap in the *src* gene family: inactivation of *hck* and *fgr* impairs natural immunity. *Genes Dev.*, **8**, 387.
20. Hanafusa, H. (1988) The fps/fes oncogene. *The oncogene handbook*. Elsevier Science Publishers B.V. (Biomedical Division).

21. Mathey-Prevot, B., Hanafusa, H., and Kawai, S. (1982) A cellular protein is immunologically crossreactive with and functionally homologous to the Fujinami sarcoma virus transforming protein. *Cell*, **28**, 897.

22. Feldman, R. A., Gabrilove, J. L., Tam, J. P., More, A. S., and Hanafusa, H. (1985) Specific expression of the human fps/fes-encoded protein NCP92 in normal and leukemic myeloid cells. *Proc. Natl. Acad. Sci. USA*, **82**, 2379.

23. MacDonald, I., Levy, J., and Pawson, T. (1985) Expression of the mammalian c-*fes* protein in hematopoietic cells and identification of a distinct *fes*-related protein. *Mol. Cell. Biol.*, **5**, 2543.

24. Greer, P., Haigh, J., Mbamalu, G., Khoo, W., Bernstein, A., and Pawson, T. (1994) The Fps/Fes protein-tyrosine kinase promotes angiogenesis in transgenic mice. *Mol. Cell. Biol.*, **14**, 6755.

25. Jücker, M., Roebroek, A. J. M., Mautner, J., Koch, K., Eick, D., Diehl, V., *et al.* (1992) Expression of truncated transcripts of the proto-oncogene c-*fps/fes* in human lymphoma and lymphoid leukemia cell lines. *Oncogene*, **7**, 943.

26. Pawson, T., Letwin, K., Lee, T., Hao, Q.-L., Heisterkamp, N., and Groffen, J. (1989) The FER gene is evolutionarily conserved and encodes a widely expressed member of the FPS/FES protein-tyrosine kinase family. *Mol. Cell. Biol.*, **9**, 5722.

27. Letwin, K., Yee, S. P., and Pawson, T. (1993) Novel protein-tyrosine kinase cDNAs related to fps/fes and eph cloned using anti-phosphotyrosine antibody. *Oncogene*, **3**, 621.

28. Yu, G., Smithgall, T. E., and Glazer, R. I. (1989) K562 leukemia cells transfected with the human c-fes gene acquire the ability to undergo myeloid differentiation. *J. Biol. Chem.*, **264**, 10276.

29. Daley, G. Q. and Ben-Neriah, Y. (1991) Implicating the bcr/abl gene in the pathogenesis of Philadelphia chromosome-positive human leukemia. *Adv. Cancer Res.*, **57**, 151.

30. Rosenberg, N. and Witte, O. (1986) Function of the abl oncogene. *Cancer Surv.*, **5**, 183.

31. Sawyers, C. L. (1992) The *bcr-abl* gene in chronic myelogenous leukaemia. *Cancer Surv.*, **15**, 37.

32. Perego, R., Ron, D., and Kruh, G. D. (1991) Arg encodes a widely expressed 145 kDa protein-tyrosine kinase. *Oncogene*, **6**, 1899.

33. Renshaw, M. W., Capozza, M. A., and Wang, J. Y. J. (1988) Differential expression of type-specific c-abl mRNAs in mouse tissues and cell lines. *Mol. Cell. Biol.*, **8**, 4547.

34. Hoffman, F. M. (1991) Drosophila Abl and genetic redundancy in signal transduction. *Trends Genet.*, **7**, 351.

35. Swartzberg, P. L., Stall, A. M., Hardin, J. D., Bowdish, K. S., Humaran, T., Boast, S., *et al.* (1991) Mice homozygous for the Abl^m1 mutation show poor viability and depletion of selected B and T cell population. *Cell*, **65**, 1165.

36. Tybulewicz, V. L. J., Crawford, C. E., Jackson, P. K., Bronson, R. T., and Mulligan, R. C. (1991) Neonatal lethality and lymphopenia in mice with homozygous disruption of the c-abl proto-oncogene. *Cell*, **65**, 1153.

37. Hanks, S. J., Quinn, A. M., and Hunter, T. (1988) The protein kinase family: conserved features and deduced phylogeny of the catalytic domains. *Science*, **241**, 42.

38. Ferracini, R. and Brugge, J. (1990) Analysis of mutant forms of the c-*src* gene product containing a phenylalanine substitution of tyrosine 416. *Oncogene Res.*, **5**, 205.

39. Hjermstad, S. J., Peters, K. L., Briggs, S. D., Glazer, R. I., and Smithgall, T. E. (1993) Regulation of the human c-*fes* protein tyrosine kinase (p93^c-fes) by its *src* homology 2 domain and major autophosphorylation site (Tyr-713). *Oncogene*, **8**, 2283.

40. Kmiecik, T. E. and Shalloway, D. (1987) Activation and suppression of pp60$^{c\text{-}src}$ transforming ability by mutation of its primary sites of tyrosine and phosphorylation. *Cell*, **49**, 65.

41. Piwnica-Worms, H., Saunders, K. B., Roberts, T. M., Smith, A. E., and Cheng, S. H. (1987) Tyrosine phosphorylation regulates the biochemical and biological properties of pp60$^{c\text{-}src}$. *Cell*, **49**, 75.

42. Weinmaster, G., Zoller, M. J., Smith, M., Hinze, E., and Pawson, T. (1984) Mutagenesis of Fujinami sarcoma virus: evidence that tyrosine phosphorylation of P130$^{gag\text{-}fps}$ modulates its biological activity. *Cell*, **37**, 559.

43. Sadowski, I., Stone, J. C., and Pawson, T. (1986) A noncatalytic domain conserved among cytoplasmic protein-tyrosine kinases modifies the kinase function and transforming activity of Fujinami sarcoma virus p130$^{gag\text{-}fps}$. *Mol. Cell. Biol.*, **6**, 4396.

44. Pawson, T. and Schlessinger, J. (1993) SH2 and SH3 domains. *Curr. Biol.*, **3**, 434.

45. van der Geer, P. and Hunter, T. (1994) Receptor protein-tyrosine kinases and their signal transduction. *Annu. Rev. Cell. Biol.*, **10**, 251.

46. Pawson, T. (1995) Protein modules and signalling networks. *Nature*, **373**, 573.

47. Songyang, Z., Shoelson, S. E., Chaudhuri, M., Gish, G., Pawson, T., Haser, W. G., *et al.* (1993) SH2 domains recognize specific phosphopeptide sequences. *Cell*, **72**, 767.

48. Waksman, G., Kominos, D., Robertson, S. C., Pant, N., Baltimore, D., Birge, R. B., *et al.* (1992) Crystal structure of the phosphotyrosine recognition domain SH2 of v-*src* complexed with tyrosine-phosphorylated peptides. *Nature*, **358**, 646.

49. Mayer, B. J., Hamaguchi, M., and Hanafusa, H. (1988) A novel viral oncogene with structural similarity to phospholipase C. *Nature*, **332**, 272.

50. Stahl, M. L., Ferenz, C. R., Kelleher, K. L., Kriz, R. W., and Knopf, J. L. (1988) Sequence similarity of phospholipase C with the non-catalytic region of src. *Nature*, **332**, 269.

51. Musacchio, A., Gibson, T., Lehto, V.-P., and Saraste, M. (1992) SH3—an abundant protein domain in search of a function. *FEBS Lett.*, **307**, 55.

52. Feller, S. M., Ren, R., Hanafusa, H., and Baltimore, D. (1994) SH2 and SH3 domains as molecular adhesives: the interaction of Crk and Abl. *Trends Biochem. Sci.*, **19**, 453.

53. Ren, R., Mayer, B. J., Cicchetti, P., and Baltimore, D. (1993) Identification of a ten-amino acid proline-rich SH3 binding site. *Science*, **259**, 1157.

54. Koyama, S., Yu, H., Dalgarno, D. C., Shin, T. B., Zydowsky, L. D., and Schreiber, S. L. (1993) Structure of the PI 3-K SH3 domain and analysis of the SH3 family. *Cell*, **72**, 945.

55. Musacchio, A., Noble, M., Pauptit, R., Wierenga, R., and Saraste, M. (1992) Crystal structure of a Src-homology 3 (SH3) domain. *Nature*, **359**, 851.

56. Musacchio, A., Saraste, M., and Wilmanns, M. (1994) High-resolution crystal structures of tyrosine kinase SH3 domains complexed with proline-rich peptides. *Struct. Biol.*, **1**, 546.

57. Bar-Sagi, D., Rotin, D., Batzer, A., Mandiyan, V., and Schlessinger, J. (1993) SH3 domains direct cellular localisation of signaling molecules. *Cell*, **74**, 83.

58. Resh, M. D. (1994) Myristylation and palmitylation of Src family members: the fats of the matter. *Cell*, **76**, 411.

59. Shaw, A. S., Whytney, C. J. A., Hammond, C., Amerin, E., Kavathas, P., Sefton, B. M., *et al.* (1990) Short related sequences in the cytoplasmic domains of CD4 and CD8 mediate binding to the amino-terminal domain of the p56^{lck} tyrosine protein kinase. *Mol. Cell Biol.*, **10**, 1853.

60. Maru, Y., Peters, K. L., Afar, D. E., Shibuya, M., Witte, O. N., and Smithgall, T. E. (1995)

Tyrosine phosphorylation of BCR by FPS/FES protein-tyrosine kinases induces associ-ation of BCR with GRB-2/SOS. *Mol. Cell. Biol.*, **15**, 835.

61. Wang, J. Y. J. (1993) Abl tyrosine kinase in signal transduction and cell-cycle regulation. *Curr. Opin. Genet. Dev.*, **3**, 35.

62. Kipreos, E. T. and Wang, J. Y. J. (1992) Cell cycle-regulated binding of c-Abl tyrosine kinase to DNA. *Science*, **256**, 382.

63. Dickstein, R., Heffetz, D., Benneriah, Y., and Shaul, Y. (1992) c-Abl has a sequence spe-cific enhancer binding activity. *Cell*, **69**, 751.

64. McWhirter, J. R. and Wang, J. Y. J. (1991) Activation of tyrosine kinase and microfila-ment-binding functions of c-*abl* by *bcr* sequences in *bcr/abl* fusion proteins. *Mol. Cell. Biol.*, **11**, 1553.

65. Cooper, J. A., Gould, K. L., Cartwright, C. A., and Hunter, T. (1986) Tyr527 is phospho-rylated in pp60^{c-src}: implications for regulation. *Science*, **231**, 1431.

66. Cartwright, C. A., Eckhart, W., Simon, S., and Kaplan, P. L. (1987) Cell transformation by pp60^{c-src} mutated in the carboxy-terminal regulatory domain. *Cell*, **49**, 83.

67. Courtneidge, S. A. (1985) Activation of pp60^{c-src} kinase by middle-T antigen binding or by dephosphorylation. *EMBO J.*, **4**, 1471.

68. Nada, S., Okada, M., MacAuley, A., Cooper, J. A., and Nakagawa, H. (1991) Cloning of a complementary DNA for a protein-tyrosine kinase that specifically phosphorylates a negative regulatory site of p60^{c-src}. *Nature*, **351**, 69.

69. Ruzzene, M., James, P., Brunati, A. M., Donell-Deana, A., and Pinna, L. A. (1994) Regu-lation of c-Fgr protein kinase by c-Src kinase (CSK) and by polycationic effectors. *J. Biol. Chem.*, **269**, 15885.

70. Murphy, S. M., Bergman, M., and Morgan, D. O. (1993) Suppression of c-Src activity by C-terminal Src kinase involves the c-Src SH2 and SH3 domains: analysis with *Saccha-romyces cerevisiae*. *Mol. Cell. Biol.*, **13**, 5290.

71. Okada, M., Howell, B., Broome, M. A., and Cooper, J. A. (1993) Deletion of the SH3 domain of SRC interferes with regulation by the phosphorylated carboxy terminal tyrosine. *J. Biol. Chem.*, **268**, 18070.

72. Superti-Furga, G., Fumagalli, S., Koegl, M., Courtneidge, S. A., and Draetta, G. (1993) Csk inhibition of Src activity requires both the SH2 and SH3 domains of Src. *EMBO J.*, **12**, 2625.

73. Erpel, T., Superti-Furga, G., and Courtneidge, S. A. (1995) Mutational analysis of the Src SH3 domain: the same residues of the ligand binding surface are important for intra- and intermolecular interactions. *EMBO J.*, **14**, 968.

74. Kypta, R. M., Goldberg, Y., Ulug, E. T., and Courtneidge, S. A. (1990) Association between the PDGF receptor and members of the *src* family of tyrosine kinases. *Cell*, **62**, 481.

75. Twamley, G., Hall, B., Kypta, R., and Courtneidge, S. A. (1992) Association of Fyn with the activated PDGF receptor: requirements for binding and phosphorylation. *Oncogene*, **7**, 1893.

76. Gould, K. and Hunter, T. (1988) Platelet-derived growth factor induces multisite phos-phorylation of pp60^{c-src} and increases its protein-tyrosine kinase activity. *Mol. Cell. Biol.*, **8**, 3345.

77. Ralston, R. and Bishop, J. M. (1985) The product of the proto-oncogene c-*src* is modified during the cellular response to platelet-derived growth factor. *Proc. Natl. Acad. Sci. USA*, **82**, 7845.

78. Mustelin, T. and Altman, A. (1990) Dephosphorylation and activation of the T cell tyrosine kinase pp56^{lck} by the leukocyte common antigen (CD45). *Oncogene*, **5**, 809.

79. Ostergaard, H. L., Shackleford, D. A., Hurley, T. R., Johnson, P., Hyman, R., Sefton, B. M., *et al.* (1989) Expression of CD45 alters phosphorylation of the *lck*-encoded tyrosine protein kinase in murine T-cell lymphoma cell lines. *Proc. Natl. Acad. Sci. USA*, **86**, 8959.

80. Veillette, A., Bookman, M. A., Horak, E. M., Samelson, L. E., and Bolen, J. B. (1989) Signal transduction through the CD4 receptor involves the activation of the internal membrane tyrosine kinase p56^{lck}. *Nature*, **338**, 257.

81. Taylor, S. J. and Shalloway, D. (1993) The cell cycle and c-Src. *Curr. Opin. Gene. Dev.*, **3**, 26.

82. Stover, D. R., Liebetanz, J., and Lydon, N. B. (1994) Cdc2-mediated modulation of pp60^{c-src} activity. *J. Biol. Chem.*, **269**, 26885.

83. Shenoy, S., Chckalaparampil, I., Bagrodia, S., Lin, P.-H., and Shalloway, D. (1992) Role of p34cdc2-mediated phosphorylations in two-step. *Proc. Natl. Acad. Sci. USA*, **89**, 7237.

84. Feldman, R. A., Lowy, D. R., and Vass, W. C. (1990) Selective potentiation of c-*fps*/*fes* transforming activity by a phosphatase inhibitor. *Oncogene Res.*, **5**, 187.

85. Hanazono, Y., Chiba, S., Sasaki, K., Mano, H., Miyajima, A., Arai, K.-I., *et al.* (1993) c-*fps*/*fes* protein-tyrosine kinase is implicated in a signaling pathway triggered by granulocyte-macrophage colony-stimulating factor and interleukin-3. *EMBO J.*, **12**, 1641.

86. Hanazono, Y., Chiba, S., Sasaki, K., Mano, H., Yasaki, Y., and Hirai, H. (1993) Erythropoietin induces tyrosine phosphorylation and kinase activity of the c-*fps*/*fes* prot-oncogene product in human erythropoietin-responsive cells. *Blood*, **81**, 3193.

87. Yu, G. and Glazer, R. I. (1987) Purification and characterization of p92^{fes} and p6^{src}-related tyrosine protein kinase activities in differentiated HL-60 leukemia cells. *J. Biol. Chem.*, **262**, 17543.

88. Koch, C. A., Moran, M., Sadowski, I., and Pawson, T. (1989) The common *src* homology region 2 domain of cytoplasmic signaling proteins is a positive effector of v-*fps* tyrosine kinase function. *Mol. Cell. Biol.*, **9**, 4131.

89. Foster, D. A., Shibuya, M., and Hanafusa, H. (1985) Activation of the transformation potential of the cellular *fps* gene. *Cell*, **42**, 105.

90. Greer, P. A., Meckling-Hansen, K., and Pawson, T. (1988) The human c-*fps*/*fes* gene product expressed ectopically in rat fibroblasts is nontransforming and has retained protein-tyrosine kinase activity. *Mol. Cell. Biol.*, **8**, 578.

91. Sodroski, J. G., Gosh, W. C., and Haseltine, W. A. (1984) Transforming potential of a human protooncogene (c-fps/fes) locus. *Proc. Natl. Acad. Sci. USA*, **81**, 3039.

92. Muller, A. J., Young, J. C., Pendergast, A.-M., Pondel, M., Littman, D. R., and Witte, O. N. (1991) Bcr first exon sequences specifically activate the Bcr/Abl tyrosine kinase oncogene of Philadelphia chromosome-positive human leukaemias. *Mol. Cell. Biol.*, **11**, 1785.

93. Pendergast, A. M., Muller, A. J., Havlik, M. H., Clark, R., McCormick, F., and Witte, O. N. (1991) Evidence for regulation of the human ABL tyrosine kinase by a cellular inhibitor. *Proc. Natl. Acad. Sci. USA*, **88**, 5927.

94. Walkenhorst, J., Goga, A., Witte, O. N., and Superti-Furga, G. (1996) Analysis of human c-Abl tyrosine kinase activity regulation in *S. pombe*. *Oncogene*, **12**, 1512.

95. Dai, Z. and Pendergast, A.-M. (1995) Abi-2, a novel SH3-containing protein interacts with the c-Abl tyrosine kinase and modulates c-Abl transforming activity. *Genes Dev.*, **9**, 2569.

96. Shi, Y. and Goff, S. P. (1995) Abl-Interactor-1, a novel SH3 protein binding to the carboxy-terminal portion of the Abl protein, supresses v-Abl transforming activity. *Genes Dev.*, **9**, 2583.

97. Goga, A., McLaughlin, J., Pendergast, A. M., Parmar, K., Muller, A., Rosenberg, N., *et al.* (1993) Oncogenic activation of c-*ABL* by mutation within its last exon. *Mol. Cell. Biol.*, **13**, 4967.

98. Pendergast, A. M., Muller, A. J., Havlik, M. H., Maru, Y., and Witte, O. N. (1991) BCR sequences essential for transformation by the *BCR-ABL* oncogene bind to the ABL SH2 regulatory domain in a non-phosphotyrosine dependent manner. *Cell*, **66**, 161.

99. David-Pfeuty, T. and Nouvian-Dooghe, Y. (1990) Immunolocalization of the cellular *src* protein in interphase and mitotic NIH c-*src* overexpressor cells. *J. Cell Biol.*, **111**, 3097.

100. Kaplan, K. B., Swedlow, J. R., Varmus, H. E., and Morgan, D. O. (1992) Association of p60$^{c\text{-}src}$ with endosomal membranes in mammalian fibroblasts. *J. Cell Biol.*, **118**, 321.

101. Resh, M. D. and Erikson, R. L. (1985) Highly specific antibody to Rous Sarcoma virus src gene product recognizes a novel population of pp60$^{v\text{-}src}$ and pp60$^{c\text{-}src}$ molecules. *J. Cell Biol.*, **100**, 409.

102. Hamaguchi, M. and Hanafusa, H. (1987) Association of pp60^{src} with Triton X-100-resistant cellular structure correlates with morphological transformation. *Proc. Natl. Acad. Sci. USA*, **84**, 2312.

103. Loeb, D. M., Woolford, J., and Beemon, K. (1987) pp60$^{c\text{-}src}$ has less affinity for the detergent-insoluble cellular matrix than do pp60$^{v\text{-}src}$ and other viral protein-tyrosine kinases. *J. Virol.*, **61**, 2420.

104. Kaplan, K. B., Bibbins, K. B., Swedlow, J. R., Arnaud, M., Morgan, D. O., and Varmus, H. E. (1994) Association of the amino-terminal half of c-Src with focal adhesions alters their properties and is regulated by phosphorylation of tyrosine 527. *EMBO J.*, **13**, 4745.

105. Moss, P., Radke, K. V. C., Young, J. C., Gilmore, T., and Martin, G. S. (1984) Cellular localization of the transforming protein of wild-type and temperature-sensitive Fujinami sarcoma virus. *J. Virol.*, **52**, 557.

106. Rohrschneider, L. R. and Najita, L. M. (1984) Detection of the v-*abl* gene product at cell-substratum contact sites in Abelson murine leukemia virus-transformed fibroblasts. *J. Virol.*, **51**, 547.

107. Young, J. C. and Martin, S. (1984) Cellular localization of c-*fps* gene product NCP98. *J. Virol.*, **52**, 913.

108. Wang, J. Y. J. (1994) Nuclear tyrosine kinases. *Trends Biochem. Sci.*, **19**, 373.

109. Welch, P. J. and Wang, J. Y. J. (1993) A C-terminal protein-binding domain in the retinoblastoma protein regulates nuclear c-Abl tyrosine kinase in the cell cycle. *Cell*, **75**, 779.

110. Baskaran, R., Dahmus, M. E., and Wang, J. Y. J. (1993) Tyrosine phosphorylation of mammalian RNA polymerase II carboxy-terminal domain. *Proc. Natl. Acad. Sci. USA*, **90**, 11167.

111. Sawyers, C. L., McLaughlin, J., Goga, A., Havlik, M., and Witte, O. (1994) The nuclear tyrosine kinase c-Abl negatively regulates cell growth. *Cell*, **77**, 121.

112. McWhirter, J. R. and Wang, J. Y. J. (1993) An actin-binding function contributes to transformation by Bcr-Abl oncoprotein of Philadelphia chromosome-positive leukemias. *EMBO J.*, **12**, 1533.

113. McWhirter, J. R., Galasso, D. L., and Wang, J. Y. J. (1993) A coiled-coil oligomerization

domain of Bcr is essential for the transforming function of Bcr-Abl oncoprotein. *Mol. Cell. Biol.*, **13**, 7587.

114. Kawakami, T., Kawakami, Y., Aaronson, S. A., and Robbins, K. C. (1988) Acquisition of transforming properties of FYN, a normal SRC-related human gene. *Proc. Natl. Acad. Sci. USA*, **85**, 3870.

115. Franz, W. M., Berger, P., and Wang, J. Y. J. (1989) Deletion of an N-terminal regulatory domain of the c-Abl tyrosine kinase activates its oncogenic potential. *EMBO J.*, **8**, 137.

116. Johnson, P. J., Coussens, P. M., Danko, A. V., and Shalloway, D. (1985) Overexpressed pp60[c-src] can induce focus formation without complete transformation of NIH3T3 fibroblasts. *Mol. Cell. Biol.*, **5**, 1073.

117. Koegl, M. and Courtneidge, S. A. (1992) The regulation of Src activity. *Semin. Virol.*, **2**, 375.

118. Mayer, B. J., Jackson, P. K., Van Etten, R. A., and Baltimore, D. (1992) Point mutations in the abl SH2 domain coordinately impair phosphotyrosine binding *in vitro* and transforming activity *in vivo*. *Mol. Cell. Biol.*, **12**, 609.

119. Ariizumi, K. and Shibuya, M. (1985) Construction and biological analysis of deletion mutants of Fujinami sarcoma virus: 5'-*fps* sequence has a role in the transforming activity. *J. Virol.*, **55**, 660.

120. Pendergast, A. M., Quilliam, L. A., Cripe, L. D., Bassing, C. H., Dai, Z., Li, N., *et al.* (1993) BCR-ABL-induced oncogenesis is mediated by direct interaction with the SH2 domain of the GRB-2 adaptor protein. *Cell*, **75**, 175.

121. Puil, L., Liu, J., Gish, G., Mbamalu, G., Bowtell, D., Pelicci, O. G., *et al.* (1994) Bcr-Abl oncoproteins bind directly to activators of the Ras signalling pathway. *EMBO J.*, **13**, 764.

122. Brizuela, L., Murphy, C., and Courtneidge, S. A. (1994) Transformation by polyomavirus middle T antigen. *Semin. Virol.*, **5**, 381.

123. Courtneidge, S. A. and Heber, A. (1987) An 81 kd protein complexed with middle-T antigen and pp60[c-src]: a possible phosphatidylinositol kinase. *Cell*, **50**, 1031.

124. Kaplan, D. R., Whitman, M., Schaffhausen, B., Pallas, D. C., White, M., Cantley, L. (1987) Common elements in growth factor stimulation and oncogenic transformation: 85 kd phosphoprotein and phosphatidylinositol kinase activity. *Cell*, **50**, 1021.

125. Talmage, D. A., Freund, R., Young, A. T., Dahl, J., Dawe, C. J., and Benjamin, T. L. (1989) Phosphorylation of middle T by pp60[c-src] a switch for binding of phosphatidylinositol 3-kinase and optimal tumorigenesis. *Cell*, **59**, 55.

126. Whitman, M., Kaplan, D. R., Schaffhausen, B., Cantley, L., and Roberts, T. M. (1985) Association of phosphatidylinositol kinase activity with polyoma middle T competent for transformation. *Nature*, **315**, 239.

127. Campbell, K. S., Ogris, E., Burke, B., Su, W., Auger, K. R., Druker, B. J., *et al.* (1994) Polyoma middle tumor antigen interacts with SHC protein via the NPTY (Asn-Pro-Thr-Tyr) motif in middle tumor antigen. *Proc. Natl. Acad. Sci. USA*, **91**, 6344.

128. Dilworth, S., Brewster, C. E., Jones, M. D., Lanfrancone, L., Pelicci, G., and Pelicci, P. G. (1994) Transformation by polyoma virus middle T antigen involves the binding and tyrosine phosphorylation of Shc. *Nature*, **367**, 87.

129. Cantley, L. C., Auger, K. R., Carpenter, C., Duckworth, B., Graziani, A., Kapeller, R., *et al.* (1991) Oncogenes and signal transduction. *Cell*, **64**, 281.

130. Feller, S. M., Knudsen, B., and Hanafusa, H. (1994) c-Abl kinase regulates the protein binding activity of c-Crk. *EMBO J.*, **13**, 2341.

131. Ren, R., Ye, Z.-S., and Baltimore, D. (1994) Abl protein-tyrosine kinase selects the Crk adapter as a substrate using SH3-binding sites. *Genes Dev.*, **8**, 783.

132. Courtneidge, S. A., Dhand, R., Pilat, D., Twamley, G. M., Waterfield, M. D., and Roussel, M. (1993) Activation of Src family kinases by colony stimulating factor-1, and their association with its receptor. *EMBO J.*, **12**, 943.

133. Osherov, N. and Levitzki, A. (1994) Epidermal growth factor dependent activation of the Src family kinases. *Eur. J. Biochem.*, **225**, 1047.

134. Roche, S., Koegl, M., Barone, V. M., Roussel, M., and Courtneidge, S. A. (1995) DNA synthesis induced by some, but not all, growth factors requires Src family protein tyrosine kinases. *Mol. Cell. Biol.*, **15**, 1102.

135. Twamley-Stein, G. M., Pepperkok, R., Ansorge, W., and Courtneidge, S. A. (1993) The Src family tyrosine kinases are required for platelet-derived growth factor-mediated signal transduction in NIH-3T3 cells. *Proc. Natl. Acad. Sci. USA*, **90**, 7696.

136. Twardzik, D. R., Todaro, G. J., Reynolds, F. H. J., and Stephenson, J. R. (1983) Similar transforming growth factors (TGFs) produced by cells transformed by different isolates of feline Sarcoma virus. *Virology*, **124**, 201.

137. Peterson, J. E., Jelinek, T., Kaleko, M., Siddle, K., and Weber, M. J. (1994) Phosphorylation and activation of the IGFI receptor in *src*-transformed cells. *J. Biol. Chem.*, **269**, 27315.

138. Sakai, R., Iwamatsu, A., Hirano, N., Ogawa, S., Tanaka, T., Mano, H., *et al.* (1994) A novel signaling molecule, p130, forms stable complexes *in vivo* with v-Crk and v-Src in a tyrosine phosphorylation-dependent manner. *EMBO J.*, **13**, 3748.

139. Bollag, G. and McCormick, F. (1991) Regulators and effectors of ras proteins. *Annu. Rev. Cell Biol.*, **7**, 601.

140. McCormick, F. (1994) Raf: the holy grail of Ras biology? *Trends Cell Biol.*, **4**, 347.

141. Smith, M. R., DeGudicibus, S. J., and Stacey, D. W. (1986) Requirement for c-*ras* proteins during viral oncogene transformation. *Nature*, **320**, 540.

142. McGlade, J., Cheng, A., Pelicci, G., Pelicci, P. G., and Pawson, T. (1992) Shc proteins are phosphorylated and regulated by the v-Src and v-Fps protein-tyrosine kinases. *Proc. Natl. Acad. Sci. USA*, **89**, 8869.

143. Tauchi, T., Boswell, H. S., Leibowitz, D., and Broxmeyer, H. E. (1994) Coupling between p210 bcr-abl and Shc and Grb2 adaptor proteins in hematopoietic cells permits growth factor receptor-independent link to ras activation pathway. *J. Exp. Med.*, **179**, 167.

144. Rozakis-Adcock, M., McGlade, J., Mbamalu, G., Pelicci, G., Li, W., Batzer, A., *et al.* (1992) Association of the Shc and Grb2/Sem5 SH2-containing proteins is implicated in activation of Ras pathway by tyrosine kinases. *Nature*, **360**, 689.

145. Fabian, J. R., Daar, I. O., and Morrison, D. K. (1993) Critical tyrosine residues regulate the enzymatic and biological activity of Raf-1 kinase. *Mol. Cell. Biol.*, **13**, 7170.

146. Marais, R., Light, Y., Paterson, H. F., and Marshall, C. J. (1995) Ras recruits Raf-1 to the plasma membrane for activation by tyrosine phosphorylation. *EMBO J.*, **14**, 3136.

147. Williams, N. G., Roberts, T. M., and Li, P. (1992) Both p21[ras] and pp60[v-src] are required, but neither alone is sufficient, to activate the Raf-1 kinase. *Proc. Natl. Acad. Sci. USA*, **89**, 2922.

148. Kizaka-Kondoh, S., Sata, K., Tamura, K., Nojima, H., and Okayama, H. (1992) Raf-1 protein kinase is an integral component of the oncogenic signal cascade shared by epidermal growth factor and platelet-derived growth factor. *Mol. Cell. Biol.*, **12**, 5078.

149. Afar, D. E. H., Goga, A., McLaughlin, J., Witte, O. N., and Sawyers, C. L. (1994) Differential complementation of Bcr-Abl point mutants with c-Myc. *Science*, **264**, 424.
150. Barone, M. V. and Courtneidge, S. A. (1995) Myc but not Fos rescue of PDGF signaling block caused by kinase inactive Src. *Nature*, **378**, 509.
151. Fry, M. J. (1994) Structure, regulation and function of phosphoinositide 3-kinases. *Biochem. Biophys. Acta*, **1226**, 237.
152. Kapeller, R. and Cantley, L. C. (1994) Phosphatidylinositol 3-kinase. *Bioessays*, **16**, 565.
153. Varticovski, L., Daley, G. Q., Jackson, P., Baltimore, D., and Cantley, L. C. (1991) Activation of phosphatidylinositol 3-kinase in cells expressing *abl* oncogene variants. *Mol. Cell. Biol.*, **11**, 1107.
154. Baker, J. M., Myers, M. G., Jr, Shoelson, S. E., Chin, D. J., Sun, X.-J., Miralpeix, M., *et al.* (1992) Phosphatidylinositol 3'-kinase is activated by association with IRS-1 during insulin stimulation. *EMBO J.*, **11**, 3469.
155. Carpenter, C. L., Auger, K. R., Chanudhuri, M., Yoakim, M., Schaffhausen, B., Shoelson, S., *et al.* (1993) Phosphoinositide-3-kinase is activated by phosphopeptides that bind to the SH2 domains of the 85-kDa subunit. *J. Biol. Chem.*, **268**, 9478.
156. Pleiman, C. M., Hertz, W. M., and Cambier, J. C. (1994) Activation of Phosphatidylinositol-3' kinase by Src-family kinase SH3 binding to the p85 subunit. *Science*, **263**, 1609.
157. Roche, S., Koegl, M., and Courtneidge, S. A. (1994) The phosphatidylinositol 3-kinase α is required for DNA synthesis induced by some, but not, all growth factors. *Proc. Natl. Acad. Sci. USA*, **91**, 9185.
158. Roche, S., Dhan, R., Waterfield, M. D., and Courtneidge, S. A. (1994) The catalytic subunit of phosphatidylinositol 3-kinase is a substrate for the platelet-derived growth factor receptor, but not for middle-T antigen-pp60c-src complexes. *Biochem. J.*, **301**, 703.
159. Cheatham, B., Vlahos, C. J., Cheatham, L., Wang, L., Blenis, J., and Kahn, C. R. (1994) Phosphatidylinositol 3-kinase activation is required for insulin stimulation of pp70 S6 kinase, DNA synthesis, and glucose transporter translocation. *Mol. Cell. Biol.*, **14**, 4902.
160. Chung, J., Grammer, T. C., Lemon, K. P., Kazlauskas, A., and Blenis, J. (1994) PDGF- and insulin-dependent pp70[S6k] activation mediated by phosphatidylinositol-3-OH kinase. *Nature*, **370**, 71.
161. Kozma, S. C. and Thomas, G. (1994) p70[s6k]/p85[s6k]: mechanism of activation and role in mitogenesis. *Semin. Cancer Biol.*, **5**, 255.
162. Lane, H. A., Fernandez, A., Lamb, N. J. C., and Thomas, G. (1993) p70[S6k] function is essential for G1 progression. *Nature*, **363**, 170.
163. Ming, X.-F., Burgering, B. M. T., Wennström, S., Claesson-Welsh, L., Heldin, C.-H., Bos, J. L., *et al.* (1994) Activation of p70/p85 S6 kinase by a pathway independent of p21[ras.] *Nature*, **371**, 426.
164. Jackowski, S., Rettenmier, C. W., Sherr, C. J., and Rock, C. O. (1986) A guanine nucleotide-dependent phosphatidylinositol 4,5-diphosphate phospholipase C in cells transformed by the v-*fms* and v-*fes* oncogenes. *J. Biol. Chem.*, **261**, 4978.
165. Jiang, H., Alexandropoulos, K., Song, J., and Foster, D. A. (1994) Evidence that v-Src-Induced phospholipase D Activity is mediated by a G protein. *Mol. Cell. Biol.*, **14**, 3676.
166. Weng, Z., Thomas, S. M., Rickles, R. J., Taylor, J. A., Brauer, A. W., Seidel-Dugan, C., *et al.* (1994) Identification of Src, Fyn, and Lyn SH3-binding proteins: implications for a function of SH3 domains. *Mol. Cell. Biol.*, **14**, 4509.
167. Courtneidge, S. A. and Fumagalli, S. (1994) A mitotic function for Src? *Trends Cell Biol.*, **4**, 345.

168. Fumagalli, S., Totty, N., Hsuan, J. J., and Courtneidge, S. A. (1994) A target for Src in mitosis. *Nature*, **368**, 871.

169. Taylor, S. T. and Shalloway, D. (1994) An RNA-binding protein associated with Src through its SH2 and SH3 domains in mitosis. *Nature*, **368**, 867.

170. Richard, S., Yu, D., Blumer, K. J., Hausladen, D., Olszowy, M. W., Connelly, P. A., *et al.* (1995) Association of p62, a multifunctional SH2- and SH3-domain-binding protein, with src family tyrosine kinases, Grb2, and phospholipase Cγ -1. *Mol. Cell. Biol.*, **15**, 186.

171. Roche, S., Fumagalli, S., and Courtneidge, S. A. (1995) Requirement for Src family protein tyrosine kinases in G2 for fibroblast cell division. *Science*, **269**, 1567.

172. David-Pfeuty, T. and Singer, S. J. (1980) Altered distribution of the cytoskeletal proteins vinculin and alpha actinin in cultured fibroblasts transformed by Rous Sarcoma Virus. *Proc. Natl. Acad. Sci. USA*, **77**, 6687.

173. Flynn, D. C., Leu, T.-H., Reynolds, A. B., and Parsons, J. T. (1993) Identification and sequence analysis of cDNAs encoding a 110-kilodalton actin filament-associated pp60^{src} substrate. *Mol. Cell. Biol.*, **13**, 7892.

174. Wu, H. and Parsons, J. T. (1993) Cortactin, an 80/85-Kilodalton pp60^{src} substrate, is a filamentous actin-binding protein enriched in the cell cortex. *J. Cell Biol.*, **6**, 1417.

175. Wu, H., Reynolds, A. B., Kanner, S. B., Vines, R. R., and Parsons, J. T. (1991) Identification and characterization of a novel cytoskeleton-associated pp60^{src} substrate. *Mol. Cell. Biol.*, **11**, 5113.

176. Zhan, X., Hu, X., Hampton, B., Burgess, W. H., Frieles, R., and Maciag, T. (1993) Murine cortactin is phosphorylated in response to fibroblasts growth factor-1 on tyrosine residues late in G1 phase of BALB/c 3T3 cell cycle. *J. Biol. Chem.*, **268**, 24427.

177. Guadagno, T. M. and Assoian, R. K. (1991) G1/S control of anchorage-independent growth in the fibroblast cell cycle. *J. Cell. Biol.*, **115**, 1419.

178. Chong, L. D., Traynor-Kaplan, A., Bokoch, G. M., and Shwartz, M. A. (1994) The small GTP-binding protein rho regulates a phosphatidylinositol 4-phosphate 5-kinase in mammalian cells. *Cell*, **79**, 507.

179. Kapron-Bras, C., Fitz-Gibbon, L., Jeevaratnam, P., Wilkins, J., and Dedhar, S. (1993) Stimulation of tyrosine phosphorylation and accumulation of GTP-bound p21^{ras} upon antibody-mediated α2β1 integrin activation in T-lymphoblastic cells. *J. Biol. Chem.*, **268**, 20701.

180. Schaller, M. D., Borgman, C. A., Cobb, B. S., Vines, R. R., Reynolds, A. B., and Parsons, J. T. (1992) pp125^{FAK}, a structurally distinctive protein-tyrosine kinase associated with focal adhesions. *Proc. Natl. Acad. Sci. USA*, **89**, 5192.

181. Schaller, M. D. and Parsons, J. T. (1994) Focal adhesion kinase and associated proteins. *Curr. Opin. Cell Biol.*, **6**, 705.

182. Cobb, B. S., Schaller, M. D., Leu, T.-H., and Parsons, J. T. (1994) Stable association of pp60^{src} and pp59^{fyn} with the focal adhesion-associated protein tyrosine kinase, pp125$^{FAK.}$ *Mol. Cell. Biol.*, **14**, 147.

183. Schlaepfer, D. D., Hanks, S. K., Hunter, T., and van der Geer, P. (1994) Integrin-mediated signal transduction linked to Ras pathway by GRB2 binding to focal adhesion kinase. *Nature*, **372**, 786.

184. Schaller, M. D., Hildebrand, J. D., Shannon, J. D., Fox, J. W., Vines, R. R., and Parsons, J. T. (1994) Autophosphorylation of the focal adhesion kinase, pp125^{FAK}, directs SH2-dependent binding of pp60$^{src.}$ *Mol. Cell. Biol.*, **14**, 1680.

185. Calalb, M. B., Polte, T. R., and Hanks, S. K. (1995) Tyrosine phosphorylation of focal

adhesion kinase at sites in the catalytic domain regulates kinase activity: a role for Src kinases. *Mol. Cell. Biol.*, **15**, 954.

186. Chen, H. C. and Guan, J. L. (1994) Association of focal adhesion kinase with its potential substrate phosphatidylinositol 3-kinase. *Proc. Natl. Acad. Sci. USA*, **91**, 10148.

187. Kotani, K., Yonezawa, K., Hara, K., Ueda, H., Kitamura, Y., Sakaue, H., *et al.* (1994) Involvement of phosphoinositide 3-kinase in insulin- or IGF|1-induced membrane ruffling. *EMBO J.*, **13**, 2313.

188. Wennström, S., Hawkins, P., Cooke, F., Hara, K., Yonezawa, K., Kasuga, M., *et al.* (1994) Activation of phosphoinositide 3-kinase is required for PDGF-stimulated membrane ruffling. *Curr. Biol.*, **4**, 385.

189. Wages, D. S., Keefer, J., Rall, T. B., and Weber, M. J. (1992) Mutation in the SH3 domain of the src oncogene which decrease association of PI-3 kinase activity with pp60$^{c\text{-}src}$ and alter cell morphology. *J. Virol.*, **66**, 1866.

190. Weng, Z., Taylor, J. A., Turner, C. E., Brugge, J. S., and Seidel-Dugan, C. (1993) Detection of Src homology 3-binding proteins, including paxillin, in normal and v-Src-transformed Balb/c 3T3 cells. *J. Biol. Chem.*, **268**, 14956.

191. Park, J., Meisler, A. L., and Cartwright, C. A. (1993) c-Yes tyrosine kinase activity in human colon carcinoma. *Oncogene*, **8**, 2627.

192. Loganzo, F. J., Dosik, J. S., Zhao, Y., Vidal, M. J., Nanus, D. M., Sudol, M., *et al.* (1993) Elevated expression of protein tyrosine kinase c-Yes, but not c-Src, in human malignant melanoma. *Oncogene*, **8**, 2637.

193. Muthuswamy, S. K. and Muller, W. J. (1994) Activation of the Src family of tyrosine kinases in mammary tumorigenesis. *Adv. Cancer Res.*, **64**, 111.

194. Guy, C. T., Cardiff, R. D., and Muller, W. J. (1992) Induction of mammary tumors by expression of polyomavirus middle T oncogene: a transgenic mouse model for metastatic disease. *Mol. Cell. Biol.*, **12**, 954.

195. Guy, C. T., Muthuswamy, S. K., Cardiff, R. D., Soriano, P., and Muller, W. (1994) Activation of the c-Src tyrosine kinase is required for the induction of mammary tumors in transgenic mice. *Gene Dev.*, **8**, 23.

196. Muthuswamy, S. K., Siegel, P. M., Dankort, D. L., Webster, M. A., and Muller, W. J. (1994) Mammary tumors expressing the *neu* proto-oncogene possess elevated c-Src tyrosine kinase activity. *Mol. Cell. Biol.*, **14**, 735.

197. Luttrell, D. K., Luttrell, L. M., and Parsons, S. J. (1988) Augmented mitogenic responsiveness to epidermal growth factor in murine fibroblasts that overexpress pp60$^{c\text{-}src.}$ *Mol. Cell. Biol.*, **8**, 497.

198. Maa, M. G.-C., Leu, T.-H., McCarley, D. J., Schatzman, R. C., and Parson, S. J. (1995) Potentiation of epidermal growth factor receptor-mediated oncogenesis by c-Src: implications for the etiology of multiple human cancers. *Proc. Natl. Acad. Sci. USA*, **92**, 6981.

199. Wright, D. D., Sefton, B. M., and Kamps, M. P. (1994) Oncogenic activation of the Lck protein accompanies translocation of the *LCK* gene in the human HSB2 T-cell leukemia. *Mol. Cell. Biol.*, **14**, 2429.

200. Kurzrock, R., Gutterman, J. U., and Talpaz, M. (1988) The molecular genetics of Philadelphia chromosome-positive leukemias. *N. Engl. J. Med.*, **319**, 990.

201. Daley, G. Q., Etten, R. A., and Baltimore, D. (1990) Induction chronic myelogenous leukemia in mice by the p210$^{bcr\text{-}abl}$ of the Philadelphia chromosome. *Science*, **247**, 824.

202. Kelliher, M. A., McLaughlin, J., Witte, O. N., and Rosenberg, N. (1990) Induction of

chronic myelogenous leukemia-like syndrome in mice with v-abl and Bcr/Abl. *Proc. Natl. Acad. Sci. USA*, **87**, 6649.

203. Heisterkamp, N., Jenster, G., ten Hoeve, J., Zovich, D., Pattengale, P. K., and Groffen, J. (1990) Acute leukaemia in bcr/abl transgenic mice. *Nature*, **344**, 251.

204. Scherle, P. A., Dorshkind, K., and Witte, O. N. (1990) Clonal lymphoid progenitor cell lines expressing the BCR/ABL oncogene retain full differentiation function. *Proc. Natl. Acad. Sci. USA*, **87**, 1908.

205. Gishizky, M. L. and Witte, O. N. (1992) Initiation of deregulated growth of multipotent progenitor cells by bcr-abl *in vitro*. *Science*, **256**, 836.

206. Rosenbaum, H., Harris, A. W., Bath, M. L., McNeall, J., Webb, E., Adams, J. M., *et al.* (1990) An Eμ-v-abl transgene elicits plasmacytomas in concert with an activated *myc* gene. *EMBO J.*, **9**, 897.

5 | The RAS/RAF/ERK signal transduction pathway

SUSAN G. MACDONALD and FRANK McCORMICK

1. Introduction

The importance of RAS proteins in human cancer was established in 1982, when the first human oncogene was recognized to be a mutant version of a normal *H-RAS* allele (1). These early observations prompted exhaustive efforts to identify effectors of RAS proteins, and so to understand their precise molecular function. These efforts have led to the conclusion that a major effector pathway for RAS proteins is the MAP kinase cascade (2–4; and Fig. 1). Recently, the existence of other effector pathways has been inferred, and will be discussed below. Here we summarize biochemical and biological properties of the mammalian RAS–RAF–MEK–MAP kinase signal transduction pathway and discuss questions about the pathway that remain to be answered.

RAS proteins function as binary switches, cycling between the ON state (GTP-bound) and the OFF state (GDP-bound). Much attention has been focused on the regulation of this switching mechanism by guanine nucleotide exchange factors (GEFs) which switch RAS proteins ON and GTPase activating proteins (GAPs) which switch them OFF (5). The biological activity of RAS in the cell reflects the level of RAS protein in the GTP state. This is determined by the relative activity of GEFs and GAPs, and by the level of RAS protein expression, issues that have been discussed extensively elsewhere. RAS–GTP can interact with a number of different proteins, with different results. Interaction with GAPs (p120–GAP, GAP^m, neurofibromin) results in hydrolysis of bound GTP to GDP. The possibility that these interactions also generate a signal has been discussed, but no clear evidence exists to implicate GAPs as effectors in pathways that we currently recognize. Still, it is possible that GAP acts as an 'effector by proxy', in that it may interact with and regulate RAC and RHO GAPs, which help regulate the cytoskeleton. Such an interpretation is consistent with the phenotype observed with RAS–GAP null mice in which a vascular plexus forms but the endothelial cells fail to migrate and organize into a vascular network (6). Several other proteins interact specifically with RAS in its GTP state and are candidates for physiologically important effectors. Of these, phosphatidyl inositol 3-kinase (PI3K) and RAL–GDS are of particular interest, and will be discussed briefly below. However, RAF isoforms are the clearest direct effectors of RAS biological action. This is because a substantial body of evidence from diverse biological systems clearly shows that

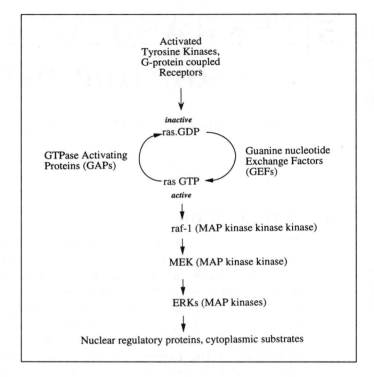

Fig. 1 Activation of RAS and the MAP kinase cascade by growth factor receptors. RAS accumulates in the GTP state through activation of exchange factors (such as SOS), or through inhibition of GAP activity (p120GAP, neurofibromin, etc).

RAF is downstream from RAS, and that RAS needs RAF and other components of the MAP kinase cascade for its transforming activity. These statements cannot be made for other putative RAS effectors.

2. The RAS–RAF interaction

The discovery that RAS–GTP and RAF interact directly (7–11), and that in cells the result of this interaction is stimulation of RAF activity and initiation of the MAP kinase cascade, represented major breakthroughs in understanding RAS biology (12, 13).

RAF is a serine/threonine kinase that was first identified in the murine sarcoma virus 3611 which encodes a fusion protein comprising the kinase domain of RAF joined to a myristylated viral gag sequence (14). Identification of the human homologue revealed that *RAF* is part of a multigene family, consisting of *RAF* itself (formally called *RAF1*), *A-RAF*, and *B-RAF* (15–18). Whereas *RAF1* is ubiquitously expressed, the tissue distribution of *A-RAF* and *B-RAF* is more restricted (19, 20), perhaps reflecting a more specialized function in these tissues. In addition, recent evidence has suggested that the *B-RAF* gene encodes several isoforms of B-RAF whose expression is regulated in a tissue-specific manner by alternative splicing (21). The structures of each isoform, however, would predict that each isoform interacts with RAS, although there are obvious implications for the intrinsic activity, regulation, and substrate recognition of the isoforms. Each RAF isoform contains an amino terminal regulatory domain, consisting of two conserved regions (CR1 and CR2), in addition to the kinase domain (CR3) found in the gag–RAF fusion (Fig. 2). CR1 contains a zinc-finger homologous to that found in PKC and CR2 is rich in serine and threonine residues prompting speculation that it contains sites of regulatory phosphorylation. Its position in a signalling pathway downstream of RAS was first inferred from the work of Stacey and co-workers (22), who showed that antibodies that neutralize RAS have no effect on RAF transformation. Similar conclusions were drawn from genetic analysis of signalling pathways in yeast, flies, and worms (23–33).

In 1993, Wolfman and co-workers, showed that RAF proteins from cell extracts bound *in vitro* to immobilized RAS proteins (34). A number of other proteins, including the GAP neurofibromin (35), also bound to RAS specifically in this experimental system, so that the precise nature of the association between RAS and RAF (direct or indirect) remained to be determined. Likewise, RAS and RAF interacted when tested in a yeast two-hybrid system (7). In both cases, association bore the required

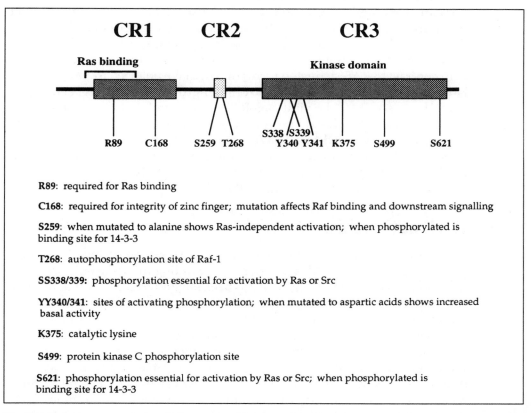

Fig. 2 Schematic representation of human RAF, featuring conserved domains and important phosphorylation sites.

characteristics of true effector interaction: only the active form of RAS interacted, and mutations in the putative effector binding site that render RAS inactive (see below) prevented RAF association. Independently, yeast two-hybrid screens for proteins that associate with RAS or RAF led to the suggestion that these proteins interact directly, and this was definitively proven using purified recombinant proteins (8–11).

A small region of RAF sufficient to bind directly to RAS was identified in the CR1 region: amino acids 51–131 appear to comprise a minimal binding region (36, 37). The structure of a similar region (amino acids 55–132) has been solved using three-dimensional NMR spectroscopy (38), whereas the 51–131 fragment has been co-crystallized with the RAS-related protein, RAP1, and the structure of the complex solved by X-ray crystallography (39). Figure 3 shows the structure of the RAS–RAF complex predicted from the RAP–RAF co-ordinates. RAS and RAP1 are identical in this region of contact (the effector binding loop) and we expect this model to be quite accurate. In the model, amino acids N64, Q66, R67, T68, and R89 of RAF form specific side chain interactions with the side chains of amino acids E37, D38, S39, and R41 of RAS. These results are striking in that several of these direct contacts were predicted from muta-genesis analysis of RAS proteins (residues 37–41 are part of the RAS effector binding domain proposed in 1986) and genetic analysis of the *sevenless* pathway in *Drosophila*; the equivalent of R89 was identified as a null mutant allelle of *D-RAF* (40, 41). Most of the interactions are polar and the two domains make up a continuous beta sheet in which the RAS binding region of RAF is folded in a ubiquitin-like structure (38).

In contrast to RAS, activated forms of RAF have not been found in human tumours. However, the importance of RAF to cellular growth control has been demonstrated in several ways. *v-RAF* (the viral gag–RAF fusion) and *A-RAF* are tumorigenic and can impart a metastatic phenotype (42), while amino terminally truncated forms of RAF (43–45) and RAF fused to a K-RAS isoprenylation motif (46) are able to transform cells. In addition, the expression of a dominant negative form of RAF1, in which the catalytic lysine is mutated, or of *RAF* antisense RNA, have shown that RAF1 is required for the growth of normal cells (47).

3. RAF activation

One of the enduring mysteries of the RAS–MAP kinase pathway continues to be the precise mechanism of RAF activation. RAS binding to RAF results in its translocation to the plasma membrane (Fig. 4). It has been suggested recently that this is actually the sole role for RAS in the process of RAF activation, since RAF proteins directed to the plasma membrane through specific targeting sequences (CAAX motifs, or myristyla-tion) become activated in a RAS-independent manner (12, 13, 43). However, it is not clear that RAF activation through RAS binding is identical to RAF activation through direct targeting. Both events could achieve the same end result (active RAF) using different biochemical means. The fact that RAF can be activated by RAS-independent means raises the possibility that addition of the CAAX motif mimics RAF activation through a RAS-independent pathway. The simple association of purified RAS and RAF *in vitro* does not appear to activate RAF (48), nor is the continued presence of

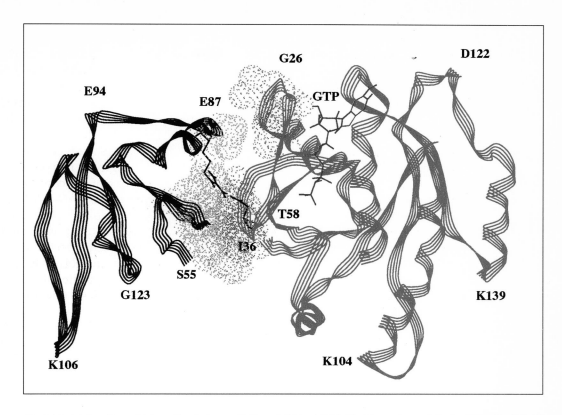

Fig.3 Model for sites of interaction between RAS and CR1 of RAF. Model courtesy of Dr Sookhee Ha (Bayer) based on the structure of the RAP1–RAF complex determined by Wittinghofer and co-workers. RAF (residues 55–130) in blue, RAS (residues 1–186) in red. The side chains of arginine 89 of RAF and aspartate 40 of RAS, which are in direct contact, are shown in black.

RAS required for the maintenance of RAF activity (12, 49), and we are left with the conclusion that the fundamental process of RAF activation by RAS is not yet fully understood.

A major obstacle in the search for the mechanism of RAF activation, and thus an activator, is the difficulty in assigning specific and definitive roles for the many phosphorylation sites identified in RAF and for the CR2 domain. Phosphorylation appears to be involved in the activation process: stimulation of growth factor receptors and expression of membrane-bound oncoproteins can result in the hyperphosphorylation of RAF and an increase in its kinase activity (50–54). In addition, one study showed that RAF immunoprecipitated from insulin-stimulated cells was inactivated by treatment with a serine/threonine-specific phosphatase (52) and more recent work has indicated the existence of a $G\alpha_{i/o}$-regulated, membrane-associated phosphatase which can inactivate RAF (55–57). Furthermore, activation of RAF *in vitro* by transformed cell membranes is ATP-dependent (58). In contrast, other work has indicated that treatment with phosphatases does not inactivate RAF (59). This apparent paradox may be explained by the ability of associated 14-3-3 proteins to prevent the dephosphorylation of RAF, as will be discussed later.

While several sites of RAF phosphorylation have been identified and their functional significance investigated (60–62; and see Fig. 2), no single phosphoamino acid accounts for RAF activation. Phosphorylation of tyrosines 340 and 341 have been implicated in activation by RAS (60, 63, 64) although these phosphorylations do not appear to represent the only mechanism by which RAF can be activated. Recently, phosphorylation of serines 338 and 339, immediately adjacent to tyrosines 340 and 341, have been identified as essential for activation of RAF by RAS or by SRC (65). It was further shown that S338 must be phosphorylated in order for phosphorylation of Y340 and Y341 to activate RAF and Y340 and Y341 need not be phosphorylated for

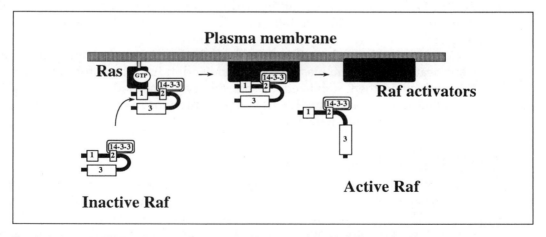

Fig. 4. Activation of RAF by recruitment to the membrane. In this model, RAF in its inactive state, bound to 14-3-3 (and presumably to other associated proteins) binds to RAS–GTP in the plasma membrane. Activation occurs as a result of a conformational change after deposition in the membrane by RAS.

the activation of RAF by membrane association. Phosphorylation of S621 appears to be necessary, but not sufficient, for the activation of RAF as mutation of this site to alanine renders the kinase insensitive to activation by any stimulus (48, 61, 65). Serine 259 has been identified as a potential site of inhibitory phosphorylation (61), since a mutation at that site allows RAS-independent activation in 293 cells and oocytes (66). Phosphorylation of both S259 and S621 is required for binding of 14-3-3, as will be discussed in the next section. The kinases that phosphorylate these sites have not yet been identified, although such a discovery would greatly aid in the identification of relative contributions of different phosphoamino acids to the activation state of RAF.

It has been suggested that protein kinase C (PKC), which phosphorylates RAF on S499, can activate RAF (62). While it can lead to RAF activation in cells, PKC does not directly activate RAF *in vitro* with respect to its substrate, MEK, although it does appear to stimulate autophosphorylation (49, 62, 67, 68). Furthermore, activation of PKC does not appear to be a prerequisite for RAF activation in all systems, suggesting PKC-stimulated events may not be the primary means of RAF activation but may instead superimpose a permissive mode of regulation on RAS- or growth factor-stimulated events, leading to the activation of RAF.

The presence of a cysteine-rich zinc-finger in RAF, which bears homology to the diacylglycerol binding site in PKC, suggests that a lipid may regulate RAF activity. It has been shown that this region binds two moles of zinc (69), that a methanol–chloroform extract from transformed cell membranes can enhance the activity of activated RAF (70), and that phosphatidylserine binds to this region (71). However, no lipid has yet been demonstrated to bind to or significantly alter basal RAF activity. The function of this region may be to maintain the ternary and quaternary structure of RAF via the co-ordinating zinc ions or to participate in the process of RAS-dependent activation. Indeed, its disruption decreases the affinity of RAS for RAF *in vitro* and compromises, but does not eliminate, its ability to be activated by RAS in cells (10, 11, 72, 73). Interestingly, phosphatidic acid has been shown to bind to a site in the CR3 domain of RAF and the inhibition of phosphatidic acid formation in MDCK cells reduces translocation to the plasma membrane (74).

Cumulatively, the data suggest a complex model of activation in which RAS translocates RAF to the plasma membrane and induces a conformational change in RAF which is then stabilized by phosphorylations and/or lipid interactions at the membrane. In addition, RAF-associated proteins may have a role in permitting activation or preventing the inactivation of RAF.

3.1 RAF-associated proteins

RAF immunoprecipitated from mammalian and insect cells co-purifies with several other proteins, including HSP50, HSP70, HSP90, tubulin, and 14-3-3 proteins (48, 49, 75–79). The functional relevance of all of these associations with RAF is not completely understood, but they have led to speculation that the activity, subcellular localization, or substrate specificity of RAF could be allosterically regulated through association or dissociation with one of these proteins or by the covalent modification of one of these proteins. HSP90 is required for and stabilizes the active conformation of the glucocorticoid receptor (80–82) and modulates the activity and expression of SRC (83; and Chapter 4) as well as regulating cellular trafficking of SRC through cycles of HSP90 phosphorylation and dephosphorylation (84). It is not surprising then, that HSP90 has been found to stabilize levels of RAF in the cell and may aid in its trafficking to the plasma membrane (85).

14-3-3 proteins are necessary for the activation of RAF, at least in a yeast system of RAF activation: strains possessing a deletion of 14-3-3 (BMH1) do not support RAS-dependent RAF activation (86). Accordingly, RAF prepared from yeast or *Xenopus* extracts has been reported to be stimulated by the addition of 14-3-3 proteins (86–88). RAF mutagenesis experiments have shown that 14-3-3 proteins bind to specific phosphoserine residues of RAF: S259 and S621 (66, 89). Their association with RAF apparently blocks dephosphorylation and subsequent inactivation of RAF (55, 89). Prevention of the 14-3-3/RAF interaction using phosphopeptides directed to S259 or S621 (89) blocked insulin-stimulated oocyte maturation. While this is consistent with observations that 14-3-3 is required for RAF activation (77, 86, 87) it is inconsistent with the observation that a serine to alanine mutation at position 259 of RAF abolishes its association with 14-3-3 and results in its RAS-independent activation in 293 cells and *Xenopus* oocytes (66). However, the same study showed that biochemical dissociation of 14-3-3 from RAF did not result in enhanced basal activity of RAF. Since biochemical dissociation of 14-3-3 from RAF should leave S259 phosphorylated, the data may suggest that RAF from which 14-3-3 proteins have been biochemically dissociated and mutated RAF unable to associate with 14-3-3 at phosphoserine 259 may not be functionally identical. The S259A mutation may mimic a conformational change in RAF which is normally induced by the binding of 14-3-3 to RAF and is required for its activation, or the association between 14-3-3 proteins and RAF may alter substrate affinity or specificity. Another explanation for the apparently anomalous results is the suggestion that 14-3-3 proteins help mediate the RAS-independent activation of RAF (87). Since phosphorylated S621 also binds 14-3-3, and its mutation to alanine renders RAF unable to be activated, perhaps its dephosphorylation is a critical event in the inactivation of RAF. In any case, because 14-3-3 proteins are associated with both active and inactive forms of RAF (77, 79), they do not appear to be sufficient for the activation of RAF.

The specificity of the different isoforms of RAF for different isoforms of MEK is of interest. Are there different combinations of RAF and MEK isoforms which transduce different signals in different tissues? Perhaps they produce a similar signal, but at altered levels, either quantitatively or temporally. Whereas RAF is ubiquitously expressed, the tissue distributions of A-RAF and B-RAF are much more restricted (19, 20). The amino acids in B-RAF corresponding to Y340 and Y341 of RAF, whose phosphorylation is activating (60), are aspartic acids (18), whose negative charges can mimic those of a phosphate group. Indeed, mutation of Y340 and Y341 of RAF to aspartic acid residues yields a molecule with elevated basal activity which is further increased by *v-RAS*, but not *v-SRC* (60, 90). Curiously, in NIH/3T3 cells, B-RAF is not further activated by RAS (64). Furthermore, in *Drosophila melanogaster* and *Caenor-*

habditis elegans, organisms in which RAF is known to be involved in differentiation, the analogous residues are EEN and ED, respectively (31, 91). Based on these data, it is tempting to speculate that, in systems in which the role of RAF is primarily one of differentiation, a higher basal level of kinase activity is required than in systems in which RAF regulates proliferation and helps to maintain cellular homeostasis. In support of this concept is the observation that the major soluble MEK activator purified from both unstimulated bovine brain and adrenal chromaffin cells appears to be B-RAF (88), while the soluble RAF purified from the same sources shows no apparent activity towards MEK1 (92). Indeed, B-RAF has been shown to possess a higher level of basal activity than RAF (64). Given this observation, one would expect to find soluble, cytosolic B-RAF, but not RAF in purifications from these cells. Furthermore, this observation is consistent with the idea that the higher basal activity of B-RAF in these unstimulated cells is related to their function in maintaining a differentiated neuronal phenotype. This does not imply that B-RAF is exclusively activated in neuronal cells. Indeed, both RAF and B-RAF can be activated in PC12 cells upon NGF stimulation in a RAS-dependent manner (93). Finally, the multiple isoforms of B-RAF allow for the possibility of regulation by factors other than RAS, as well as for alternative substrate recognition (21).

4. MEK

The identification of MEK (MKK) as a substrate of RAF provided a sought-after link between the activation of RAS and the activation of ERK (49, 94–96). MEK is a dual specificity kinase, phosphorylating ERK on both a tyrosine and a threonine residue, rendering it active (97). It is predominantly cytoplasmic (98). However, approximately 10% of total transfected MEK associates with the membrane in cells stimulated with RAS–G12V (the activated form of RAS in which glycine 12 is replaced with valine; ref. 48). This is consistent with the observation that RAF from rat brain which was able to form a complex with immobilized RAS–GTP also contains MEK activity and that RAF and MEK1 are able to form a complex in cells (34, 99, 100). The mechanism by which MEK translocates between activated, membrane-bound RAF and the cytoplasm is not yet known.

Three MEKs have since been cloned that are susceptible to phosphorylation by RAF (97, 101–104). MEK3, however, may not be catalytically active, as it has sustained a 26 amino acid deletion in an essential kinase domain and is not able to activate ERK *in vitro*, despite its ability to bind to it, nor does it have any effect on the activation of ERK1 or ERK2 by MEK1 or MEK2 *in vitro* (105). MEK is activated by RAF-mediated phosphorylation on S218 and S222 (106–109). While the activation of MEK can be mediated by MOS, MEKK, or RAF *in vitro* or in heterologous cell systems (49, 109, 110), it may be that only RAF activates MEK in response to growth factors that signal through RAS (see Section 7).

It is not known how MEK is inactivated following cessation of a stimulatory extra-cellular signal. While one group has reported that p34^{cdc2} inactivates MEK1 by phosphorylating it on threonines 286 and 292 (111), to date, no MEK-specific phosphatases have been identified. It has, however, been shown that treatment with the broad specificity phosphatase, phosphatase 2A, inactivates MEK *in vitro* (112–114). In addition, sequestration of phosphatase 2A by SV40 small t antigen in CV-1 cells results in increased MEK and ERK activities (115). Finally, a phosphatase 2C, which appears to act specifically on the MEK homologue WIS1, has been recently cloned from *S. pombe* and appears to function in an osmoregulatory pathway (116). Still, the inactivation of MEK may not be a simple process, as MonoQ fractionation of cell extracts containing activated MEK yields two peaks of active MEK, the second of which is more sensitive to inactivation by phosphatase 2A (117). This second peak of activity increases in response to prolonged growth factor stimulation and may be related to the persistent MEK activity which is seen following NGF stimulation. Identification of MEK-specific phosphatases which are themselves activated by extracellular signals may help provide some insight into the inactivation of MEK, and perhaps impart some specificity upon it.

MEK can also be phosphorylated by its substrate, ERK (105, 118),leading to speculation that this event represents feedback inhibition of MEK. While it is possible that this phosphorylation constitutes feedback inhibition of the RAS signalling pathway, it is more likely that these are *in vitro* artefacts. Indeed, we and others have found that phosphorylation of MEK1 by ERK *in vitro* has no effect on its activity after activation by RAF, nor on its ability to be activated by RAF (48, 105). The possibility remains, however, that ERK phosphorylation of MEK regulates MEK localization and therefore access by RAF or other regulatory molecules in the cell. These data do not, of course, rule out other forms of feedback inhibition of MEK.

The degree to which each MEK isozyme is susceptible to activation by RAF, A-RAF, or B-RAF is of interest. One study has suggested that B-RAF may be a major MEK activator in NIH/3T3 fibroblasts (119) and another has shown that B-RAF phosphorylates MEK1 on serines 218 and 222 (120). In HeLa cells stimulated with EGF, A-RAF is able to activate MEK1 but not MEK2, whereas RAF can activate both MEK1 and MEK2 (121). *In vitro* analyses of MEK1 activation by the kinase domains of RAF isoforms show that the efficacy of activation, in decreasing order, is B-RAF, RAF, and A-RAF (122). More recently it has been suggested that different stimuli lead to transient or sustained activation of different RAF isoforms (123). Thus, in addition to intrinsic specificities of RAF isoforms for MEK isoforms, the *in vivo* specificities may ultimately be determined by the relative concentration of each molecule in a given cell and their relative affinities for one another and their temporal period of activation.

For instance, MEK1 appears to be expressed ubiquitously (104) and at higher levels than those of MEK2, leading to the prediction that, in the absence of other regulators, MEK1 might be the preferred RAF substrate. There are, however, some tissues in which MEK2 is expressed at high levels compared to that of MEK1 (101, 104), leading to speculation that MEK2 may be the predominant MEK substrate in those tissues. The tissue distribution of MEK2 also suggests possible roles in development, differentiation, or maintenance of the differentiated phenotype. If this is true, one might expect that MEK2 is the preferred substrate for B-RAF, although despite the finding that MEK2 is highly expressed in brain relative to MEK1, it has been reported that MEK1 is the preferred substrate for B-RAF in brain and PC12 cells (124–126). It has also been reported that MEK1, but not MEK2, is found in a signalling complex with RAS and RAF in NIH/3T3 cells (99). One explanation for these apparently anomalous results is the possibility that accessory or tethering proteins equivalent to the yeast STE5 protein (127–129) regulate enzyme–substrate interactions in a cell-specific manner. In order for these apparent discrepancies to be resolved, well-controlled *in vivo* experiments need to be performed to ascertain the physiological specificities of the different RAF isoforms for the different MEK isoforms.

Just as unregulated forms of RAF have been shown to be transforming, constitutively activated forms of MEK1 have also been shown to transform cells and induce the formation of solid tumours in nude mice (130–132). Interestingly, however, the transformed phenotype is slightly different morphologically from that induced by activated RAS and it is only partially blocked by microinjection of the RAS neutralizing antibody Y13–259 (131), suggesting an additional component acting in transformation by RAS. Alternatively, the data might be explained by the presence of an autocrine loop which signals independently of RAS. Also like RAF, constitutively active forms of MEK have not yet been found in human tumours. However, the ability of unregulated forms of MEK to transform cells in culture and induce tumours in nude mice reveals its importance in cell growth. The linear placement of MEK in this proliferative pathway, downstream of an oncogene known to be mutated in human tumours (RAS), suggests MEK as a target for the development of anti-proliferative cancer therapies.

5. ERK

The only identified substrates of MEKs are the MAP kinases or ERKs (extracellular regulated kinase/microtubule-associated kinase/mitogen-activated kinase), which are required for RAS-mediated DNA synthesis (133–136), which in turn is a requirement for transformation. MEK phosphorylates ERK on both T183 and Y185, thereby activating the molecule. As is the case with RAF and MEK, the ERKs consist of a family of homologous proteins, including p44 MAP kinase (ERK1), p42 MAP kinase (ERK2), and p63 (ERK3) (137, 138). ERK3 contains a 180 amino acid carboxy terminal extension not found in ERK1 or ERK2 and substitutions in two conserved kinase subdomains (138). In the kinase subdomain VIII, the A–P–E sequence is substituted with S–P–R, and in the activation motif, T–E–Y is replaced with S–E–G, suggesting some difference in regulation relative to ERKs 1 and 2. In contrast to ERKs 1 and 2, ERK3 is constitutively nuclear and is phosphorylated on serine by a kinase that is immunologically distinct from MEKs 1 and 2 (139). Its activation may also be mediated through PKCβ (140), leaving open the question of whether ERK3 is part of a RAS-regulated pathway.

While MEK is a cytoplasmic protein (98), ERK is activated in the cytoplasm but, in some cases, is translocated into the nucleus upon activation (117, 141–143). This property endows ERK with the ability to affect the activity of both cytoplasmic and nuclear proteins. ERK activity in the nucleus primarily results in the activation of transcription factors which leads to the expression of immediate early genes, while the phosphorylation of cytoplasmic ERK substrates results in the stimulation of cytoplasmic signalling and protein synthesis (135, 136). The mechanism by which nuclear translocation of ERK occurs is not known, although it may involve an accessory protein, as no obvious nuclear localization signals have been identified on ERK.

The phenomenon of nuclear translocation of ERK has been associated with mitogenesis (144), the differentiation of PC12 cells by NGF (117, 145), and the differentiation of thymocytes (146) and pre-adipocytes (147). In these cells, growth factor stimulation leads to a rapid, transient phase of ERK activation which is followed by a lower, sustained phase. It is during the sustained phase of activation that ERK is observed to translocate into the nucleus. That the processes of proliferation and differentiation are very well-regulated is demonstrated by the fact that NGF, which causes differentiation of PC12 cells, activates both a transient and sustained phase of ERK activity, while EGF, which is weakly mitogenic and does not induce differentiation, exhibits only a transient phase of ERK activation, and does not induce its translocation into the nucleus (148, 149). These observations provide direct evidence that the location of ERK is essential to its function in a cell.

It is not known how the biphasic ERK response is regulated, but vanadate treatment of fibroblasts has been shown to result in biphasic ERK activity, suggesting that it may be controlled by phosphatases (148). Certainly, an attractive hypothesis is the existence of specifically localized phosphatases which can mediate transient or sustained ERK activity. Indeed, several ERK-specific phosphatases have recently been identified and may provide insights into the temporal levels of ERK activation (150–157). MKP1 (also known as 3CH134 or CL100) is an ERK phosphatase that acts on both ERKs 1 and 2 by dephosphorylating activating tyrosine and threonine residues (152). Its co-expression in cells with activated RAS blocks mitogenesis, suggesting that ERK activation is a necessary event in mitogenesis. Interestingly, MKP1 is an immediate early gene whose transcription is transiently induced by serum growth factors (150, 152) and regulators of the structurally homologous SAP kinase pathway (158; and see Section 7) and is strictly localized to the nucleus in both quiescent and stimulated cells (159). Similarly, PAC1 is a haematopoietic cell-specific ERK phosphatase which is expressed only in the nucleus and inhibits ERK-regulated gene transcription (151, 154). These data imply that some of the specificity in the ERK pathway, at least at the level of ERK, may be imparted by the expression of tissue-specific and localization-specific ERK phosphatases.

Since three different MEKs exist, an obvious question is whether the MEKs activate ERKs equally well or if there is any specificity in their interactions. *In vitro*, MEK1 and MEK2 have been shown to complex with ERK2 and MEK2 with ERK1. However, MEK2 activates both ERK1 and ERK2 better than does MEK1 which suggests that MEK2 is intrinsically more active than MEK1 (105). Since there is apparently more MEK1 than MEK2 in many cells (104), it is possible that the effective activity of MEK1 equals that of MEK2. Furthermore, if RAF preferentially associates with MEK1 in cells (99), perhaps the primary ERK signal is elicited through MEK1.

Table 1 ERK substrates

Substrate	Localization[a]	Effects of phosphorylation
Oestrogen receptor	C	Activates transcription (223)
RSK	C, N	Activates kinase; stimulates protein synthesis (224–226)
SH-PTP2	C	Inhibits phosphatase activity (227)
PLA2	C	Activates phospholipase (228, 229)
SOS	C, PM	Promotes disassembly of EGFR, SOS, GRB2 complex (230, 231)
EGFR	PM	Unknown (232–234)
MEK	C	Unknown (105, 118)
RAF	C, PM	Unknown (48, 235–237)
PHAS-1	C	Stimulates protein synthesis (238, 239)
C-JUN	N	Regulation complex; regulates transcription from SRE (207, 240, 241)
C-FOS	N	Regulates transcription from SRE (141, 242)
ELK-1/p62TCF	N	Promotes transcription from the c-FOS SRE and from an ETS site (243–246, 248)
SAP1a,1b	N	Promotes transcription from the c-FOS SRE and from an ETS site (244, 247)
NF-IL6	N	Promotes transcription from the IL-1 responsive element in the IL-6 gene (249)
p53	N	Unknown (250)

[a] C = cytoplasm; N = nucleus; PM = plasma membrane.

The final cellular response mediated by activated ERK is dependent upon the cell in which it is acting, but in general leads to immediate early gene transcription and the activation of other kinases, which themselves alter cellular function. Unlike RAF and MEK, the immediate substrates through which ERKs produce cellular responses, such as proliferation and differentiation, are many and varied. The physiological relevance and effects of some of these phosphorylations are still under investigation. Table 1 outlines some of the substrates of ERKs and their effects.

6. Other effectors of RAS

Transformation is accompanied by a plethora of cellular changes and activities. The observation that the constitutive activation of a single molecule, such as RAS, can effect many or all of these changes suggests that it is responsible for the control of several cellular pathways. The ERK pathway is clearly one of these pathways. However, it seems unlikely that physiological activation of the ERK pathway alone effects cell transformation. Indeed, transformed cells exhibit altered cytoskeletal architecture, which cannot be accounted for by the activation of the ERK pathway. It is becoming increasingly evident that the activation of RAS initiates the activation of several other pathways which may contribute to the RAS-transformed phenotype. Some recent work has used H-RAS effector loop mutations to help distinguish the ability of RAS to activate different effector pathways (160). In using these mutants to compare the activation of JNK (a member of the MAP kinase family which will be discussed in the following section) and ERK in HeLa cells, it was found that an E37G mutation in H-RAS preferentially activated JNK over ERK, but did not activate either protein to control levels. Interestingly, that mutant was unable to transform NIH/3T3 or Rat-1 cells, leading to the conclusion that at least two cellular pathways, each activated by RAS, are required for efficient transformation of cells. Further evidence that RAS activates multiple pathways is the identification of one effector mutant (Y40C) that induces membrane ruffling, but does not activate ERK or stimulate DNA synthesis and another (T35S) that activates ERK, but does not stimulate membrane ruffling of DNA synthesis (161). However, mutants such RAS–G12V affect all three cellular activities. While all of the pathways and proteins that directly interact with RAS have not yet been definitively identified and characterized, several candidates exist.

6.1 AF-6

The human AF-6 protein has recently been shown to bind to GTP-bound RAS through the RAS effector domain and this binding is effectively competed by RAF (162). The downstream function of AF-6 and how it is regulated by RAS is unknown, but AF-6 is homologous to the *Drosophila* Canoe protein, which functions downstream of Notch and has been genetically linked to RAS1 in eye development. Through examination of its domain structure, it is speculated that AF-6 may regulate the cytoskeleton at the junction of the plasma membrane and the cytoskeleton. However, further studies are required to define the precise role of AF-6 in RAS-mediated signal transduction.

6.2 RAL–GDS

RAL–GDS has been identified by several groups as possessing characteristics consistent with that of a RAS effector (163–165). That is, it interacts with the effector-binding domain of RAS in a GTP-dependent manner. RAL–GDS specifically catalyses guanine nucleotide exchange on the RAS-related GTP-binding protein, RAL (166). *In vitro* binding studies show a strong preference of RAL–GDS for RAP over H-RAS (167, 168), indicating that RAL–GDS may also interact with RAP in cells, although no cellular effect of the RAP/RAL–GDS interaction has yet been defined. In contrast, it has been reported that RAS activates RAL–GDS and proposed that RAS-activated RAL–GDS brings RAL bound to phospholipase D to the plasma membrane for activation by an as yet undefined factor (169). In addition, since a RAL-binding protein has been identified which is able to stimulate hydrolysis of GTP on RAC1 and CDC42, it has been postulated that the RAS/RAL–GDS interaction mediates modulation of the cytoskeletion through RAC (170). Further studies are necessary to define the functional significance of the RAL–GDS interaction with RAS and with RAP.

6.3 Phosphatidylinositol 3-kinase

Transfection of activated RAS into cells stimulates phosphatidylinositol 3-kinase (PI3K) activity, as judged by the increase in the products of this enzyme. Recently, it has been reported to be an effector of RAS (171). The interaction has been demonstrated by *in vitro* binding of purified components and is GTP-dependent and effector loop-dependent, implying a direct effector function. However, *in vitro*, RAS stimulates only a twofold increase in PI3K activity (172). It is not known whether this level of activity is sufficient to transduce an intracellular effect. Thus, the physiological significance of this interaction remains to be defined. If a twofold activation is not sufficient to transduce a cellular effect, it might imply that RAS serves to localize or sequester activated PI3K to an appropriate subcellular location or that efficient activation of PI3K by RAS *in vitro* requires additional components.

These data are in apparent contradiction to evidence which suggests that PI3K lies upstream of RAS (173) and can activate the RAS pathway (174). The ability of a constitutively active mutant of PI3K expressed in fibroblasts to activate a *FOS* reporter construct was blocked by the co-expression of a dominant interfering mutant of RAS (174). In addition, the expression of the constitutively active PI3K mutant in *Xenopus* oocytes induced maturation and led to an increase in the levels of RAS–GTP. Both results suggest that PI3K can activate the RAS pathway, but cannot be easily reconciled with the finding that PI3K is an effector of RAS. It does remain possible, however, that there are isoforms of PI3K which act upstream or downstream of RAS. This possibility is supported by the recent identifications of a regulatory subunit of PI3K that specifically associates with IRS1 during insulin signalling (175) and a PI3K which is activated by heterotrimeric G proteins (176).

Yet another study suggested that RAS and PI3K activities bifurcate at the level of the receptor, and thus act in distinct pathways (177). In NIH/3T3 cells overexpressing the insulin receptor, the introduction of dominant negative RAS was able to block ERK2 activation induced by insulin, but not PI3K activation. The issue of PI3K and its relationship to RAS is a compelling question which remains to be answered.

6.4 RAC/RHO

The transformation of cells by RAS not only involves the proliferation of cells but also involves cytoskeletal rearrangements. RAS–GAP binds a protein called p190, which, in its amino terminal region, contains domains homologous to those of RAC–GAPs and RHO–GAPs (178, 179). Since these domains could regulate cytoskeletal reorganization, the association of RAS–GAP and p190 with RAS suggests some role of RAS in the regulation of the cytoskeleton. Likewise, SOS encodes a DBL-homology domain which may regulate guanine nucleotide exchange on RAC, RHO, or CDC42Hs (5). Evidence of direct regulation of RAC or RHO by RAS has not been forthcoming, perhaps due to specialized interactions of these proteins with the cytoskeleton, which may be difficult to reconstruct *in vitro*. Recently, however, evidence has been presented suggesting that the RAC pathway, which regulates membrane ruffling through reorganization of the actin cytoskeleton (180), functions downstream of RAS. It has been shown that the introduction of a dominant negative form of RAC (RAC–N17) inhibits focus formation by RAS–G12V in NIH/3T3 cells, but not by RAF–CAAX (46). In addition, RAC–G12V synergizes with RAF–CAAX in focus formation assays and cells expressing RAC–G12V form tumours when injected subcutaneously into nude mice. Activated RAC (and CDC42Hs, but not RHO) have been linked to the activation of kinase cascades which are structurally homologous to but functionally distinct from the ERK cascade that is regulated by RAS (181, 182). Interestingly, these GTPases, like RAS, also seem to regulate their kinase cascades by direct association with, and activation of, a kinase (183–186).

RHO, which when activated leads to the formation of actin stress fibres and focal adhesions (187), has also been implicated in RAS transformation. In focus forming assays, RHO was required for RAS transformation, but not for RAF transformation, although it could potentiate transformation by RAS or RAF (188, 189). Cumulatively, the studies conclude that the RAF/ERK, RHO, and RAC pathways are all required for full RAS transformation (190) and suggest a bifurcation or trifurcation of signalling pathways emanating from RAS, all of which are required for transformation.

7. How many MAP kinase pathways does RAS regulate?

Recently, several mammalian proteins have been identified and linked to homologous signalling pathways in yeast (Fig. 5). While the elements of the pathways are structurally homologous, they appear to operate in response to distinct upstream signals and mediate distinct downstream responses (191–203). These pathways appear to be activated in response to cellular stress instead of growth factors. Termed JNKs (for JUN kinases) (204) or SAPKs (for stress-activated protein kinases) (205), p38 and ERK5 (195, 203), they are activated by such extracellular stimuli as UV light (204), ischaemia (206), heat shock (205), cycloheximide (205), cytokines (204, 205), hyperosmolarity (200), and TNFα (205, 207), and result in the phosphorylation of c-JUN at sites within the transactivation domain (see Chapter 6). In some instances the phosphorylation of c-JUN is RAS-independent and in other instances RAS may at least partially regulate some of these pathways (204, 208–210).

It has been proposed that RAS activates MEKK under certain circumstances (211) and that MEKK initiates the activation of a pathway which is parallel to the RAF–MEK–ERK pathway, but instead mediates cellular stress responses (210, 212). This may be mediated via RAS-activated RAC (181) or by MEKK directly, since MEKK has also been shown to bind to RAS in a GTP-dependent manner (213). The extent to which this occurs *in vivo* and the physiological relevance of these observations is not yet clearly understood.

Activated MEKK may also activate MEK to a limited extent. Interestingly, one study has shown that a constitutively active form of MEKK prefers to phosphorylate S218, while a constitutively active form of RAF phosphorylates both S218 and S222 with equal efficacy (109). This observation may explain the *in vivo* data which suggests that MEKK is not an activator of MEK, but rather activates a related kinase, SEK1 (212, 214), which phosphorylates and activates JNKs/SAPKs. The recently identified MEKK2 and MEKK3 have been shown to preferentially activate JNK and ERKs 1 and 2, respectively, but not p38, in 293 cells (215). If different upstream kinases do show different *in vivo* preferences for different MEKs or sites of MEK phosphory-

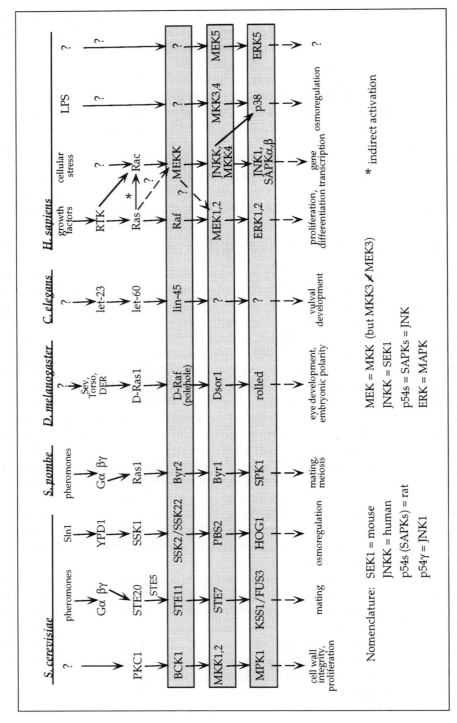

Fig. 5 Comparison of MAP kinase cascades and their functions in different species. The core of the kinase cascade, as exemplified by RAF (a MEK kinase), MEK and MAP kinase, is conserved throughout evolution. The activation of the cascade and its cellular responses, however, are remarkably different. Direct activation of the MEK kinases is achieved by other kinases (PKC1, STE20) or GTPases (RAS1, D-RAS1, LET-60. RAS). Transduction of an extracellular signal through the membrane is effected by heterotrimeric G proteins, receptor tyrosine kinases (RTK), such as SEV, LET-23, and the EGF receptor or histidine kinases (SLN1). Activation of the cascades results in specific cellular responses. Thus, the divergent responses must derive from the specific signal at the plasma membrane.

lation, which in turn activate MEK to differing extents, this quantitative level of activation may provide a qualitative change in cellular signalling. In support of this is the observation that the proline-rich sequence unique to MEKs 1 and 2 is required for activation by RAF, but not by a partially purified novel MEK1 activator (216). More regulation of pathway specificity may be inferred from a study in which expression of MEKK in mammalian cells activated MEK1 and MEK2 but did not lead to efficient activation of ERK2 (217). This may be explained by the observation that the MEKK-activated SEK pathway induces the expression of MKP1 (158), which may rapidly inactivate ERK. However, activated MEKK induces the transactivation of c-MYC and ELK1 (see Chapter 6), whereas activated RAF stimulates only ELK1 transactivation, suggesting MEKK does activate the MEK1 and MEK2 pathway (218). Although more research on the interactions between the pathways needs to be done, it can be expected that cross-talk exists between the pathways at some level.

Some extracellular signals may initiate the activation of more than one kinase cascade. For instance, it has been shown that RAS–G12V can stimulate JNK (160) and that growth factor stimulation is able to stimulate JNK in a RAS-dependent manner (210). While this may proceed through RAC and MEKK, it is important to note that TNFα is able to stimulate JNK, but not ERK, and does so in a RAS-independent manner (210). Is this a reflection of the concept that a cell in which the proliferative response is active may also require the stress response to maintain cellular homeostasis? Perhaps the answers for mammalian cells will come from examination of homologous systems in yeast, *Drosophila* or *C. elegans*. In *Drosophila*, three receptor tyrosine kinases appear to converge upon and share central elements of the ERK pathway before diverging at the level of transcription to provide unique growth signals (27). The specificity in that system may be imparted by spatial and temporal expression of the receptor tyrosine kinases and transcription factors. Cross-talk and integration of signals may also be imposed by the expression and activity of specific phosphatases: PAC1 recognizes ERK and p38, MKP2 recognizes ERK and JNK, MKP1 recognizes ERK, p38, and JNK (219, 220), and the nuclear threonine–tyrosine phosphatase TYP1 inhibits ERK2 and JNK (221).

The question is then raised: how do bona fide RAS effectors compete for the GTP-bound form of RAS to produce their individual signals? Do they 'share' RAS? Do they need to share RAS? Is the process regulated by mass action or by specific protein regulators, or by temporal or spatial considerations? Indeed, with the number of proteins having been shown to bind to RAS, is there a limit to the number of effectors RAS may effectively regulate?

8. Conclusions

The framework of the RAS–RAF–MEK–ERK signalling pathway has been well defined. However, many critical questions remain about the regulation of its individual components, the isozyme specificity of some of those components and the integration of the multiple signals with which the pathway generates a specific cellular response, in some cases culminating in transformation and oncogenesis. The finding that RAS is able to activate multiple pathways, all of which may be required to elicit an appropriate cellular response to external stimuli, has provided new ways to investigate and interpret the pleiotropic responses elicited by RAS in a given cell. Perhaps it is the interaction of these pathways which defines the aggressiveness and malignancy of a tumour. This could explain why only RAS mutations are found in human tumours even though unregulated RAF, MEK, and ERK can lead to transformation in cultured cells and induce tumours in immunocompromised mice. Since RAS, on the other hand, is apparently central to the activation of at least two pathways that synergize with the ERK pathway in the transformation of cells, a mutation in RAS would be expected to have profound effects on cell growth. The ability to draw upon diverse genetic, biochemical, and cellular techniques will allow the evaluation of the importance of each protein in these pathways and their interactions with other proteins in the transduction of the final signal.

The existence of homologous kinase cascades in mammalian cells begs the questions of specificity and cross-talk. Are functionally homologous elements of each pathway promiscuous? Or have they developed mechanisms by which they are effectively segregated from each other, thereby ensuring specificity in signalling? Evidence suggests that in mammalian cells, MEKK1 does not lead to effective activation of ERK2 (217). In *Saccharomyces cerevisiae*, the product of the *STE5* gene specifically and simultaneously binds to STE5, STE7, and FUS3, serving as a scaffold upon which catalytic efficiency of the kinase cascade is increased and preventing cross-talk between members of homologous cascades (127–129). The existence of a functionally homologous protein in mammalian cells has been suggested by the identification of a functional complex of RAS, RAF, MEK, and ERK (34). Again in *S. cerevisiae*, the phosphatase MSG5 specifically inactivates the ERK homologue, FUS3, which is involved in pheromone-induced growth arrest (222). It does not, however, affect the two other ERK homologues or their pathways, suggesting that more homologue-specific ERK phosphatases will be found in mammalian systems.

The core of the RAS–RAF–MEK–ERK pathway, consisting of the MEK kinases (including RAF), MEKs, and ERKs, is employed by different extracellular signals to yield specific cellular responses. How is this achieved? Since the pathways are activated by a diverse set of signals, the specificity must lie in the additional responses (perhaps both synergistic and antagonistic) initiated by activated transmembrane receptors. These additional responses must help to direct the cytoplasmic and nuclear events which define stimulus-specific responses in a given cell. More investigations are necessary into cell- and signal-specific regulation of individual kinase pathway components and integrated responses at the nuclear level.

References

1. Barbacid, M. (1987) ras Genes. *Annu. Rev. Biochem.*, **56**, 779.
2. Leevers, S. J. and Marshall, C. J. (1992) Activation of extracellular signal-regulated kinase, ERK2, by p21 *ras* oncoprotein. *EMBO J.*, **11**, 569.

3. Thomas, S. M., DeMarco, M., D'Arcangelo, G., Halegoua, S., and Brugge, J. S. (1992) Ras is essential for nerve growth factor- and phorbol ester-induced tyrosine phosphorylation of MAP kinases. *Cell*, **68**, 1031.

4. Wood, K. W., Sarnecki, C., Roberts, T. M., and Blenis, J. (1992) *ras* mediates nerve growth factor receptor modulation of three signal-transducing protein kinases: MAP kinase, Raf-1 and RSK. *Cell*, **68**, 1041.

5. Boguski, M. S. and McCormick, F. (1993) Proteins regulating Ras and its relatives. *Nature*, **366**, 643.

6. Henkemeyer, M., Rossi, D. J., Holmyard, D. P., Puri, M. C., Mbamalu, G., Harpal, K., *et al.* (1995) Vascular system defects and neuronal apoptosis in mice lacking ras GTPase-activating protein. *Nature*, **377**, 695.

7. Van Aelst, L., Barr, M., Marcus, S., Polverino, A., and Wigler, M. (1993) Complex formation between RAS and RAF and other protein kinases. *Proc. Natl. Acad. Sci. USA*, **90**, 6213.

8. Vojtek, A. B., Hollenberg, S. M., and Cooper, J. A. (1993) Mammalian Ras interacts directly with the serine/threonine kinase Raf. *Cell*, **74**, 205.

9. Koide, H., Satoh, T., Nakafuku, M., and Kaziro, Y. (1993) GTP-dependent association of Raf-1 with Ha-Ras: identification of Raf as a target downstream of Ras in mammalian cells. *Proc. Natl. Acad. Sci. USA*, **90**, 8683.

10. Zhang, X.-F., Settleman, J., Kyriakis, J. M., Takeuchi-Suzuki, E., Elledge, S. J., Marshall, M. S., *et al.* (1993) Normal and oncogenic p21[ras] proteins bind to the amino-terminal regulatory domain of c-Raf-1. *Nature*, **364**, 308.

11. Warne, P. H., Rodriguez-Viciana, P., and Downward, J. (1993) Direct interaction of Ras and the amino-terminal region of Raf-1 *in vitro*. *Nature*, **364**, 352.

12. Leevers, S. J., Paterson, H. F., and Marshall, C. J. (1994) Requirement for Ras in Raf activation is overcome by targeting Raf to the plasma membrane. *Nature*, **369**, 411.

13. Stokoe, D., Macdonald, S. G., Cadwallader, K., Symons, M., and Hancock, J. F. (1994) Activation of Raf as a result of recruitment to the plasma membrane. *Science*, **264**, 1463.

14. Moelling, K., Heimann, B., Beimling, P., Rapp, U. R., and Sander, T. (1984) Serine- and threonine-specific protein kinase activities of purified gag-*mil* and gag-*raf* proteins. *Nature*, **312**, 558.

15. Bonner, T. I., Kerby, S. B., Sutrave, P., Gunnell, M. A., Mark, G., and Rapp, U. R. (1985) Structure and biological activity of human homologs of the *raf/mil* oncogene. *Mol. Cell. Biol.*, **5**, 1400.

16. Bonner, T. I., Oppermann, H., Seeburg, P., Kerby, S. B., Gunnell, M. A., Young, A. C., *et al.* (1986) The complete coding sequence of the human *raf* oncogene and the corresponding structure of the c-*raf*-1 gene. *Nucleic Acids Res.*, **14**, 1009.

17. Huleihel, M., Goldsborough, M., Cleveland, J., Gunnell, M., Bonner, T., and Rapp, U. R. (1986) Characterization of the murine A-*raf*, a new oncogene related to the v-*raf* oncogene. *Mol. Cell. Biol.*, **6**, 2655.

18. Ikawa, S., Fukui, M., Ueyama, Y., Tamaoki, N., Yamamoto, T., and Toyoshima, K. (1988) B-*raf*, a new member of the *raf* family, is activated by DNA rearrangement. *Mol. Cell. Biol.*, **8**, 2651.

19. Storm, S. M., Brennscheidt, U., Sithanandam, G., and Rapp, U. R. (1990) Raf oncogenes in carcinogenesis. *Crit. Rev. Oncogenesis*, **2**, 1.

20. Storm, S. M., Cleveland, J. L., and Rapp, U. R. (1990) Expression of *raf* family proto-oncogenes in normal mouse tissues. *Oncogene*, **5**, 345.

21. Barnier, J. V., Papin, C., Eychene, A., Lecoq, O., and Calothy, G. (1995) The mouse B-raf gene encodes multiple protein isoforms with tissue-specific expression. *J. Biol. Chem.*, **270**, 23381.

22. Smith, M. R., DeGudicibus, S. J., and Stacey, D. W. (1986) Requirement for c-ras proteins during viral oncogene transformation. *Nature*, **320**, 540.

23. Levin, D. E. and Errede, B. (1995) The proliferation of MAP kinase signaling pathways in yeast. *Curr. Opin. Cell Biol.*, **7**, 197.

24. Ambrosio, L., Mahowald, A. P., and Perrimon, N. (1989) Requirement of the *Drosophila raf* homologue for *torso* function. *Nature*, **342**, 288.

25. Biggs, W. H., Zavitz, K. H., Dickson, B., van der Straten, A., Brunner, D., Hafen, E., and Zipursky, S. L. (1994). The Drosophila rolled locus encodes a MAP kinase required in the sevenless signal transduction pathway. *EMBO J.*, **13**, 1628.

26. Fortini, M. E., Simon, M. A., and Rubin, G. M. (1992) Signalling by the *sevenless* protein tyrosine kinase is mimicked by Ras1 activation. *Nature*, **355**, 559.

27. Perrimon, N. (1994) Signalling pathways initiated by receptor protein tyrosine kinases in Drosophila. *Curr. Opin. Cell Biol.*, **6**, 260.

28. Tsuda, L., Inoue, Y., Yoo, M.-A., Mizuno, M., Hata, M., Lim, Y.-M., *et al.* (1993) A protein kinase similar to MAP kinase activator acts downstream of the Raf kinase in Drosophila. *Cell*, **72**, 407.

29. Aroian, R. V., Koga, M. M., Mendel, J. E., Ohshima, Y., and Sternberg, P. W. (1990) The *let-23* gene necessary for *Caenorhabditis elegans* vulval induction encodes a tyrosine kinase of the EGF receptor subfamily. *Nature*, **348**, 693.

30. Eisenmann, D. M. and Kim, S.K. (1994) Signal transduction and cell fate specification during Caenorhabditis elegans vulval development. *Curr. Opin. Genet. Dev.*, **4**, 508.

31. Han, M., Golden, A., Han, Y., and Sternberg, P. W. C. (1993) *elegans lin-45 raf* gene participates in *let-60 ras*-stimulated vulval differentiation. *Nature*, **363**, 133.

32. Kornfeld, K., Guan, K. L., and Horvitz, H.R. (1995) The Caenorhabditis elegans gene mek-2 is required for vulval induction and encodes a protein similar to the protein kinase MEK. *Genes Dev.*, **9**, 756.

33. Wu, Y., Han, M., and Guan, K. L. (1995) MEK-2, a Caenorhabditis elegans MAP kinase kinase, functions in Ras-mediated vulval induction and other developmental events. *Genes Dev.*, **9**, 742.

34. Moodie, S. A., Willumsen, B. M., Weber, M. J., and Wolfman, A. (1993) Complexes of Ras•GTP with Raf-1 and mitogen-activated protein kinase kinase. *Science*, **260**, 1658.

35. DiBattiste, D., Golubic, M., Stacey, D., and Wolfman, A. (1993) Differences in the interaction of p21c-Ha-ras-GMP-PNP with full-length neurofibromin and GTPase-activating protein. *Oncogene*, **8**, 637.

36. Scheffler, J. E., Waugh, D. S., Bekesi, E., Kiefer, S. E., LoSardo, J. E., Neri, A. *et al.* (1994) Characterization of a 78-residue fragment of c-Raf-1 that comprises a minimal binding domain for the interaction with Ras-GTP. *J. Biol. Chem.*, **269**, 22340.

37. Pumiglia, K., Chow, Y. H., Fabian, J., Morrison, D., Decker, S., and Jove, R. (1995) Raf-1 N-terminal sequences necessary for Ras-Raf interaction and signal transduction. *Mol. Cell. Biol.*, **15**, 398.

38. Emerson, S. D., Waugh, D. S., Scheffler, J. E., Tsao, K. L., Prinzo, K. M., and Fry, D. C. (1994) Chemical shift assignments and folding topology of the Ras-binding domain of human Raf-1 as determined by heteronuclear three-dimensional NMR spectroscopy. *Biochemistry*, **33**, 7745.

39. Nassar, N., Horn, G., Herrmann, C., Scherer, A., McCormick, F., and Wittinghofer, A. (1995) The 2.2 Å crystal structure of the Ras-binding domain of the serine/threonine kinase c-Raf1 in complex with RAP1A and a GTP analogue. *Nature*, **375**, 554.

40. Fabian, J. R., Vojtek, A. B., Cooper, J. A., and Morrison, D. K. (1994) A single amino acid change in Raf-1 inhibits Ras binding and alters Raf-1 function. *Proc. Natl. Acad. Sci. USA*, **91**, 5982.

41. Lu, X., Melnick, M. B., Hsu, J. C., and Perrimon, N. (1994) Genetic and molecular analyses of mutations involved in Drosophila raf signal transduction. *EMBO J.*, **13**, 2592.

42. Egan, S. E., Wright, J. A., Jarolim, L., Yanagihara, K., Bassin, R. H., and Greenberg, A. H. (1987) Transformation by oncogenes encoding protein kinases induces the metastatic phenotype. *Science*, **238**, 202.

43. Heidecker, G., Huleihel, M., Cleveland, J. L., Kolch, W., Beck, T. W., Lloyd, P., et al. (1990) Mutational activation of c-raf-1 and definition of the minimal transforming sequence. *Mol. Cell. Biol.*, **10**, 2503.

44. Ishikawa, F., Sakai, R., Ochiai, M., Takaku, F., Sugimura, T., and Nagao, M. (1988) Identification of a transforming activity suppressing sequence in the *c-raf* oncogene. *Oncogene*, **3**, 653.

45. Stanton, V. P., Jr., Nichols, D. W., Laudano, A. P., and Cooper, G. M. (1989) Definition of the human *raf* amino-terminal regulatory region by deletion mutagenesis. *Mol. Cell. Biol.*, **9**, 639.

46. Qiu, R. G., Chen, J., Kirn, D., McCormick, F., and Symons, M. (1995) An essential role for Rac in Ras transformation. *Nature*, **374**, 457.

47. Kolch, W., Heidecker, G., Lloyd, P., and Rapp, U. R. (1991) Raf-1 protein kinase is required for growth of induced NIH/3T3 cells. *Nature*, **349**, 426.

48. Macdonald, S. G. and McCormick, F. Unpublished observations.

49. Macdonald, S. G., Crews, C. M., Wu, L., Driller, J., Clark, R., Erikson, R. L., et al. (1993) Reconstitution of the raf-1-MEK-ERK signal transduction pathway *in vitro*. *Mol. Cell Biol.*, **13**, 6615.

50. App, H., Hazan, R., Zilberstein, A., Ullrich, A., Schlessinger, J., and Rapp, U. (1991) Epidermal growth factor (EGF) stimulates association and kinase activity of *raf-1* with the EGF receptor. *Mol. Cell. Biol.*, **5**, 1400.

51. Izumi, T., Tamemoto, H., Nagao, M., Kadowaki, T., Takaku, F., and Kasuga, M. (1991) Insulin and platelet-derived growth factor stimulate phosphorylation of the *c-raf* product at serine and threonine residues in intact cells. *J. Biol. Chem.*, **266**, 7933.

52. Kovacina, K. S., Yonezawa, K., Brautigan, D. L., Tonks, N. K., Rapp, U. R., and Roth, R. A. (1990) Insulin activates the kinase activity of the raf-1 proto-oncogene by increasing its serine phosphorylation. *J. Biol. Chem.*, **265**, 12115.

53. Morrison, D. K., Kaplan, D. R., Rapp, U., and Roberts, T. M. (1988) Signal transduction from membrane to cytoplasm: growth factors and membrane-bound oncogene products increase Raf-1 phosphorylation and associated protein kinase activity. *Proc. Natl. Acad. Sci. USA*, **85**, 8855.

54. Morrison, D. K., Kaplan, D. R., Escobedo, J. A., Rapp, U. R., Roberts, T. M., and Williams, L. T. (1989) Direct activation of the serine/threonine kinase activity of Raf-1 through tyrosine phosphorylation by the PDGF β-receptor. *Cell*, **58**, 649.

55. Dent, P., Jelenik, T., Morrison, D. K., Weber, M. J., and Sturgill, T. W. (1995) Reversal of Raf-1 activation by purified and membrane-associated protein phosphatases. *Science*, **268**, 1902.

56. Dent, P., Reardon, D. B., Wood, S. L., Lindorfer, M. A., Graber, S. G., Garrison, J. C., *et al.* (1996) Inactivation of Raf-1 by a protein-tyrosine phosphatase stimulated by GTP and reconstituted by $G_{\alpha i/o}$ subunits. *J. Biol. Chem.*, **271**, 3119.

57. Reardon, D. B., Wood, S. L., Brautigan, D. L., Bell, G. I., Dent, P., and Sturgill, T. W. (1996) Activation of a protein tyrosine phosphatase and inactivation of Raf-1 by somatostatin. *Biochem J.*, **314**, 401.

58. Dent, P. and Sturgill, T. W. (1994) Activation of $(His)_6$-Raf-1 *in vitro* by partially purified plasma membranes from v-Ras-transformed and serum-stimulated fibroblasts. *Proc. Natl. Acad. Sci. USA*, **91**, 9544.

59. Traverse, S., Cohen, P., Paterson, H., Marshall, C., Rapp, U. and Grand, R. J. A. (1993) Specific association of activated MAP kinase kinase kinase (Raf) with the plasma membranes of *ras*-transformed retinal cells. *Oncogene*, **8**, 3175.

60. Fabian, J. R., Daar, I. O., and Morrison, D. K. (1993) Critical tyrosine residues regulate the enzymatic activity and biological activity of Raf-1 kinase. *Mol. Cell. Biol.*, **13**, 7170.

61. Morrison, D. K., Heidecker, G., Rapp, U. R., and Copeland, T. D. (1993) Identification of the major phosphorylation sites of the Raf-1 kinase. *J. Biol. Chem.*, **268**, 17309.

62. Kolch, W., Heidecker, G., Koch, G., Hummel, R., Vahidi, H, Mischak, H., *et al.* (1993) Protein kinase Cα activates RAF-1 by direct phosphorylation. *Nature*, **364**, 249.

63. Marais, R., Light, Y., Paterson, H. F., and Marshall, C. J. (1995) Ras recruits Raf-1 to the plasma membrane for activation by tyrosine phosphorylation. *EMBO J.*, **14**, 3136.

64. Jelinek, T., Dent, P., Sturgill, T. W., and Weber, M. J. (1996) Ras-induced activation of Raf-1 is dependent on tyrosine phosphorylation. *Mol. Cell. Biol.*, **16**, 1027.

65. Diaz, B., Barnard, D., Filson, A., King, A., Macdonald, S., and Marshall, M. (1996) Phosphorylation of Raf-1 serine 338/339 is an essential regulatory event for activation and biological signaling, in press.

66. Michaud, N. R., Fabian, J. R., Mathes, K. D., and Morrison, D. K. (1995) 14-3-3 is not essential for Raf-1 function: identification of Raf-1 proteins that are biologically activated in a 14-3-3- and Ras-independent manner. *Mol. Cell. Biol.*, **15**, 3390.

67. Sozeri, O., Vollmer, K., Liyanage, M., Frith, D., Kour, G., Mark, G. E. I., *et al.* (1992) Activation of the c-Raf protein kinase by protein kinase C phosphorylation. *Oncogene*, **7**, 2259.

68. Marquardt, B., Frith, D., and Stabel, S. (1994) Signalling from TPA to MAP kinase requires protein kinase C, raf and MEK: reconstitution of the signalling pathway *in vitro. Oncogene*, **9**, 3213.

69. Kazanietz, M. G., Bustelo, X. R., Barbacid, M., Kolch, W., Mischak, H., Wong, G., *et al.* (1994) Zinc finger domains and phorbol ester pharmacophore. Analysis of binding to mutated form of protein kinase C zeta and the vav and c-raf proto-oncogene products. *J. Biol. Chem.*, **269**, 11590.

70. Dent, P., Reardon, D. B., Morrison, D. K., and Sturgill, T. W. (1995) Regulation of Raf-1 and Raf-1 mutants by Ras-dependent and Ras-independent mechanisms *in vitro. Mol. Cell. Biol.*, **15**, 4125.

71. Ghosh, S., Xie, W. Q., Quest, A. F. G., Mabrouk, G. M., Strum, J. C., and Bell, R. M. (1994) The cysteine-rich region of Raf-1 kinase contains zinc, translocates to liposomes, and is adjacent to a segment that binds GTP-Ras. *J. Biol. Chem.*, **269**, 10000.

72. Bruder, J. T., Heidecker, G., and Rapp, U. R. (1992) Serum-, TPA, and ras-induced expression from AP-1/Ets-driven promoters requires Raf-1 kinase. *Genes Dev.*, **6**, 545.

73. Stokoe, D., Macdonald, S. G., and McCormick, F. Unpublished observations.

74. Ghosh, S., Strum, J. C., Sciorra, V. A., Daniel, L., and Bell, R. M. (1996) Raf-1 kinase possesses distinct binding domains for phosphatidylserine and phosphatidic acid. *J. Biol. Chem.*, **271**, 8472.

75. Stancato, L. F., Chow, Y. H., Hutchison, K. A., Perdew, G. H., Jove, R., and Pratt, W. B. (1993) Raf exists in a native heterocomplex with hsp90 and p50 that can be reconstituted in a cell-free system. *J. Biol. Chem.*, **268**, 21711.

76. Wartmann, M. and Davis, R. (1994) The native structure of the activated raf protein kinase is a membrane-bound multi-subunit complex. *J. Biol. Chem.*, **269**, 6695.

77. Freed, E., Symons, M., Macdonald, S. G., McCormick, F., and Ruggieri, R. (1994) Binding of 14-3-3 proteins to the protein kinase Raf and effects on its activation. *Science*, **265**, 1713.

78. Fantl, W. J., Muslin, A. J., Kikuchi, A., Martin, J. A., MacNicol, A. M., Gross, R. W., *et al.* (1994) Activation of Raf-1 by 14-3-3 proteins. *Nature*, **371**, 612.

79. Fu, H., Pallas, D. C., Cui, C., Conroy, K., Narsimhan, R. P., Mamon, H., *et al.* (1994) Interaction of the protein kinase Raf-1 with 14-3-3 proteins. *Science*, **266**, 126.

80. Bohen, S. P. (1995) Hsp90 mutants disrupt glucocorticoid receptor ligand binding and destabilize aporeceptor complexes. *J. Biol. Chem.*, **270**, 29433.

81. Nathan, D. F. and Lindquist, S. (1995) Mutational analysis of Hsp90 function: interactions with a steroid receptor and a protein kinase. *Mol. Cell. Biol.*, **15**, 3917.

82. Sabbah, M., Radanyi, C., Redeuilh, G., and Baulieu, E.-E. (1996) The 90 kDa heat-shock protein (hsp90) modulates the binding of the oestrogen receptor to its cognate DNA. *Biochem J.*, **314**, 205.

83. Xu, Y. and Lindquist, S. (1993) Heat-shock protein hsp90 governs the activity of pp60v-src kinase. *Proc. Natl. Acad. Sci. USA*, **90**, 7074.

84. Mimnaugh, E. G., Worland, P. J., Whitesell, L., and Neckers, L. M. (1995) Possible role for serine/threonine phosphorylation in the regulation of the heteroprotein complex between the hsp90 stress protein and the pp60v-src tyrosine kinase. *J. Biol. Chem.*, **270**, 28654.

85. Schulte, T. W., Blagosklonny, M. V., Ingui, C., and Neckers, L. (1995) Disruption of the Raf-1-Hsp90 molecular complex results in destabilization of Raf-1 and loss of Raf-1-Ras association. *J. Biol. Chem.*, **270**, 24585.

86. Irie, K., Gotoh, Y., Yashar, B. M., Errede, B., Nishida, E., and Matsumoto, K. (1994) Stimulatory effects of yeast and mammalian 14-3-3 proteins on the Raf protein kinase. *Science*, **265**, 1716.

87. Li, S., Janosch, P., Tanji, M., Rosenfeld, G. C., Waymire, J. C., Mischak, H., *et al.* (1995) Regulation of Raf-1 kinase activity by the 14-3-3 family of proteins. *EMBO J.*, **14**, 685.

88. Yamamori, B., Kuroda, S., Shimizu, K., Fukui, K., Ohtsuka, T., and Takai, Y. (1995) Purification of a Ras-dependent mitogen-activated protein kinase kinase kinase from bovine brain cytosol and its identification as a complex of B-Raf and 14-3-3 proteins. *J. Biol. Chem.*, **270**, 11723.

89. Muslin, A. J., Tanner, J. W., Allen, P. M., and Shaw, A. S. (1996) Interaction of 14-3-3 with signaling proteins is mediated by the recognition of phosphoserine. *Cell*, **84**, 889.

90. Macdonald, S. G., Stokoe, D., and McCormick, F. Unpublished observations.

91. Nishida, Y., Hata, M., Ayaki, T., Ryo, H., Yamagata, M., and Shimizu, K. (1988) Proliferation of both somatic and germ cells is affected in the Drosophila mutants of raf proto-oncogene. *EMBO J.*, **7**, 775.

92. Catling, A. D., Reuter, C. W., Cox, M. E., Parsons, S. J., and Weber, M. J. (1994) Partial

purification of a mitogen-activated protein kinase kinase activator from bovine brain. Identification as B-Raf or a B-Raf-associated activity. *J. Biol. Chem.*, **269**, 30014.

93. Wood, K. W., Qi, H., D'Arcangelo, G., Armstrong, R. C., Roberts, T. M., and Halegoua, S. (1993) The cytoplasmic raf oncogene induces a neuronal phenotype in PC12 cells: a potential role for cellular raf kinases in neuronal growth factor signal transduction. *Proc. Natl. Acad. Sci. USA*, **90**, 5016.

94. Howe, L. R., Leevers, S. J., Gomez, N., Nakielny, S., Cohen, P., and Marshall, C. J. (1992) Activation of the MAP kinase pathway by the protein kinase raf. *Cell*, **71**, 335.

95. Kyriakis, J. M., App, H., Zhang, X.-F., Banerjee, P., Brautigan, D. L., Rapp, U. R., *et al.* (1992) Raf-1 activates MAP kinase-kinase. *Nature*, **358**, 417.

96. Dent, P., Haser, W., Haystead, T. A. J., Vincent, L. A., Roberts, T. M., and Sturgill, T. W. (1992) Activation of Mitogen-Activated Protein Kinase Kinase by v-raf in NIH 3T3 Cells and *in vitro*. *Science*, **257**, 1404.

97. Crews, C. M., Alessandrini, A., and Erikson, R. L. (1992) The primary structure of MEK, a protein kinase that phosphorylates the *ERK* gene product. *Science*, **258**, 478.

98. Zheng, C.-F. and Guan, K.-L. (1994) Cytoplasmic localization of the mitogen-activated protein kinase activator MEK. *J. Biol. Chem.*, **269**, 19947.

99. Jelenik, T., Catling, A. D., Reuter, C. W. M., Moodie, S. A., Wolfman, A., and Weber, M. J. (1994) Ras and Raf-1 form a signalling complex with MEK-1 but not MEK-2. *Mol. Cell. Biol.*, **14**, 9212.

100. Huang, W., Alessandrini, A., Crews, C. M., and Erikson, R. L. (1993) Raf-1 forms a stable complex with Mek1 and activates Mek1 by serine phosphorylation. *Proc. Natl. Acad. Sci. USA*, **90**, 10947.

101. Brott, B. K., Alessandrini, A., Largaespada, D. A., Copeland, N. G., Jenkins, N. A., Crews, C. M., *et al.* (1993) MEK2 is a kinase related to MEK1 and is differentially expressed in murine tissues. *Cell Growth Diff.*, **4**, 921.

102. Zheng, C.-F. and Guan, K.-L. (1993) Cloning and characterization of two distinct human extracellular signal-regulated kinase activator kinases, MEK1 and MEK2. *J. Biol. Chem.*, **268**, 11435.

103. Wu, J., Harrison, J. K., Vincent, L. A., Haystead, C., Haystead, T. A. J., Michel, H., *et al.* (1993) Molecular structure of a protein-tyrosine/threonine kinase activating p42 mitogen-activated protein (MAP) kinase: MAP kinase kinase. *Proc. Natl. Acad. Sci. USA*, **90**, 173.

104. Wu, J., Harrison, J. K., Dent, P., Lynch, K. R., Weber, M. J., and Sturgill, T. W. (1993) Identification and characterization of a new mammalian mitogen-activated protein kinase kinase, MKK2. *Mol. Cell. Biol.*, **13**, 4539.

105. Zheng, C.-F. and Guan, K.-L. (1993) Properties of MEKs, the kinases that phosphorylate and activate the extracellular signal-regulated kinases. *J. Biol. Chem.*, **268**, 23933.

106. Alessi, D. R., Saito, Y., Campbell, D. G., Cohen, P., Sithanandam, G., Marshall, C. J. *et al.* (1994) Identification of the sites in MAP kinase kinase-1 phosphorylated by p74[raf-1.] *EMBO J*, **13**, 1610.

107. Pages, G., Brunet, A., L'Allemain, G., and Pouyssegur, J. (1994) Constitutive mutant and putative regulatory serine phosphorylation site of mammalian MAP kinase kinase (MEK1). *EMBO J.*, **13**, 3003.

108. Zheng, C.-F. and Guan, K.-L. (1994). Activation of MEK family kinases requires phosphorylation of two conserved Ser/Thr residues. *EMBO J.*, **13**, 1123.

109. Yan, M. and Templeton, D. J. (1994) Identification of 2 serine residues of MEK-1 that are

differentially phosphorylated during activation by raf and MEK kinase. *J. Biol. Chem.*, **269**, 19067.

110. Posada, J., Yew, N., Ahn, N. G., Woude, G. F. V., and Cooper, J. A. (1993) Mos stimulates MAP kinase in *Xenopus* oocytes and activates a MAP kinase kinase *in vitro*. *Mol. Cell. Biol.*, **13**, 2546.

111. Rossomando, A. J., Dent, P., Sturgill, T. W., and Marshak, D. R. (1994) Mitogen-activated protein kinase kinase 1 (MKK1) is negatively regulated by threonine phosphorylation. *Mol. Cell. Biol.*, **14**, 1594.

112. Matsuda, S., Kosako, H., Takenaka, K., Moriyama, K., Sakai, H., Akiyama, T., *et al.* (1992) Xenopus MAP kinase activator: identification and function as a key intermediate in the phosphorylation cascade. *EMBO J.*, **11**, 973.

113. Nakielny, S., Cohen, P., Wu, J., and Sturgill, T. (1992) MAP kinase activator from insulin-stimulated skeletal muscle is a protein threonine/tyrosine kinase. *EMBO J.*, **11**, 2123.

114. Rossomando, A., Wu, J., Weber, M. J., and Sturgill, T. W. (1992) The phorbol ester-dependent activator of the mitogen-activated protein kinase p42mapk is a kinase with specificity for the threonine and tyrosine regulatory sites. *Proc. Natl. Acad. Sci. USA*, **89**, 5221.

115. Sontag, E., Fedorov, S., Kamibayashi, C., Robbins, D., Cobb, M., and Mumby, M. (1993) The interaction of SV40 small tumor antigen with protein phosphatase 2A stimulates the map kinase pathway and induces cell proliferation. *Cell*, **75**, 887.

116. Shiozaki, K. and Russell, P. (1995) Counteractive roles of protein phosphatase 2C (PP2C) and a MAP kinase kinase homolog in the osmoregulation of fission yeast. *EMBO J.*, **14**, 492.

117. Traverse, S., Gomez, N., Paterson, H., Marshall, C., and Cohen, P. (1992) Sustained activation of the mitogen-activated protein (MAP) kinase cascade may be required for differentiation of PC12 cells. *Biochem. J.*, **288**, 351.

118. Gotoh, Y., Matsuda, S., Takenaka, K., Hattori, S., Iwamatsu, A., Ishikawa, M., *et al.* (1994) Characterization of recombinant Xenopus MAP kinase kinases mutated at potential phosphorylation sites. *Oncogene*, **9**, 1891.

119. Reuter, C. W., Catling, A. D., Jelinek, T., and Weber, M. J. (1995) Biochemical analysis of MEK activation in NIH3T3 fibroblasts. Identification of B-Raf and other activators. *J. Biol. Chem.*, **270**, 7644.

120. Papin, C., Eychene, A., Brunet, A., Pages, G., Pouyssegur, J., Calothy, G., *et al.* (1995) B-Raf protein isoforms interact with and phosphorylate MEK-1 on serine residues 218 and 222. *Oncogene*, **10**, 1647.

121. Wu, X., Noh, S. J., Zhou, G., Dixon, J. E., and Guan, K.-L. (1996) Selective activation of MEK1 but not MEK2 by A-Raf from epidermal growth factor-stimulated Hela cells. *J. Biol. Chem.*, **271**, 3265.

122. Pritchard, C. A., Samuels, M. L., Bosch, E., and McMahon, M. (1995) Conditionally oncogenic forms of the A-Raf and B-Raf protein kinases display different biological and biochemical properties in NIH 3T3 cells. *Mol. Cell. Biol.*, **15**, 6430.

123. Bogoyevitch, M. A., Marshall, C. J., and Sugden, P. H. (1995) Hypertrophic agonists stimulate the activities of the protein kinases c-RAF and A-Raf in cultured ventricular myocytes. *J. Biol. Chem.*, **270**, 26303.

124. Jaiswal, R. K., Moodie, S. A., Wolfman, A., and Landreth, G. E. (1994) The mitogen-activated protein kinase cascade is activated by B-Raf in response to nerve growth factor through interaction with p21ras. *Mol. Cell. Biol.*, **14**, 6944.

125. Moodie, S. A., Paris, M. J., Kolch, W., and Wolfman, A. (1994) Association of MEK1 with p21ras.GMPPNP is dependent on B-Raf. *Mol. Cell. Biol.*, **14**, 7153.

126. Vaillancourt, R. R., Gardner, A. M., and Johnson, G. L. (1994) B-Raf-dependent regulation of the MEK-1/mitogen-activated protein kinase pathway in PC12 cells and regulation by cyclic AMP. *Mol. Cell. Biol.*, **14**, 6522.

127. Choi, K. Y., Satterberg, B., Lyons, D. M., and Elion, E. A. (1994) Ste5 tethers multiple protein kinases in the MAP kinase cascade required for mating in *S. cerevisiae*. *Cell*, **78**, 499.

128. Marcus, S., Polverino, A., Barr, M., and Wigler, M. (1994) Complexes between STE5 and components of the pheromone-responsive mitogen-activated protein kinase module. *Proc. Natl. Acad. Sci. USA*, **91**, 7762.

129. Printen, J. A. and Sprague, G. J. (1994) Protein-protein interactions in the yeast pheromone response pathway: Ste5p interacts with all members of the MAP kinase cascade. *Genetics*, **138**, 609.

130. Mansour, S. J., Matten, W. T., Hermann, A. S., Candia, J. M., Rong, S., Fukasawa, K., *et al.* (1994) Transformation of mammalian cells by constitutively active MAP kinase kinase. *Science*, **265**, 966.

131. Cowley, S., Paterson, H., Kemp, P., and Marshall, C. J. (1994) Activation of MAP kinase kinase is necessary and sufficient for PC12 differentiation and for transformation of NIH 3T3 cells. *Cell*, **77**, 841.

132. Brunet, A., Pages, G., and Pouyssegur, J. (1994) Constitutively active mutants of MAP kinase kinase (MEK1) induce growth factor-relaxation and oncogenicity when expressed in fibroblasts. *Oncogene*, **9**, 3379.

133. Cobb, M. H. and Goldsmith, E. J. (1995) How MAP kinases are regulated. *J. Biol. Chem.*, **270**, 14843.

134. Cobb, M. H., Hepler, J. E., Cheng, M., and Robbins, D. (1994) The mitogen-activated protein kinases, ERK1 and ERK2. *Semin. Cancer Biol.*, **5**, 261.

135. Marshall, C. J. (1994) MAP kinase kinase kinase, MAP kinase kinase and MAP kinase. *Curr. Opin. Genet. Dev.*, **4**, 82.

136. Marshall, C. J. (1995) Specificity of receptor tyrosine kinase signaling: transient versus sustained extracellular signal-regulated kinase activation. *Cell*, **80**, 179.

137. Charest, D. L., Mordret, G., Harder, K. W., Jirik, F., and Pelech, S. L. (1993) Molecular cloning, expression, and characterization of the human mitogen-activated protein kinase p44erk1. *Mol. Cell. Biol.*, **13**, 4679.

138. Gonzalez, F. A., Raden, D. L., Rigby, M. R., and Davis, R. J. (1992) Heterogeneous expression of four MAP kinase isoforms in human tissues. *FEBS Lett.*, **304**, 170.

139. Cheng, M., Zhen, E., Robinson, M. J., Ebert, D., Goldsmith, E., and Cobb, M. H. (1996) Characterization of a protein kinase that phosphorylates serine 189 of the mitogen-activated protein kinase homolog ERK3. *J. Biol. Chem.*, **271**, 12057.

140. Sauma, S. and Friedman, E. (1996) Increased expression of protein kinase Cβ activates ERK3. *J. Biol. Chem.*, **271**, 11422.

141. Chen, R.-H., Sarnecki, C., and Blenis, J. (1992) Nuclear localization and regulation of *erk*- and *rsk*-encoded protein kinases. *Mol. Cell. Biol.*, **12**, 915.

142. Sanghera, J. S., Peter, M., Nigg, E. A., and Pelech, S. L. (1992) Immunological characterization of avian MAP kinases: evidence for nuclear localization. *Mol. Biol. Cell*, **3**, 775.

143. Mamajiwalla, S. N. and Burgess, D. R. (1995) Differential regulation of the activity of the 42 kD mitogen activated protein kinase (p42^{mapk}) during enterocyte differentiation *in vivo*. *Oncogene*, **11**, 377.

144. Pages, G., Lenormand, P., L'Allemain, G. L., Chambard, J.-C., Meloche, S., and Pouyssegur, J. (1993) Mitogen-activated protein kinases p42^{mapk} and p44^{mapk} are required for fibroblast proliferation. *Proc. Natl. Acad. Sci. USA*, **90**, 8319.

145. Qiu, M. S. and Green, S. H. (1992) PC12 cell neuronal differentiation is associated with prolonged p21ras activity and consequent prolonged ERK activity. *Neuron*, **9**, 705.

146. Alberola-Ila, J., Forbush, K. A., Seger, R., Krebs, E. G., and Perlmutter, R. M. (1995) Selective requirement for MAP kinase activation in thymocyte differentiation. *Nature*, **373**, 620.

147. Sale, E. M., Atkinson, P. G., and Sale, G. J. (1995) Requirement of MAP kinase for differentiation of fibroblasts to adipocytes, for insulin activation of p90 S6 kinase and for insulin or serum stimulation of DNA synthesis. *EMBO J.*, **14**, 674.

148. Nguyen, T. T., Scimeca, J. C., Filloux, C., Peraldi, P., Carpentier, J. L., and Van, O. E. (1993) Co-regulation of the mitogen-activated protein kinase, extracellular signal-regulated kinase 1, and the 90-kDa ribosomal S6 kinase in PC12 cells. Distinct effects of the neurotrophic factor, nerve growth factor, and the mitogenic factor, epidermal growth factor. *J. Biol. Chem.*, **268**, 9803.

149. Traverse, S., Seedorf, K., Paterson, H., Marshall, C. J., Cohen, P., and Ullrich, A. (1994) EGF triggers neuronal differentiation of PC12 cells that overexpress the EGF receptor. *Curr. Biol.*, **4**, 694.

150. Charles, C. H., Abler, A. S., and Lau, L. F. (1992) cDNA sequence of a growth factor-inducible immediate early gene and characterization of its encoded protein. *Oncogene*, **7**, 187.

151. Rohan, P. J., Davis, P., Moskaluk, C. A., Kearns, M., Krutzsch, H., Siebenlist, U., *et al.* (1993) PAC-1: a mitogen-induced nuclear protein tyrosine phosphatase. *Science*, **259**, 1763.

152. Sun, H., Charles, C., Lau, L, and Tonks, N. (1993) MKP-1 (3CH134), an immediate early gene product, is a dual specificity phosphatase that dephosphorylates MAP kinase *in vivo*. *Cell* **75**, 487.

153. Ishibashi, T., Bottaro, D. P., Michieli, P., Kelley, C. A., and Aaronson, S. A. (1994) A novel dual specificity phosphatase induced by serum stimulation and heat shock. *J. Biol. Chem.*, **269**, 29897.

154. Ward, Y., Gupta, S., Jensen, P., Wartmann, M., Davis, R. J., and Kelly, K. (1994) Control of MAP kinase activation by the mitogen-induced threonine/tyrosine phosphatase PAC1. *Nature*, **367**, 651.

155. Guan, K. L. and Butch, E. (1995) Isolation and characterization of a novel dual specific phosphatase, HVH2, which selectively dephosphorylates the mitogen-activated protein kinase. *J. Biol. Chem.*, **270**, 7197.

156. Misra-Press, A., Rim, C. S., Yao, H., Roberson, M. S., and Stork, P. J. (1995) A novel mitogen-activated protein kinase phosphatase. Structure, expression, and regulation. *J. Biol. Chem.*, **270**, 14587.

157. Zheng, Y., Olson, M. F., Hall, A., Cerione, R. A., and Toksoz, D. (1995) Direct involvement of the small GTP-binding protein Rho in lbc oncogene function. *J. Biol. Chem.*, **270**, 9031.

158. Bokemeyer, D., Sorokin, A., Yan, M., Ahn, N. G., Templeton, D. J., and Dunn, M. J. (1996) Induction of mitogen-activated protein kinase phosphatase 1 by the stress-activated protein kinase signaling pathway but not by extracellular signal-regulated kinase in fibroblasts. *J. Biol. Chem.*, **271**, 639.

159. Brondello, J. M., McKenzie, F. R., Sun, H., Tonks, N. K., and Pouyssegur, J. (1995) Constitutive MAP kinase phosphatase (MKP-1) expression blocks G1 specific gene transcription and S-phase entry in fibroblasts. *Oncogene*, **10**, 1895.

160. White, M. A., Nicolette, C., Minden, A., Polverino, A., Van, A. L., Karin, M., *et al.* (1995) Multiple Ras functions can contribute to mammalian cell transformation. *Cell*, **80**, 533.

161. Joneson, T., White, M. A., Wigler, M. H., and Bar-Sagi, D. (1996) Stimulation of membrane ruffling and MAP kinase activation by distinct effectors of RAS. *Science*, **271**, 810.

162. Kuriyama, M., Harada, N., Kuroda, S., Yamamoto, T., Nakafuku, M., Iwamatsu, A., *et al.* (1996) Identification of AF-6 and canoe as putative targets for Ras. *J. Biol. Chem.*, **271**, 607.

163. Hofer, F., Fields, S., Schneider, C., and Martin, G. S. (1994) Activated Ras interacts with the Ral guanine nucleotide dissociation stimulator. *Proc. Natl. Acad. Sci. USA*, **91**, 11089.

164. Kikuchi, A., Demo, S. D., Ye, Z. H., Chen, Y. W., and Williams, L. T. (1994) ralGDS family members interact with the effector loop of ras p21. *Mol. Cell. Biol.*, **14**, 7483.

165. Spaargaren, M. and Bischoff, J. R. (1994) Identification of the guanine nucleotide dissociation stimulator for Ral as a putative effector molecule of R-ras, H-ras, K-ras, and Rap. *Proc. Natl. Acad. Sci. USA*, **91**, 12609.

166. Albright, C. F., Giddings, B. W., Liu, J., Vito, M., and Weinberg, R. A. (1993) Characterization of a guanine nucleotide dissociation stimulator for a ras-related GTPase. *EMBO J.*, **12**, 339.

167. Herrmann, C., Horn, G., Spaargaren, M., and Wittinghofer, A. (1996) Differential interaction of the Ras family GTP-binding proteins H-Ras, Rap1A, and R-Ras with the putative effector molecules Raf kinase and Ral-guanine nucleotide exchange factor. *J. Biol. Chem.*, **271**, 6794.

168. Erickson, J. and Powers, S. Unpublished observations.

169. Jiang, H., Luo, J. Q., Urano, T., Frankel, P., Lu, Z., Foster, D. A., *et al.* (1995) Involvement of Ral GTPase in v-Src-induced phospholipase D activation. *Nature*, **378**, 409.

170. Jullien, F. V., Dorseuil, O., Romero, F., Letourneur, F., Saragosti, S., Berger, R., *et al.* (1995) Bridging Ral GTPase to Rho pathways. RLIP76, a Ral effector with CDC42/Rac GTPase-activating protein activity. *J. Biol. Chem.*, **270**, 22473.

171. Rodriguez-Viciana, P., Warne, P., Dhand, R., Vanhaesebroeck, B., Gout, I., Fry, M. J., *et al.* (1994) Phosphatidylinositol-3-OH kinase as a direct target of Ras. *Nature*, **370**, 527.

172. Kodaki, T., Woscholski, R., Hallberg, B., Rodriguez, V. P., Downward, J., and Parker, P. J. (1994) The activation of phosphatidylinositol 3-kinase by Ras. *Curr. Biol.*, **4**, 798.

173. Yamauchi, K., Holt, K., and Pessin, J. E. (1993) Phosphatidylinositol 3-kinase functions upstream of Ras and Raf in mediating insulin stimulation of c-fos transcription. *J. Biol. Chem.*, **268**, 14597.

174. Hu, Q., Klippel, A., Muslin, A. J., Fantl, W. J., and Williams, L. T. (1995) Ras-dependent induction of cellular responses by constitutively active phosphatidylinositol-3 kinase. *Science*, **268**, 100.

175. Pons, S., Asano, T., Glasheen, E., Miralpeix, M., Zhang, Y., Fisher, T. L., *et al.* (1995) The structure and function of p55[PIK] reveal a new regulatory subunit for phosphatidylinositol 3-kinase. *Mol. Cell. Biol.*, **15**, 4453.

176. Stoyanov, B., Volinia, S., Hanck, T., Rubio, I., Loubtchenkov, M., Malek, D., *et al.* (1995) Cloning and characterization of a G protein-activated human phosphoinositide-3 kinase. *Science*, **269**, 690.

177. de Vries-Smits, A. M., Burgering, B. M., Leevers, S. J., Marshall, C. J., and Bos, J. L. (1992) Involvement of p21ras in activation of extracellular signal-regulated kianse 2. *Nature*, **357**, 602.

178. Settleman, J., Albright, C. F., Foster, L. C., and Weinberg, R. A. (1992) Association between GTPase activators for Rho and Ras families. *Nature*, **359**, 153.

179. Settleman, J., Narasimhan, V., Foster, L. C., and Weinberg, R. A. (1992) Molecular cloning of cDNAs encoding the GAP-associated protein p190: implications for a signaling pathway from ras to the nucleus. *Cell*, **69**, 539.

180. Ridley, A. J., Paterson, H. F., Johnston, C. L., Diekmann, D., and Hall, A. (1992) The small GTP-binding protein rac regulates growth factor-induced membrane ruffling. *Cell*, **70**, 401.

181. Minden, A., Lin, A., Claret, F. X., Abo, A., and Karin, M. (1995) Selective activation of the JNK signaling cascade and c-Jun transcriptional activity by the small GTPases Rac and Cdc42Hs. *Cell*, **81**, 1147.

182. Zhang, S., Han, J., Sells, M. A., Chernoff, J., Knaus, U. G., Ulevitch, R. J., *et al.* (1995) Rho family GTPases regulate p38 mitogen-activated protein kinase through the downstream mediator Pak1. *J. Biol. Chem.*, **270**, 23934.

183. Martin, G. A., Bollag, G., McCormick, F., and Abo, A. (1995) A novel serine kinase activated by rac1/CDC42Hs-dependent autophosphorylation is related to PAK65 and STE20. *EMBO J.*, **14**, 1970.

184. Bagrodia, S., Taylor, S. J., Creasy, C. L., Chernoff, J., and Cerione, R. A. (1995) Identification of a mouse p21Cdc42/Rac activated kinase. *J. Biol. Chem.*, **270**, 22731.

185. Leung, T., Manser, E., Tan, L., and Lim, L. (1995) A novel serine/threonine kinase binding the Ras-related RhoA GTPase which translocates the kinase to peripheral membranes. *J. Biol. Chem.*, **270**, 29051.

186. Matsui, T., Amano, M., Yamamoto, T., Chihara, K., Nakafuku, M., Ito, M., *et al.* (1996) Rho-associated kinase, a novel serine/threonine kinase, as a putative target for the small GTP binding protein Rho. *EMBO J.*, **15**, 2208.

187. Ridley, A. J. and Hall, A. (1992) The small GTP-binding protein rho regulates the assembly of focal adhesions and actin stress fibers in response to growth factors. *Cell*, **70**, 389.

188. Prendergast, G. C., Khosravi, F. R., Solksi, P. A., Kurzawa, H., Lebowitz, P. F., and Der, C. J. (1995) Critical role of Rho in cell transformation by oncogenic Ras. *Oncogene*, **10**, 2289.

189. Qiu, R. G., Chen, J., McCormick, F., and Symons, M. (1995) A role for Rho in Ras transformation. *Proc. Natl. Acad. Sci. USA*, **92**, 11781.

190. Khosravi, F. R., Solski, P. A., Clark, G. J., Kinch, M. S., and Der, C. J. (1995) Activation of Rac1, RhoA, and mitogen-activated protein kinases is required for Ras transformation. *Mol. Cell. Biol.*, **15**, 6443.

191. Blumer, K. J. and Johnson, G. L. (1994) Diversity in function and regulation of MAP kinase pathways. *Trends Biochem. Sci.*, **19**, 236.

192. Brewster, J. L, de, V. T., Dwyer, N. D., Winter, E., and Gustin, M. C. (1993) An osmosensing signal transduction pathway in yeast. *Science*, **259**, 1760.

193. Cano, E. and Mahadevan, L. C. (1995) Parallel signal processing among mammalian MAPKs. *Trends Biochem. Sci.*, **20**, 117.

194. Gotoh, Y., Nishida, E., Shimanuki, M., Toda, T., Imai, Y., and Yamamoto, M. (1993) Schizosaccharomyces pombe spk1 is a tyrosine-phosphorylated protein functionally related to Xenopus mitogen-activated protein kinase. *Mol. Cell. Biol.*, **13**, 6427.

195. Han, J., Lee, J. D., Bibbs, L., and Ulevitch, R. J. (1994) A MAP kinase targeted by endo-toxin and hyperosmolarity in mammalian cells. *Science*, **265**, 808.
196. Herskowitz, I. (1995) MAP kinase pathways in yeast: for mating and more. *Cell*, **80**, 187.
197. Irie, K., Takase, M., Lee, K. S., Levin, D. E., Araki, H., Matsumoto, K., *et al.* (1993) *MKK1* and *MKK2*, which encode *Saccharomyces cerevisiae* mitogen-activated protein kinase-kinase homologs, function in the pathway mediated by protein kinase C. *Mol. Cell. Biol.*, **13**, 3076.
198. Lee, K. S., Irie, K., Gotoh, Y., Watanabe, Y., Araki, H., Nishida, E., *et al.* (1993) A yeast mitogen-activated protein kinase homolog (Mpk1p) mediates signalling by protein kinase C. *Mol. Cell. Biol.*, **13**, 3067.
199. Maeda, T., Wurgler, M. S., and Saito, H. (1994) A two-component system that regulates an osmosensing MAP kinase cascade in yeast. *Nature*, **369**, 242.
200. Matsuda, S., Kawasaki, H., Moriguchi, T., Gotoh, Y., and Nishida, E. (1995) Activation of protein kinase cascades by osmotic shock. *J. Biol. Chem.*, **270**, 12781.
201. Neiman, A. M. and Herskowitz, I. (1994) Reconstitution of a yeast protein kinase cas-cade *in vitro*: activation of the yeast MEK homologue STE7 by STE11. *Proc. Natl. Acad. Sci. USA*, **91**, 3398.
202. Zhou, Z., Gartner, A., Cade, R., Ammerer, G., and Errede, B. (1993) Pheromone-induced signal transduction in *Saccharomyces cerevisiae* requires the sequential function of three protein kinases. *Mol. Cell. Biol.*, **13**, 2069.
203. Zhou, G., Bao, Z. Q., and Dixon, J. E. (1995) Components of a new human protein kinase signal transduction pathway. *J. Biol. Chem.*, **270**, 12665.
204. Derijard, B., Hibi, M., Wu, I. H., Barrett, T., Su, B., Deng, T., *et al.* (1994) JNK1: a protein kinase stimulated by UV light and Ha-Ras that binds and phosphorylates the c-Jun acti-vation domain. *Cell*, **76**, 1025.
205. Kyriakis, J. M., Banerjee, P., Nikolakaki, E., Dai, T., Rubie, E. A., Ahmad, M. F., *et al.* (1994) The stress-activated protein kinase subfamily of c-Jun kinases. *Nature*, **369**, 156.
206. Pombo, C. M., Bonventre, J. V., Avruch, J., Woodgett, J. R., Kyriakis, J. M., and Force, T. (1994) The stress-activated protein kinases are major c-Jun amino-terminal kinases activated by ischemia and reperfusion. *J. Biol. Chem.*, **269**, 26546.
207. Westwick, J. K., Weitzel, C., Minden, A., Karin, M., and Brenner, D. A. (1994) Tumor necrosis factor alpha stimulates AP-1 activity through prolonged activation of the c-Jun kinase. *J. Biol. Chem.*, **269**, 26396.
208. Fanklin, C. C., Unlap, T., Adler, V., and Kraft, A. S. (1993) Multiple signal transduction pathways mediate c-Jun protein phosphorylation. *Cell Growth Diff.*, **4**, 377.
209. Engelberg, D., Klein, C., Martinetto, H., Struhl, K., and Karin, M. (1994) The UV response involving the Ras signaling pathway and AP-1 transcription factors is con-served between yeast and mammals. *Cell*, **77**, 381.
210. Minden, A., Lin, A., McMahon, M., Lange, C. C., Derijard, B., Davis, R. J. *et al.* (1994) Differential activation of ERK and JNK mitogen-activated protein kinases by Raf-1 and MEKK. *Science*, **266**, 1719.
211. Lange-Carter, C. A. and Johnson, G. L. (1994) Ras-dependent growth factor regulation of MEK kinase in PC12 cells. *Science*, **265**, 1458.
212. Yan, M., Dai, T., Deak, J. C., Kyriakis, J. M., Zon, L. I., Woodgett, J. R., *et al.* (1994) Activation of stress-activated protein kinase by MEKK1 phosphorylation of its activator SEK1. *Nature*, **372**, 798.
213. Russell, M., Lange-Carter, C., and Johnson, G. L. (1995) Direct interaction between Ras

and the kinase domain of mitogen-activated protein kinase kinase kinase (MEKK1). *J. Biol. Chem.*, **270**, 11757.

214. Sanchez, I., Hughes, R. T., Mayer, B. J., Yee, K., Woodgett, J. R., Avruch, J., *et al.* (1994) Role of SAPK/ERK kinase-1 in the stress-activated pathway regulating transcription factor c-Jun. *Nature*, **372**, 794.

215. Blank, J. L., Gerwin, P., Elliott, E. M., Sather, S., and Johnson, G. L. (1996) Molecular cloning of mitogen-activated protein/ERK kinase kinases (MEKK) 2 and 3. *J. Biol. Chem.*, **271**, 5361.

216. Catling, A. D., Schaeffer, H. J., Reuter, C. W., Reddy, G. R., and Weber, M. J. (1995) A proline-rich sequence unique to MEK1 and MEK2 is required for raf binding and regulates MEK function. *Mol. Cell. Biol.*, **15**, 5214.

217. Xu, S., Robbins, D., Frost, J., Dang, A., Lange-Carter, C., and Cobb, M. H. (1995) MEKK1 phosphorylates MEK1 and MEK2 but does not cause activation of mitogen-activated protein kinase. *Proc. Natl. Acad. Sci. USA*, **92**, 6808.

218. Zinck, R., Cahill, M. A., Kracht, M., Sachsenmaier, C., Hipskind, R. A., and Nordheim, A. (1995) Protein synthesis inhibitors reveal differential regulation of mitogen-activated protein kinase and stress-activated protein kinase pathways that converge on Elk-1. *Mol. Cell. Biol.*, **15**, 4930.

219. Liu, Y., Gorospe, M., Yang, C., and Holbrook, N. J. (1995) Role of mitogen-activated protein kinase phosphatase during the cellular response to genotoxic stress. Inhibition of c-June N-terminal kinase activity and AP-1-dependent gene activation. *J. Biol. Chem.*, **270**, 8377.

220. Chu, Y., Solski, P. A., Khosravi-Far, R., Der, C. J., and Kelly, K. (1996) The mitogen-activated protein kinase phosphatases PAC1, MKP-1, and MKP-2 have unique substrate specificities and reduced activity *in vivo* toward the ERK2 *sevenmaker* mutation. *J. Biol. Chem.*, **271**, 6497.

221. King, A. G., Ozanne, B. W., Smythe, C., and Ashworth, A. (1995) Isolation and characterisation of a uniquely regulated threonine, tyrosine phosphatase (TYP 1) which inactivates ERK2 and p54jnk. *Oncogene*, **11**, 2553.

222. Doi, K., Gartner, A., Ammerer, G., Errede, B., Shinkawa, H., Sugimoto, K., *et al.* (1994) MSG5, a novel protein phosphatase promotes adaptation to pheromone response in *S. cerevisiae*. *EMBO J.*, **13**, 61.

223. Bunone, G., Briand, P.-A., Miksicek, R. J., and Picard, D. (1996) Activation of the unliganded estrogen receptor by EGF involves the MAP kinase pathway and direct phosphorylation. *EMBO J.*, **15**, 2174.

224. Blenis, J., Chung, J., Erikson, E., Alcorta, D. A., and Erikson, R. L. (1991) Distinct mechanisms for the activation of the RSK kinases/MAP2 kinase/pp90rsk and pp70-S6 kinase signaling systems are indicated by inhibition of protein synthesis. *Cell Growth Diff.*, **2**, 279.

225. Chung, J., Pelech, S. L., and Blenis, J. (1991) Mitogen-activated Swiss mouse 3T3 RSK kinases I and II are related to pp44mpk from sea star oocytes and participate in the regulation of pp90rsk activity. *Proc. Natl. Acad. Sci. USA*, **88**, 4981.

226. Sturgill, T. W., Ray, L. B., Erikson, E., and Maller, J. L. (1988) Insulin-stimulated MAP-2 kinase phosphorylates and activates ribosomal protein S6 kinase II. *Nature*, **334**, 715.

227. Peraldi, P., Zhao, Z., Filloux, C., Fischer, E. H., and Van, O. E. (1994) Protein-tyrosine-phosphatase 2C is phosphorylated and inhibited by 44-kDa mitogen-activated protein kinase. *Proc. Natl. Acad. Sci. USA*, **91**, 5002.

228. Lin, L. L., Wartmann, M., Lin, A. Y., Knopf, J. L., Seth, A., and Davis, R. J. (1993) cPLA2 is phosphorylated and activated by MAP kinase. *Cell*, **72**, 269.

229. Qiu, Z. H. and Leslie, C. C. (1994) Protein kinase C-dependent and -independent pathways of mitogen-activated protein kinase activation in macrophages by stimuli that activate phospholipase A2. *J. Biol. Chem.*, **269**, 19480.

230. Cherniack, A. D., Klarlund, J. K., and Czech, M. P. (1994) Phosphorylation of the Ras nucleotide exchange factor son of sevenless by mitogen-activated protein kinase. *J. Biol. Chem.*, **269**, 4717.

231. Cherniack, A. D., Klarlund, J. K., Conway, B. R., and Czech, M. P. (1995) Disassembly of Son-of-sevenless proteins from Grb2 during p21ras desensitization by insulin. *J. Biol. Chem.*, **270**, 1485.

232. Griswold-Prenner, I., Carlin, C. R., and Rosner, M. R. (1993) Mitogen-activated protein kinase regulates the epidermal growth factor receptor through activation of a tyrosine phosphatase. *J. Biol. Chem.*, **268**, 13050.

233. Northwood, I. C., Gonzalez, F. A., Wartmann, M., Raden, D. L., and Davis, R. J. (1991) Isolation and characterization of two growth factor-stimulated protein kinases that phosphorylate the epidermal growth factor receptor at threonine 669. *J. Biol. Chem.*, **266**, 15266.

234. Takishima, K., Griswold-Prenner, I., Ingebritsen, T., and Rosner, M. R. (1991) Epidermal growth factor (EGF) receptor T669 peptide kinase from 3T3-L1 cells is an EGF-stimulated 'MAP' kinase. *Proc. Natl. Acad. Sci. USA*, **88**, 2520.

235. Anderson, N. G., Li, P., Marsden, L. A., Williams, N., Roberts, T. M., and Sturgill, T. W. (1991) Raf-1 is a potential substrate for mitogen-activated protein kinase *in vivo*. *Biochem. J.*, **277**, 573.

236. Lee, R.-M., Cobb, M. H., and Blackshear, P. J. (1992) Evidence that extracellular signal-regulated kinases are the insulin-activated Raf-1 kinase kinases. *J. Biol. Chem.*, **267**, 1088.

237. Kyriakis, J. M., Force, T. L., Rapp, U. R., Bonventre, J. V., and Avruch, J. (1993) Mitogen regulation of c-Raf-1 protein kinase activity toward mitogen-activated protein kinase-kinase. *J. Biol. Chem.*, **268**, 16009.

238. Haystead, T. A. J., Haystead, C. M. M., Hu, C., Lin, T.-A., and Lawrence, J. C., Jr. (1994) Phosphorylation of PHAS-I by mitogen-activated protein (MAP) kinase. *J. Biol. Chem.*, **269**, 23185.

239. Lin, T. A., Kong, X., Haystead, T. A., Pause, A., Belsham, G., Sonenberg, N., *et al.* (1994) PHAS-I as a link between mitogen-activated protein kinase and translation initiation. *Science*, **266**, 653.

240. Pulverer, B. J., Kyriakis, J. M., Avruch, J., Nikolakaki, E., and Woodgett, J. R. (1991) Phosphorylation of c-*jun* mediated by MAP kinases. *Nature*, **353**, 670.

241. Chou, S. Y., Baichwal, V., and Ferrell, J. J. (1992) Inhibition of c-Jun DNA binding by mitogen-activated protein kinase. *Mol. Biol. Cell.*, **3**, 1117.

242. Deng, T. and Karin, M. (1994) c-Fos transcriptional activity stimulated by H-Ras-activated protein kinase distinct from JNK and ERK. *Nature*, **371**, 171.

243. Gille, H., Kortenjann, M., Thomae, O., Moomaw, C., Slaughter, C., Cobb, M. H., *et al.* (1995) ERK phosphorylation potentiates Elk-1-mediated ternary complex formation and transactivation. *EMBO J.*, **14**, 951.

244. Hipskind, R. A., Buscher, D., Nordheim, A., and Baccarini, M. (1994) Ras/MAP kinase-dependent and -independent signaling pathways target distinct ternary complex factors. *Genes Dev.*, **8**, 1803.

245. Janknecht, R., Ernst, W. H., Pingoud, V., and Nordheim, A. (1993) Activation of ternary complex factor Elk-1 by MAP kinases. *EMBO J.*, **12**, 5097.

246. Marais, R., Wynne, J., and Treisman, R. (1993) The SRF accessory protein Elk-1 contains a growth factor-regulated transcriptional activation domain. *Cell*, **73**, 381.

247. Janknecht, R., Ernst, W. H., and Nordheim, A. (1995) SAP1a is a nuclear target of signaling cascades involving ERKs. *Oncogene*, **10**, 1209.

248. Gille, H., Sharrocks, A. D., and Shaw, P. E. (1992) Phosphorylation of transcription factor p62TCF by MAP kinase stimulates ternary complex formation at c-fos promoter. *Nature*, **358**, 414.

249. Nakajima, T., Kinoshita, S., Sasagawa, T., Sasaki, K., Naruto, M., Kishimoto, T., *et al.* (1993) Phosphorylation at threonine-235 by a ras-dependent mitogen-activated protein kinase cascade is essential for transcription factor NF-IL6. *Proc. Natl. Acad. Sci. USA*, **90**, 2207.

250. Milne, D. M., Campbell, D. G., Caudwell, F. B., and Meek, D. W. (1994) Phosphorylation of the tumor suppressor protein p53 by mitogen-activated protein kinases. *J. Biol. Chem.*, **269**, 9253.

6 | Oncogenic transcription factors: FOS, JUN, MYC, MYB, and ETS

SUZANNE J. BAKER and TOM CURRAN

1. Introduction

Many oncogenes encode important components of the cellular machinery that are responsible for the translation of growth and differentiation signals in response to a diverse array of extra- and intracellular stimuli. Included in this broad range of oncogenic molecules are growth factor receptors (see Chapters 2 and 3), cytoplasmic signalling molecules (Chapters 4 and 5), and nuclear transcription factors. Transcription factors are critical components of signal transduction pathways that can transmit a regulatory signal to altered patterns of gene expression. It is not surprising that the disruption of normal regulation of such important control points can contribute to tumorigenesis. This chapter will focus on several transcription factors originally discovered as transforming genes carried by retroviruses (for a historical review see ref. 1). The intention is to provide a generalized view of the mode of action and regulation of these genes and their relationship to cellular growth and differentiation rather than a comprehensive review of the extensive literature.

It is becoming increasingly clear that although transcription factors bind to specific DNA target sequences, they do not function in isolation. A common theme for the regulation of these proteins is the effect of protein–protein interactions on biological activity. Many transcription factors interact, through homologous domains, with related dimerization partners that regulate the activity of the protein. However, additional higher order interactions with unrelated transcription factors and components of the basal transcription machinery are likely to play an important role in modulating activity and target gene specificity.

2. FOS and JUN

The FOS and JUN family of transcription factors provided some of the earliest insights into the potential for complex regulation and diverse responses through combinatorial interactions among transcription factors. The *v-FOS* and *v-JUN* oncogenes were originally isolated from the Finkel–Biskis–Jinkins murine sarcoma virus (FBJ–MSV) and the avian sarcoma virus 17 (ASV 17) respectively. The discovery that *c-FOS* and *c-JUN* encode components of the transcription factor activator protein 1 (AP-1) (reviewed in ref. 2) led to the extensive molecular analysis of the signal transduction pathways that mediate AP-1 activation in response to a wide range of extracellular stimuli.

2.1 Dimerization of FOS and JUN

Members of the *FOS* and *JUN* gene families are transcription factors that contain the highly conserved basic region and leucine zipper (bZIP) motifs that mediate dimerization and DNA binding (Fig. 1). The leucine zipper dictates dimerization specificity. Proteins encoded by the *FOS* family of genes form heterodimers with JUN family members, but they cannot form homodimers or heterodimers with other FOS family members. JUN family members can form homodimers or heterodimers with other JUN family members as well as with FOS family members. Homodimers and

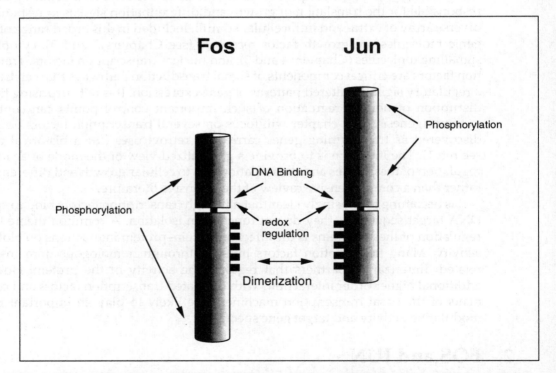

Fig. 1 FOS and JUN structure. Dimerization of FOS and JUN is mediated by the leucine zipper, a hydrophobic coiled-coil structure that dictates the specificity of interactions with other zipper proteins. DNA binding activity is contained in the basic region adjacent to the zipper. Phosphorylation and redox state also contribute to regulation of activity.

heterodimers formed by combinations of FOS- and JUN-related proteins bind to a variety of AP-1 (TGACTCA) and cyclic AMP responsive element (CRE) (TGACGTCA) type recognition sequences with similar DNA binding specificities. FOS and JUN family proteins form dimers with members of the bZIP activating transcription factor (ATF)/CRE-binding (CREB) family that interact with CRE or AP-1 sites (for review see ref. 3). The MAF subfamily of bZIP proteins also form dimers with FOS and JUN family proteins and recognize a non-palindromic consensus DNA binding sequence $TGAC(N)_{3-4}GCA$. Each half of the dimer is responsible for recognition of half of the binding sequence (4, 5). FOS and JUN can also interact with additional proteins that do not contain a leucine zipper. Table 1 lists the proteins that

Table 1 Proteins that interact directly with FOS or JUN

	Transcription factor[a]	FOS	JUN	DNA recognition site[b]	Reference
A.	c-FOS	−	+	AP-1, CRE	For review see ref. 3
	FOS B	−	+		For review see ref. 3
	FRA1	−	+		For review see ref. 3
	FRA2	−	+		For review see ref. 3
	c-JUN	+	+		For review see ref. 3
	JUN B	+	+		For review see ref. 3
	JUN D	+	+		For review see ref. 3
B.	ATFa	+	+	AP-1, CRE	161
	ATF2	+	+		162
	ATF3	−	+		162
	ATF4	+	+		162
	TAXREB67	+	+/−		163
C.	c-MAF	+	+	MARE	4, 5, 164
	MAF B	+	−	MARE	165
	MAF F	+	−	MARE	166
	MAF G	+	−	MARE	166
	MAF K	+	−	MARE	166
	NRL	+	+	MARE	164
D.	NF-IL-6	+	+	AP-1	167
	FIP	+	−	ND	168
E.	QM	−	+	Inhibits binding to AP-1	169
	NF-AT	+	+	AP-1	170
	GR	+	+	Inhibits binding to AP-1	171
	NFκBp65	+	+	κB and AP-1	172
	TBP	+	+	AP-1	173, 174
	TFIIE-30	+	+	AP-1	M. L. Martin and T. Curran
	TFII-34	+	+	AP-1	unpublished data
	TFIIE-74	+	+	AP-1	unpublished data
	MYO D	ND	+	ND	175

[a] A: FOS–JUN family. B: ATF/CREB family. C: MAF family. D. Other bZIP proteins. E. Non-zipper proteins.
[b] ATFa–JUN heterodimers bind efficiently to AP-1 and CRE sites, but ATFa–FOS heterodimers do not bind DNA. AP-1 (also TRE or TPA-responsive element): TGACTCA. CRE (cyclic AMP responsive element): TCACGTCA. MARE (MAF responsive element): $TGAC(N)_{3-4}GCA$. kB binding site: GGGRNNYYCC. ND: not determined.

have been shown to directly contact FOS and JUN through higher order interactions. Many other proteins are believed to act in concert with FOS and JUN by binding other sites in promoter regions, but this may not involve direct protein–protein contacts.

2.2. Regulation of FOS and JUN activity

c-FOS and *c-JUN* are members of the group of genes known as cellular immediate early genes. In the majority of cell types, basal expression of these genes is low, but expression may be induced rapidly and transiently by extracellular stimulation (Fig. 2). Several *FOS*- and *JUN*-related genes exhibit distinct patterns of induction. The levels of FOS and JUN family proteins vary depending on the cell type as well as the inducing stimulus. Thus, the composition, specificity, and activity of AP-1 are dynamic, changing over time in response to the cellular pool of available dimerization or interaction partners. There is a vast literature regarding the induction of *FOS* and *JUN* family genes in response to a broad range of stimuli including depolarization of neurons, exposure to tumour promoting agents, and even association with the normal process of cell death during development. It is clear that this gene family is

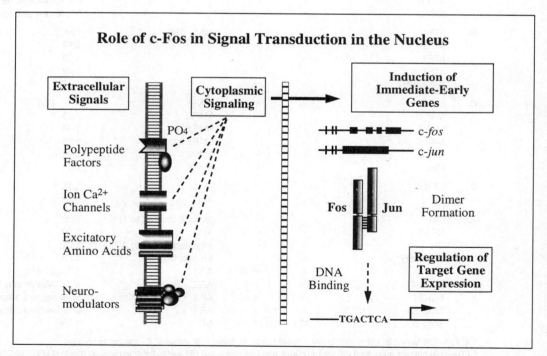

Fig. 2 The role of FOS and JUN in signal transduction in the nucleus. A broad range of extracellular stimuli transduced through different cytoplasmic signalling cascades can induce the rapid and transient expression of *c-FOS* and *c-JUN*, and the subsequent transient increase in AP-1 activity.

highly inducible, and able to integrate a wide array of cellular signals into distinct transcriptional responses through complex interactions (6).

In addition, AP-1 activity can be induced in the absence of protein synthesis by several post-translational control mechanisms (see Fig. 1). For example, the cellular protein REF1 is capable of reducing a conserved cysteine in the DNA binding domain of all FOS and JUN family proteins. Reduction of this cysteine is required for high affinity DNA binding activity *in vitro* (7). Both FOS and JUN are phosphorylated in response to several stimuli including serum stimulation, TPA (tetradecanoylphorbol 13-acetate), and ultraviolet radiation. A number of different kinases have been shown to phosphorylate serines 63, 73, or 246 of c-JUN *in vitro*. It has become generally accepted that phosphorylation of serines 63 and 73 increases c-JUN transcriptional activity based on co-transfection experiments. However, *in vitro* analysis with purified JUN protein showed no effect of phosphorylation on DNA binding or transcriptional activity of JUN homodimers or FOS–JUN heterodimers (8). The state of FOS and JUN as FOS–JUN heterodimers, JUN homodimers, bound to DNA or free, can substantially influence their ability to serve as substrates for protein kinases *in vitro* (9). Clearly, the regulation will be even more complex in the context of an intact cell responding to different extracellular stimuli. Finally, JUN is phosphorylated on serines 63 and 73 in response to diverse signals with very different outcomes for the cell, such as mitogenic signals that lead to proliferation (8) and stress signals that lead to growth arrest (10, 11). Therefore, many additional changes within the cell, such as the expression and activation of other interacting proteins, must be required to provide specificity for the cellular response to any particular signal.

2.3 FOS in tumorigenesis

The *v-FOS* gene was originally isolated from a virus-induced osteosarcoma. Other *in vivo* models for *c-FOS* in transformation include transgenic animals that constitutively express *c-FOS* and develop chondrosarcomas (12) or osteosarcomas with a short latency period (13). The regions of FOS that are required for transforming activity have been characterized by a number of independent studies with varying conclusions (14–16). Activation through AP-1 sites does not seem to be sufficient for transformation, as overexpression of the yeast transcription factor GCN4, which also activates transcription through AP-1 sites, does not transform fibroblasts even in co-operation with an activated *RAS* gene. However, chimeric proteins of JUN or FOS fused to the GCN4 DNA binding domain can independently induce transformation (17). There is also some suggestion that *JUNB* expression is required for transformation by *v-FOS* (18). In an inducible cell culture assay for transformation using rat fibroblasts, transformed morphology is seen only after several days of continuous FOS expression, and reversion to normal morphology requires several days after FOS expression is turned off. This change in morphology can occur in the absence of cell division. This model system suggests that the target(s) for FOS in transformation may require time to accumulate to a critical level, and that morphological transformation is independent of cell cycle progression (19).

2.4   Transformation by JUN

The JUN protein is most transforming in chicken embryo fibroblasts (CEF) rather than in the classic rodent fibroblast assay. The retroviral *v-JUN* contains several point mutations and a deletion relative to *c-JUN* that may augment its transforming potential (20), but *c-JUN* also has transforming activity (21). Although GCN4 is not transforming, a chimera between the VP16 activation domain, and the bZip region of JUN, which is closely related to GCN4, is transforming (22). This somewhat contradictory difference may be the result of factors that interact with JUN in the parental cell line. It seems that JUN may interact with other FOS or JUN family members to exert its transforming activity, as CEF transformed by *c-JUN* contain high levels of the FOS-related protein FRA2 (21).

In addition to direct transformation by overexpression of FOS or JUN, it appears that FOS and JUN family members may play an important downstream role in transformation by other activated oncogenes. For example, activation of an inducible *v-SRC* in CEF resulted in cellular transformation and a concomitant increase in *c-FOS* expression and AP-1 binding (23). In another study, a dominant negative FOS or JUN suppressed transformation of CEF by *FOS* and *JUN* family members as well as *v-SRC*, *v-YES*, *v-FPS*, *c-H-RAS*, and truncated *c-RAF*. This effect was specific, as CEF transformed by *v-ROS* or *v-MYC* were unaffected by these dominant negative forms. A dominant negative *FOS* or *JUN* could act to repress the activity of a number of FOS and JUN family members as well as other dimerization partners. In this system, a FRA2/JUN heterodimer is responsible for the increased AP-1 DNA binding activity, suggesting a critical role of FRA2 and JUN in transformation by other oncogenes (24).

The retrovirus carrying *v-JUN* was isolated from a chicken sarcoma. Transgenic mice that constitutively express *v-JUN* develop dermal fibrosarcomas and rhabdomyosarcomas following wounding suggesting that the state of proliferation or specific growth factor environment determines the tumorigenic capacity of *v-JUN* (25). *c-JUN* and *JUNB* can also act as progression factors in papillomavirus induced fibrosarcomas (26).

There have been a large number of studies characterizing *FOS* and *JUN* expression in human tumours and tumour cell lines. However, control of *FOS* and *JUN* expression is highly responsive to multiple stimuli, and tumours often display abberant expression of many genes. Thus, despite the abundance of literature concerning transformation by *FOS* and *JUN* in culture, and in animals through retroviral infection or transgenic studies, there is no substantial evidence that they play a causative role in human cancer.

2.5   Gene targets for FOS and JUN

A large number of promoters contain sequences similar to the consensus AP-1 or CRE site, but only a subset of them may be valid targets of AP-1 induction. Candidate target genes include metallothionein, stromelysin, collagenase, ODC, FRA1, and proenkephalin. AP-1 activity may be induced in response to a number of different stimuli, each of which is likely to activate a subset of target genes. Thus, the promoter context of an AP-1 site, as well as other transcriptional regulatory proteins present following a specific stimulus, will govern which genes are targets for AP-1 activity in different circumstances and cell types.

3. MYC

The *MYC* oncogene was originally discovered as the cellular sequence contained within the acute transforming virus MC29 which was isolated from a chicken myelo-cytoma (Chapter 1). MC29 also induced carcinoma of the liver and kidney, sarcomas, and mesotheliomas (27). In addition to *c-MYC*, there are two other highly related family members, *L-MYC* and *N-MYC*. The MYC family proteins are comprised of several motifs that are commonly associated with transcription factors (Fig. 3). A basic region, which often mediates DNA binding activity, is located immediately adjacent to a

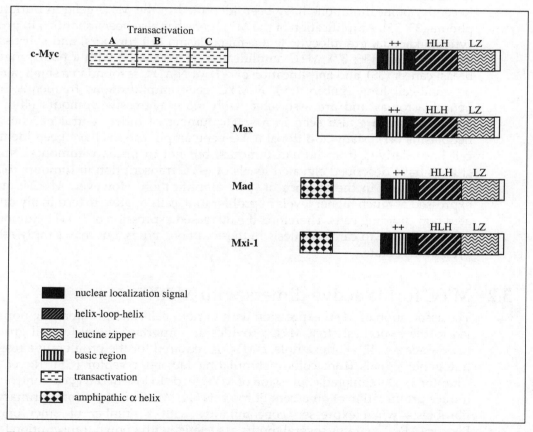

Fig. 3 Structure of MYC and interacting proteins. MYC, MAX, MAD, and MXI1 all contain related basic HLH–LZ domains which are used for dimerization and DNA binding. MAX may dimerize with MYC, MAD, or MXI1. The amphipathic α helix at the amino terminus of MAD and MXI1 mediate their interaction with mSIN2 (see Fig. 4).

helix–loop–helix domain and a leucine zipper domain, motifs that are frequently involved in protein–protein interactions (28).

3.1 MYC in transformation and tumorigenesis

MYC has been rigorously studied due to its involvement in a number of neoplastic conditions as well as its apparent contribution to cell growth regulation. In animal systems, *MYC* was found to be involved in spontaneous myelocytomatosis and mouse plasmacytomas involving a t(15;12) chromosomal translocation (27). There is strong evidence for the involvement of the *MYC* family of genes in a number of different human neoplasias (for review see refs 29, 30 and Chapter 1). In Burkitt's lymphoma, chromosomal translocations cause deregulated expression of *MYC* by joining the regulatory regions for immunoglobulin genes on chromosome 14, 2, or 22 to chromosome 8 adjacent to the *MYC* gene. Overexpression of *MYC* due to translocation is also found in AIDS-associated lymphomas and in T cell leukaemias (31, 32). Recently, point mutations have been identified in the *MYC* gene in Burkitt's lymphoma (33–35). Amplification of the *MYC* gene has also been identified in promyelocytic leukaemia, granulocytic leukaemia, plasma cell tumours, and soft tissue and bone sarcomas (36, 37). *MYC* amplification is associated with a poor prognosis in breast cancer (38), and amplification of *c-* *L-* or *N-MYC* is found in a small percentage of small-cell lung cancers (39). *N-MYC* gene amplifications frequently occur in neuroblastomas and are associated with more aggressive tumours (40). *N-MYC* amplifications are also seen in a small number of other central nervous system neoplasms (41). Many additional *MYC* gene amplifications have been identified in cell lines derived from human tumours, but not in primary tumours. Numerous studies have described elevated levels of *MYC* transcription in tumours relative to normal tissues in the absence of gene amplification. However, *MYC* is normally expressed at much higher levels in proliferating cells relative to terminally differentiated non-dividing cells. Therefore, the increased expression of *MYC* in tumours may not be relevant to carcinogenesis in these tumour types, but may simply reflect the proliferative state.

3.2 MYC forms active dimers with MAX

The association of *MYC* expression with tumour cells and proliferating normal cells led to the hypothesis that *MYC* provides an important signal for cell growth (for review see ref. 42). For example, *c-MYC* is required for the proliferative response to mitogenic signals from colony stimulating factor-1 receptor (CSF1R; ref. 43 and Chapter 3). Deregulated expression of *MYC* leads to loss of cell cycle control and can induce proliferation of quiescent fibroblasts (44). *MYC* can transform primary rodent fibroblasts when expressed concomitantly with a number of other oncogenes. Because MYC contains several motifs associated with known transcription factors, it was believed to exert its biological effect through the regulation of other genes. For many years, however, there was no evidence that MYC could directly bind DNA and activate transcription (for review see ref. 28). MYC homodimers only formed *in vitro* at extremely high concentrations that were unlikely to reflect a physiologically relevant state (45, 46).

Over the past several years, the identification of a network of interacting proteins that modulate MYC activity has provided exciting new insights into MYC regulation and function (for review see ref. 47). The MAX protein, a dimerization partner for MYC, is homologous to MYC in the basic, HLH, and leucine zipper regions, but lacks an obvious transactivation domain (48, 49) (Fig. 3). Several alternatively spliced forms of MAX exist, all of which contain the bHLHLZ domains and appear to be functionally equivalent in their effect on MYC function. MYC and MAX form heterodimers that bind the DNA consensus sequence CACGTG, also termed the E-box, and can activate transcription through this sequence (50). This activation requires the amino terminus of MYC and the bHLHLZ domains of both proteins (51). Several other transcription factors including USF, TFE3, and TFEB are capable of binding to the E-box sequence. However, MYC-MAX heterodimers can also bind to several variations of the E-box consensus that the others can not bind, thus providing some specificity (52).

3.3 MAD and MXI1: dimerization partners for MAX

Further regulation is provided by MAD and MXI1, related bHLHLZ proteins that dimerize with MAX, but not MYC (53, 54) (Fig. 3). MAX, which is expressed constitutively and at high levels, dimerizes with MYC, MAD, and MXI1 with equal affinity, but forms homodimers with a lower affinity. The expression patterns of these proteins govern the dimerization state of MAX *in vivo*. MYC is a short-lived protein that is expressed only in response to specific growth signals while MAD and MXI1 are expressed in response to differentiation-inducing agents (55, 56). Thus, MYC–MAX dimers that activate transcription are predominant in proliferating cells while MAD–MAX and MXI1–MAX dimers which repress transcription are present in differentiated cells.

3.4 mSIN3A and mSIN3B repress transcription through interaction with MAD and MXI1

It was initially thought that MAD–MAX and MXI1–MAX complexes repressed transcription because they bind to E-box sites, but lack transcriptional activation domains. It is now clear that these complexes actively repress transcription through an additional protein–protein interaction. A yeast two-hybrid screen to identify proteins that interact with MAD or MXI1 led to the discovery of two related mammalian cDNAs, mSIN3A and mSIN3B, that represent mammalian homologues of the yeast transcriptional repressor SIN3. mSIN3 proteins contain a paired amphipathic helix that can bind specifically to an amphipathic alpha helix at the amino terminus of MAD or MXI1. This interaction is required for transcriptional repression by

MAD–MAX or MXI1–MAX. Although mSIN3 proteins do not interact directly with MAX, a ternary complex of MAX–MAD–mSIN3 or MAX–MXI1–mSIN3 binds to E-box sites. MAX and mSIN3 appear to be constitutively expressed, so that the regulation of MYC activity may be primarily determined by the availability of MAD and MXI1 or MYC to dimerize with MAX (57, 58) (Fig. 4).

3.5 Additional regulation of MYC activity

Further fine tuning of MYC, MAX, and MAD activity is likely to occur from additional modifications and higher order protein–protein interactions. Phosphorylation of MYC has been reported to enhance its transactivation activity (59), or alternatively to have no effect on transactivation activity, but to potentially inhibit the transforming activity of MYC (60). MAX is phosphorylated on serines 2 and 11 *in vivo* and by casein kinase II (CKII) *in vitro*. One study suggested that CKII phosphorylation of MAX inhibited the binding of MAX homodimers, but not MYC–MAX heterodimers (61). A subsequent study demonstrated that phosphorylation increased the exchange rate of DNA binding of both MAX homodimers and MYC–MAX dimers (62). It is likely that the effect on MAX homodimers is less significant, as MAX forms heterodimers with MYC, MAD, or MXI1 with higher affinity than homodimers.

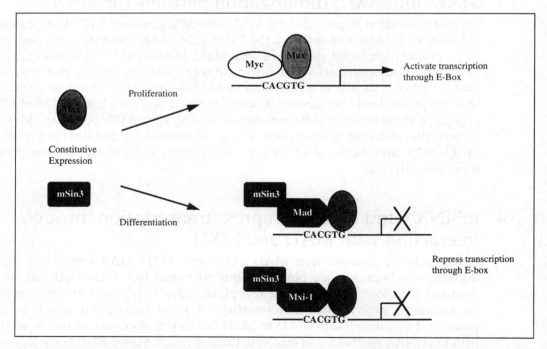

Fig. 4 Regulation of MYC transcriptional activity. MAX and mSIN3 are expressed constitutively. MYC expression is induced in proliferating cells, allowing the formation of MYC–MAX dimers which activate transcription through E-box sequences. In differentiated cells, mSIN3 interacts with MAD or MXI1. This dimer confers transcriptional repression through E-box sequences when it forms a complex with MAX. mSIN3 does not contact MAX directly.

Interactions with other proteins may also modulate the activity of MYC in different circumstances. The amino terminal transcriptional activation domain of MYC interacts with the retinoblastoma protein (pRB) (63) and with the pRB-like binding pocket of p107 (64 and Chapter 8). Transcriptional activity of MYC is enhanced by interaction with pRB (65) and repressed by interaction with p107 (66). The TATA binding protein (TBP) also binds to MYC in the same region that p107 and pRB interact (67). Also, MYC and the basal transcription factor TFII-I act through initiator elements to inhibit RNA polymerase II-dependent transcription (68). MYC, but not MYC–MAX heterodimers, can bind to and inhibit the repression and activation activities of the transcription factor Yin-Yang-1 (YY-1) (69).

Some of these interactions may contribute to the ability of MYC to induce entry into the cell cycle. p107 and the D-cyclins can act at the G1/S transition to block progression of the cell cycle (for review see ref. 70 and Chapter 7). MYC expression can overcome p107-mediated growth arrest, perhaps by binding to and saturating the available p107 with MYC. MYC represses expression of cyclin D1 at the level of transcription initiation (71).

3.6 Targets of MYC activity

It appears clear that the transcriptional activation function of MYC is essential for its biological role as a transforming protein because the amino terminal transactivation domain, basic region, HLH, and LZ are all required for transformation. However, it is extremely difficult to define the genes that are directly regulated by MYC, as it may send signals that trigger several additional cascades of gene expression through alternative pathways. Furthermore, MYC may exert different biological effects on the cell depending on the subset of genes it activates. In fact, in some circumstances, including serum starvation of transformed cells, MYC expression induces apoptosis or programmed cell death rather than proliferation (for review see ref. 47). MYC induction of apoptosis requires wild-type p53 protein (see Chapter 9) and ornithine decarboxylase (ODC) (72, 73). MYC directly activates several genes through an E-box sequence in their control regions including α-prothymosin, the embryonically expressed gene ECA 39, ODC, and p53 (74–77). MYC expression has also been shown to increase the transcription of cyclin A and cyclin E (78). These are appealing targets of MYC activation, as their expression would be expected to drive entry into the cell cycle and promote cell growth and division (see Chapter 7). This activation may occur indirectly through uncharacterized pathways. Additional indirect targets of MYC expression include several cell surface markers of differentiation (for review see ref. 28). MYC has also been shown to repress gene expression through initiator elements in several genes including the adenovirus 2 major late promoter, CEBP α and albumin (79).

4. MYB

MYB is the transforming gene carried by avian myeloblastosis virus (AMV), and the avian leukosis virus E26, in which *MYB* is fused to another oncogene, *ETS* and to a portion of viral *gag* sequences. The E26 virus induces mixed erythroid–myeloid leukaemia in quails, erythroblastic leukaemia in chickens, and can transform myeloblasts and erythroblasts *in vitro* (for historical review see ref. 80). The *MYB* and *ETS* genes encode transcription factors that are representatives of distinct families of genes that recognize different DNA target sequences.

4.1 MYB structure

The amino terminus of c-MYB contains three imperfect repeats of 51–53 amino acids termed R1, R2 and R3, each possessing the potential to form α helical structures and containing three conserved tryptophan residues at intervals of 18 or 19 amino acids. R2 and R3 are sufficient for specific binding to the DNA consensus sequence C/T AAC G/T G, termed MRE (MYB responsive element; for review see ref. 81). NMR solution structure showed that R2 and R3 each contain three helices; the third helix of each repeat is a DNA recognition helix (82). A hydrophilic and slightly acidic 50 amino acid transactivation domain is located carboxy terminal to the DNA binding repeats. The carboxy terminus of the protein contains a negative regulatory domain that includes an isoleucine and three leucine residues with a heptad spacing constituting a non-consensus leucine zipper motif (81 and Fig. 5).

4.2 MYB in tumorigenesis

The oncogenic contribution of MYB may be to block differentiation (83). Expression of MYB stimulates growth of myeloid colony-forming cells and can block terminal differentiation in mouse erythroleukaemia (MEL) cells (84). The involvement of MYB in virally-induced tumours usually involves deregulated expression under the direction of a viral promoter as well as deletion of negative regulatory domains. In the E26

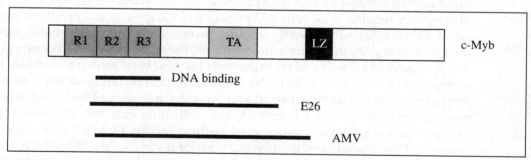

Fig. 5 Structure of c-MYB. The amino terminus of MYB contains three imperfect repeats shown as R1–R3. Only R2 and R3 are required for DNA binding activity. TA represents the slightly acidic transcriptional activation domain, and LZ represents the weak leucine zipper motif at the carboxy terminus, which also contains a negative regulatory domain. The lines labelled E26 and AMV show the portion of the MYB gene retained in the E26 avian leukosis virus and the avian myeloblastosis virus (AMV) respectively. The E26 virus encodes the DNA binding and transactivation domain of MYB and the DNA binding domain of ETS1 fused to viral gag sequences, and transcribed under the direction of the viral LTR. Both *MYB* and *ETS* sequences are required for its transforming activity. *MYB* is the only cellular gene contained in AMV

transforming virus, the first amino terminal repeat of c-MYB was deleted and replaced by sequences from the viral *gag* gene. In addition, much of the sequence encoding the carboxy terminus, including the negative regulatory domain, was deleted and replaced by sequences from the *ETS1* gene (Fig. 5). *MYB* alone acts as the transforming gene of AMV (avian myeloblastosis virus) in which the first amino terminal repeat and the carboxy terminal negative regulatory domain are deleted (Fig. 5). In avian leukosis virus-induced lymphomas, ABPL tumours, and pre-B-cell tumours induced with Abelson and Moloney murine leukaemia virus (MuLV), the provirus integrates upstream of *MYB* deleting the first three exons of *MYB*, as in E26, and directing high levels of expression using the viral promoter. Although, the *in vitro* transforming activity of *MYB* was thought to be limited to haematopoietic cells, a *MYB* gene encoding a carboxy terminal, but not an amino terminal truncation, is transforming in non-haematopoietic mesenchymal cells in chicken (85).

c-*MYB* is located on human chromosome 6q22-24, a region frequently altered by translocations or allelic deletions in leukaemias, lymphomas, and cutaneous melanomas. Thus, it was suggested that the *MYB* gene was the target of these genetic alterations. There is no clear evidence that *MYB* plays an important role in the genesis of these neoplasms. Although there is a report of *MYB* gene amplification in one leukaemia (86), and one rearrangement that does not affect the coding region of the *MYB* gene in a melanoma tumour cell line (87), there is no evidence that the *MYB* gene is altered at high frequency in primary human tumours. Conversely, there is evidence that the *MYB* locus is not involved in the common genetic rearrangements on chromosome 6q in lymphoid tumours (88).

4.3 Regulation of MYB activity

MYB expression is normally limited to cells of lymphoid, erythroid, and myeloid lineages and is down-regulated during differentiation. NFκB family members appear to play an important role in the regulation of c-*MYB* expression (89). Further regulation of expression occurs through differential splicing. One alternatively spliced form includes an additional exon that interrupts the negative regulatory domain (90, 91). A second alternatively spliced form encodes an amino and carboxy terminally truncated protein that retains the DNA binding domain, but deletes the transactivation domain. This alternate protein may act as a dominant negative effector; it is capable of inducing MEL cell differentiation in direct opposition to the activity of full-length MYB (92).

MYB binds to DNA as a monomer, unlike the FOS, JUN, and MYC proteins, which must dimerize in order to bind to DNA. In fact, it appears that protein–protein interactions may serve to inhibit rather than enhance MYB activity. A number of studies have examined the mechanism of negative regulation exerted by the carboxy terminus of c-MYB which contains a non-consensus leucine zipper motif. v-MYB contains deletions of the carboxy terminus, and is a stronger transcriptional activator than c-MYB. In transfected mammalian cells, low level expression of c-MYB produces greater transactivation than high levels of c-MYB. The repression of activity at high levels of MYB expression was abrogated by a mutation of the leucine zipper in the carboxy terminus (93). Further, co-transfection of the carboxy terminal domain can enhance activation by full-length MYB (94). Taken together, these studies suggest that the carboxy terminal domain of c-MYB mediates interaction with a protein that may inhibit MYB DNA binding or transactivation. A recent study reported the identification of two proteins that interact with the leucine zipper in the carboxy terminal negative regulatory region (95). Cloning of these proteins revealed a potential weak leucine zipper in the region of MYB interaction (T. J. Gonda, personal communication).

Phosphorylation of c-MYB may provide an additional mode of regulation. Phosphorylation of serines 11 and 12 inhibits DNA binding of MYB to an MRE *in vitro* (96). These phosphorylation sites are frequently deleted in oncogenically active MYB, perhaps eliminating one mode of regulation. Recent studies suggest that phosphorylation of the amino terminal serines may act to enhance DNA binding by modulating the effect of the negative regulatory domain in the carboxy terminus (R. Ramsey, personal communication). The DNA binding activity of c-MYB is also sensitive to redox state (97).

4.4 Targets of MYB activation

There are examples of MYB functioning through its recognition sequence, the MRE, as well as independently of MRE binding. A MYB-responsive gene named *MIM1* contains three MREs in its promoter region and is expressed at high levels in promyelocytes. The *MIM1* gene encodes a 326 amino acid cysteine-rich secreted protein. Although it is likely that *MIM1* is a valid target gene for MYB, it is unlikely that it is responsible for MYB transforming activity, as it is not expressed in AMV-transformed cells and it does not stimulate growth of cells that are targets for MYB transformation (98). The MYB–ETS fusion encoded by the E26 virus activates the transcription of the erythroid-specific transcription factor GATA-1 (99). Additional targets of MYB activation are CD2, CD4, CD34, and several viral promoters (100–103). MYB can activate transcription of the HSP70 gene through the TATA element rather than the standard MRE via an unknown mechanism (104). MYB expression also activates the *MYC* promoter through cell type-specific sites that require MYB DNA binding (105). Recently, it has been shown that MYB can act in combination with the myeloid-specific transcription factor NF-M through adjacent DNA binding sites to regulate the transcription of myeloid-specific genes in heterologous cell types (98). The co-operation between MYB and other tissue-specific transcription factors may help to explain why MYB can only transform cell types in which it is normally expressed.

4.5 MYB family members

Additional family members A-MYB and B-MYB share a high degree of homology with c-MYB in the R2/R3 regions of the protein, while the remainder of the protein differs (for review see ref. 106). Although *A-MYB* expression was reported in T cells, kidney, colon, and lymphoid tissues, a recent study of *A-MYB* in mouse showed predominant expression in the undifferentiated cells of the testis, with low level expression in several other tissues (107). B-MYB is similar to c-MYB in DNA binding specificity, but may have distinct target site preference and activity (108, 109). B-*MYB* is also likely to be involved in cell growth, as its expression is regulated at the G1/S boundary of the cell cycle by p107/E2F complexes (110 and see Chapter 8).

5. ETS

5.1 Structure of the ETS family proteins

As mentioned above, the E26 virus carried portions of *MYB* and *ETS* fused to viral sequences to constitute the complete transforming virus capable of inducing erythroblastic leukaemia in chickens (see Fig. 5). The *ETS1* gene is one of a large family of genes with varying degrees of sequence similarity. All genes of the *ETS* family share a highly conserved 85 amino acid motif termed the ETS domain that defines the gene family and mediates DNA binding to the core consensus sequence GGAA/T. The carboxy terminal portion of the ETS domain is rich in basic residues while the amino terminal portion contains a conserved tryptophan triplet with a spacing of 17–18 amino acids reminiscent of the tryptophan triplets found in the DNA binding domain of c-MYB (for review see ref. 111) (Fig. 6). Introduction of mutations throughout the ETS domain can disrupt DNA binding activity, suggesting that the proper folding of this domain may play an important role in its function (112). Structural analysis of the ETS domain from murine ETS1 suggests that ETS proteins can be classified as members of the superfamily of winged helix–turn–helix DNA-binding proteins in which winged refers to a large β sheet region and any associated loops in addition to the helix–turn–helix domain. This classification is based entirely upon structural analysis in the absence of strong sequence similarity with other family members (113). The carboxy terminus of ETS1 mediates an intramolecular repression of DNA binding activity (114).

5.2 Expression patterns of ETS genes

Currently at least 30 *ETS* family genes have been identified. The large size of this gene family allows for a high degree of specificity in *ETS*-mediated transcriptional control. First, expression patterns of *ETS* genes are diverse, with some genes expressed in cell type-specific and developmentally-specific patterns while others are more broadly expressed. Secondly, many family members encode several alternatively spliced forms. Additionally, although ETS family members bind the same purine-rich core consensus sequence, different proteins have variable preferences for 5' and 3' flanking sequences, and therefore are likely to activate different target genes. T cells provide an excellent example of complexity of gene regulation by ETS family members. Multiple ETS proteins are expressed in T cells including ETS1, ETS2, GA binding protein α (GABPα), ELF1, and FLI1. ETS-responsive genes expressed in T cells have related, but

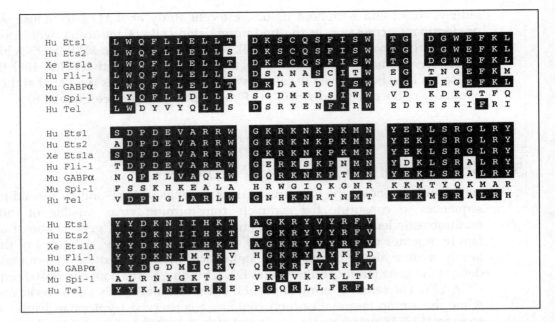

Fig. 6 Homology in the ETS domain. The ETS domain is a highly conserved DNA binding domain that is included in over 30 related genes. It is generally at the carboxy terminus of the protein, although in some proteins, such as ELK1, the ETS domain lies in the amino terminus. The sequence alignment shows the ETS domain of several representative family members; sequence identity to the human ETS1 consensus is shown with black boxes. Hu = human; Mu = mouse; Xe = Xenopus.

slightly different ETS binding sites. ETS1 activates transcription of the T cell receptor (TCR) α and β, but not interleukin-2 (IL-2), whereas ELF1 binds to ETS sites in IL-2 and the HIV enhancer, but not TCR α and β (115).

5.3 Regulation of ETS activity

Unlike the MYC–MAX and FOS–JUN interactions, ETS proteins bind to DNA as monomers and they do not dimerize with family members. However, protein–protein interactions are likely to play important roles in the regulation of activity. Several family members have been shown to form associations with heterologous factors and activate transcription synergistically through adjacent binding sites. Examples of these interactions include ETS1/CBF (core binding factor), ELK1/SRF (serum response factor) in the activation of the *FOS* promoter in response to growth factor stimulation, PU.1/NFEM5, ELF1/TAX in the activation of the HTLV1 LTR, and GABP α/GABPβ (116–120).

Further regulation is likely to occur through post-translational modification. The clearest example of such regulation has been shown for the ternary complex factors (TCF) that include ELK1, SAP1, SAP2, and NET. These proteins are ETS family members that interact with the SRF and bind to an ETS site in the *FOS* promoter adjacent to the serum response element (SRE). The activity of these proteins is strongly regulated by growth factor stimulation and activation of kinase-mediated signal transduction pathways such as the MAP kinase cascade (Chapter 5). Expression of activated oncogenes including *SRC*, *RAS*, *MOS*, and *RAF* also induce phosphorylation and activation of ELK1 and SAP1 (for review see ref. 117). Dominant negative forms of the ETS proteins SPI1/PU.1, ETS1, and ETS2 can individually induce reversion of *RAS*-transformed cells, presumably through blocking an ETS-mediated signal downstream of RAS (121). This provides an intriguing link between deregulated growth induced by oncogenes and the activation of ETS family proteins.

5.4 Involvement of ETS genes in viral tumorigenesis

Induction of chicken erythroleukaemias by the E26 virus requires a chimeric gene in which viral *gag* sequences and sequences encoding the DNA binding domain of MYB and the DNA binding domain of ETS1 are fused and transcribed under the control of the viral LTR. Both *MYB* and *ETS* are required and they must be fused for leukaemogenesis and transformation of multipotent erythroid progenitor cells (MEP) *in vitro* (122). A temperature-sensitive mutant of E26 has shown that the DNA binding domain of ETS1 is required to block the differentiation of E26-transformed MEPs (123). The expression of a cellular target gene, REM1 (regulated by ETS in MEPs) is induced by the ETS DNA binding domain in E26. However, REM1 expression does not block MEP differentiation (124), so that the specific target gene(s) for E26 in transformation are still unclear.

ETS1 is a common integration site in Moloney MuLV-induced T cell lymphomas in mice. Two *ETS* genes, *FLI1* (Friend leukaemia virus integration-1) and *SPI1* (SFFV integration-1), also named PU.1, were discovered in Friend virus-induced erythroleukaemias. The viral integration resulted in the deregulated expression of SPI1-/PU.1 or FLI1. These tumours also contained a mutated p53 gene created by an additional viral integration or by point mutation (for review see ref. 125).

5.5 Translocations activate ETS genes in human tumours

Recently, several very exciting links between *ETS* family genes and human tumorigenesis have been established by the characterization of specific chromosomal translocations associated with particular tumour types (Figure 7 and Chapter 1). These genomic rearrangements create chimeric fusion proteins between the DNA binding domain of an ETS protein and a heterologous protein. The first of these chimeras, a fusion of the 5' end of the *EWS* gene, encoding an activation domain, to the 3' end of the *FLI1* gene, encoding the ETS domain, was identified by cloning the breakpoint from the t(11;22) translocation in Ewing's sarcoma (126). Subsequently, similar fusions of the two ETS genes *ERG* and *ETV1* to *EWS* were identified in Ewing's sarcomas (127, 128) and *TLS–ERG* fusions were identified in myeloid leukaemia (129). *EWS* and *TLS* encode homologous and ubiquitously expressed RNA binding proteins (130). Although the normal functions of the two wild-type proteins are not yet under-

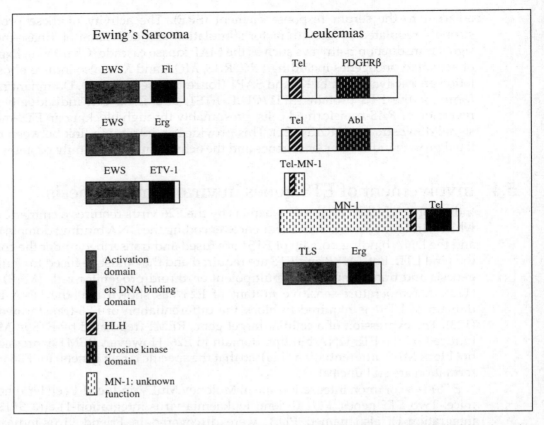

Fig. 7 Translocations fuse *ETS* genes with heterologous genes in human tumours. In Ewing's sarcoma, the amino terminus of EWS, which contains an activation domain, is fused to the ETS domain of FLI1, ERG, or ETV1 creating chimeric transcription factors. A similar fusion between TLS, which is homologous to EWS, and ERG is found in myeloid leukaemia. The ETS gene *TEL* is involved in several different leukaemias. The fusion of the HLH domain of TEL with the tyrosine kinases PDGFRβ and ABL may cause dimerization and constitutive kinase activity in the chimzeras. The mechanism of action of TEL–MN1 fusions are unclear, but the HLH domain is disrupted by the translocation.

stood, their amino terminal domains are retained in the chimeras and possess potent transcriptional activity (131, 132).

The chimeric transcription factors generated by chromosomal translocation in these tumours are capable of transforming fibroblasts in culture. In the case of EWS–FLI1 fusions, transforming activity requires both the transactivation domain provided by EWS and the ETS DNA binding domain from the FLI1 protein (133). It is unlikely that the ETS domains are recognizing novel target sequences, as the DNA binding specificity of the chimera is the same as the wild-type proteins *in vitro* (131). However, the synergistic effect of higher order interactions between ETS proteins and heterologous proteins at adjacent binding sites may dictate which genes are targeted for transcription. Thus, replacement of the interaction domain from the ETS family gene with a heterologous domain could target a different gene(s) without changing *in vitro* DNA binding specificity. Furthermore, the introduced activation domain may co-operate with other factors, or respond to signal transduction pathways that do not ordinarily affect the activity of the wild-type transcription factor. The activation domains of the EWS and TLS proteins have also been fused to the DNA binding domains of other transcription factors including leucine zipper and zinc-finger proteins in other human tumours (134, 135 and Chapter 1). Such translocations may represent a common mechanism for the conversion of transcription factors to onco-genic proteins.

Additional translocation events involving the *ETS*-family member *TEL* (trans-location, ets, leukaemia), creates a different class of fusion protein. In chronic myelomonocytic leukaemia, a translocation fuses the amino terminus of TEL, which contains some homology to HLH domains, to the transmembrane and tyrosine kinase domains of platelet-derived growth factor receptor β (PDGFRβ; 136 and Chapter 3). The ETS domain of TEL is lost in the translocation. Similarly, in human leukaemia, translocations generate ABL-TEL fusions with increased tyrosine kinase activity compared to wild-type ABL (Chapter 4). It is possible that the HLH domain of TEL mediates dimerization in PDGFRβ and ABL fusions (137). Translocation of *TEL* is also involved in myeloid leukaemias and myelodysplastic syndrome. Reciprocal translocation creates a fusion protein between the meningioma associated gene *MN1* and *TEL*, similar to the fusions seen in Ewing's sarcoma. The reciprocal translocation creates a *TEL–MN1* fusion that is also expressed in the tumours. It is presently unclear if only one or both of the two fusion proteins is required for the formation of the tumour. In a subset of the tumours, the HLH domain of TEL is disrupted by the translocation, so that the contribution of TEL to the resulting chimera may be differ-ent than in the tyrosine kinase fusions (138). However, it seems clear that transloca-tions involving *TEL* are involved in several different myelodysplastic disorders.

6. Conclusions

Oncogenes involved in viral tumorigenesis in chickens or mice are not always direct targets for genetic alteration in human neoplasia. However, the characterization of upstream and downstream modulators of transcription factor activity shows extensive overlap among gene families as targets and/or effectors of signalling path-ways. For example, there have been reports that ETS, MYB, and AP-1 stimulate *MYC* expression in different situations (139–142). An activated *RAF* or *RAS* gene leads to activation of the ETS family member ELK1, which in turn stimulates transcription from the *c-FOS* promoter. It is likely that a number of oncogenes exert their trans-forming activity through the regulation of, or interaction with, other oncogenes.

The intricacies of transcription factor function and regulation in the context of *in vivo* biology become more apparent through the evaluation of transgenic and knock-out animal models that mutate or delete specific genes. Transgenic mice carrying a *c-MYC* gene under the control of the Eµ immunoglobulin enhancer, functionally recreating the frequent t(8;14) translocation in human Burkitt's lymphoma, have a predisposition to develop B cell malignancies (143–145). Transgenic mice carrying the N- or L-MYC gene under the control of the Eμ enhancer are also predisposed to lymphomas, albeit with a longer latency and at a lower incidence (146, 147). The cyclin D1 gene has also been implicated in human B cell neoplasia through a t(11;14) translocation that brings the cyclin D1 gene under the control of the Eμ enhancer, similar to the translocations involving c-MYC in Burkitt's lymphoma (148 and Chapter 1). In contrast to Eμ–MYC mice, transgenic mice carrying an Eμ–cyclin D transgene do not develop lymphoid tumours. However, when Eμ–cyclin D mice are bred with Eμ N- or L-MYC mice, the double transgenic mice develop B cell lymphomas with significantly higher incidence and decreased latency relative to mice bearing an N- or L-MYC transgene alone. There is no enhancement in T cell lymphomagenesis (149). Thus, transgenic mice can provide a model system to study tissue-specificity and synergistic interactions among oncogenes.

'Knock-out mice', or mice containing a homozygous null mutation of a gene, have also provided novel insights into the requirement for a gene in growth and development. Mice that are homozygous for null mutations in c-FOS are less viable than wild-type littermates and develop defects in bone formation, gametogenesis, and haematopoiesis (150, 151). A subset of AP-1 target genes could not be induced in c-FOS deficient fibroblasts, but c-FOS deficient mice display normal peripheral T cell function (152, 153). Thus, despite the central role that FOS appears to play in the response to diverse signalling pathways in multiple tissues, the complete organism is able to compensate for the loss of FOS in some circumstances. It is unclear what extent of that compensation is provided through redundancy in the form of other FOS–JUN family members. The existence of related genes does not ensure the ability to overcome the deletion of a gene. A homozygous null mutation at the c-JUN, c-MYC, or N-MYC locus causes embryonic lethality by mid-gestation (154–157). The specific contribution of a gene throughout development can be further understood by creating partial loss of function mutations such as 'leaky mutations', which allow synthesis of decreased levels of wild-type protein, or conditional knock-outs, in which the normal gene is disrupted only in a specific tissue or stage of development (158). In the case of the N-MYC gene, a leaky mutation allowed the embryos to survive past the block in gestation seen in the null mice, and revealed dramatic defects in heart and lung development (159, 160).

One of the major challenges currently facing the field of molecular oncology is to understand the complexity of signalling networks. Traditional approaches to cell biology generally involve reductionist strategies that cannot elucidate signalling pathways that have redundant components permitting flexible responses and compensation mechanisms. A combination of molecular biology, genetics, cell biology, biochemistry, and the development of animal models will be required to elucidate the role of oncogenic transcription factors in tumorigenesis, and hopefully, the development of novel strategies for therapeutic intervention.

References

1. Reddy, E. P., Skalka, A. M., and Curran, T. (ed.) (1988) *The oncogene handbook 1* Elsevier Science Publishers: Amsterdam.
2. Curran, T. and Franza, B., Jr. (1988) Fos and Jun: the AP-1 connection. *Cell*, 55, 395.
3. Kerppola, T. K. and Curran, T. (1991) Transcription factor interactions: basics on zippers. *Curr. Opin. Struct. Biol.*, 1, 71.
4. Kerppola, T. K. and Curran, T. (1994) A conserved region adjacent to the basic domain is required for recognition of an extended DNA binding site by Maf/Nrl family proteins. *Oncogene*, 9, 3149.
5. Kataoka, K., Noda, M., and Nishizawa, M. (1994) Maf nuclear oncoprotein recognizes sequences related to an AP-1 site and forms heterodimers with both Fos and Jun. *Mol. Cell. Biol.*, 14, 700.
6. Morgan, J. I. and Curran, T. (1991) Stimulus-transcription coupling in the nervous system: involvement of the inducible proto-oncogenes fos and jun. *Annu. Rev. Neurosci.*, 14, 421.
7. Xanthoudakis, S. and Curran, T. (1994) Analysis of c-Fos and c-Jun redox-dependent DNA binding activity. *Methods Enzymol.*, 234, 163.
8. Baker, S. J., Kerppola, T. K., Luk, D., Vandenberg, M. T., Marshak, D. R., Curran, T., *et al.* (1992) Jun is phosphorylated by several protein kinases at the same sites that are modified in serum-stimulated fibroblasts. *Mol. Cell. Biol.*, 12, 4694.
9. Abate, C., Baker, S. J., Lees-Miller, S. P., Anderson, C. W., Marshak, D. R., and Curran, T. (1993) Dimerization and DNA binding alter phosphorylation of Fos and Jun. *Proc. Natl. Acad. Sci. USA*, 90, 6766.
10. Sluss, H. K., Barrett, T., Derijard, B., and Davis, R. J. (1994) Signal transduction by tumor necrosis factor mediated by JNK protein kinases. *Mol. Cell. Biol.*, 14, 8376.
11. Sanchez, I., Hughes, R. T., Mayer, B. J., Yee, K., Woodgett, J. R., Avruch, J., *et al.* (1994) Role of SAPK/ERK kinase-1 in the stress-activated pathway regulating transcription factor c-Jun. *Nature*, 372, 794.
12. Wang, Z. Q., Grigoriadis, A. E., Mohle-Steinlein, U., and Wagner, E. F. (1991) A novel target cell for c-fos-induced oncogenesis: development of chondrogenic tumours in embryonic stem cell chimeras. *EMBO J.*, 10, 2437.
13. Grigoriadis, A. E., Schellander, K., Wang, Z. Q., and Wagner, E. F. (1993) Osteoblasts are target cells for transformation in c-fos transgenic mice. *J. Cell Biol.*, 122, 685.
14. Wisdon, R. and Verma, I. M. (1993) Transformation by Fos proteins requires a C-terminal transactivation domain. *Mol. Cell. Biol.*, 13, 7429.
15. Jooss, K. U., Funk, M., and Muller, R. (1994) An autonomous N-terminal transactivation domain in Fos protein plays a crucial role in transformation. *EMBO J.*, 13, 1467.
16. Yoshida, T., Shindo, Y., Ohta, K., and Iba, H. (1989) Identification of a small region of the v-fos gene product that is sufficient for transforming potential and growth-stimulating activity. *Oncogene Res.*, 5, 79.
17. Oliviero, S., Robinson, G. S., Struhl, K., and Spiegelman, B. M. (1992) Yeast GCN4 as a probe for oncogenesis by AP-1 transcription factors: transcriptional activation through AP-1 sites is not sufficient for cellular transformation. *Genes Dev.*, 6, 1799.
18. Van Amsterdam, J. R., Wang, Y., Sullivan, R. C., and Zarbl, H. (1994) Elevated expression of the junB proto-oncogene is essential for v-fos induced transformation of Rat-1 cells. *Oncogene*, 9, 2969.

19. Miao, G. G. and Curran, T. (1994) Cell transformation by c-fos requires an extended period of expression and is independent of the cell cycle. *Mol. Cell. Biol.*, 14, 4295.

20. Curran, T. and Vogt, P. K. (1992) Dangerous liaisons: Fos and Jun, oncogenic transcription factors. In *Transcriptional regulation*, p. 797. Cold Spring Harbor Laboratory Press.

21. Suzuki, T., Hashimoto, Y., Okuno, H., Sato, H., Nishina, H., and Iba, H. (1991) High-level expression of human c-jun gene causes cellular transformation of chicken embryo fibroblasts. *Japan J. Cancer Res.*, 82, 58.

22. Schuur, E. R., Parker, E. J., and Vogt, P. K. (1993) Chimeras of herpes simplex viral VP16 and jun are oncogenic. *Cell Growth Diff.*, 4, 761.

23. Catling, A. D., Wyke, J. A., and Frame, M. C. (1993) Mitogenesis of quiescent chick fibroblasts by v-Src: dependence on events at the membrane leading to early changes in AP-1. *Oncogene*, 8, 1875.

24. Suzuki, T., Murakami, M., Onai, N., Fukuda, E., Hashimoto, Y., Sonobe, M. H. *et al.* (1994) Analysis of AP1 function in cellular transformation pathways. *J. Virol.*, 68, 3527.

25. Schuh, A. C., Keating, S. J., Yeung, M. C., and Breitman, M. L. (1992) Skeletal muscle arises as a late event during development of wound sarcomas in v-jun transgenic mice. *Oncogene*, 7, 667.

26. Bossy-Wetzel, E., Bravo, R., and Hanahan, D. (1992) Transcription factors junB and c-jun are selectively up-regulated and functionally implicated in fibrosarcoma development. *Genes Dev.*, 6, 2340.

27. Erisman, M. D. and Astrin, S. M. (1988) The myc oncogene. In *The oncogene handbook* (ed. E. P. Reddy, A. M. Skalka, and T. Curran), p. 341. Elsevier Science Publishers, Amsterdam.

28. Luscher, B. and Eisenman, R. N. (1990) New light on Myc and Myb. Part I. Myc. *Genes Dev.*, 4, 2025.

29. Koskinen, P. J. and Alitalo, K. (1993) Role of myc amplification and overexpression in cell growth, differentiation and death. *Semin. Cancer Biol.*, 4, 3.

30. Garte, S. J. (1993) The c-myc oncogene in tumor progression. *Crit. Rev. Oncog.* 4, 435.

31. Bhatia, K., Spangler, G., Gaidano, G., Hamdy, N., Dalla-Favera, R., and Magrath, I. (1994) Mutations in the coding region of c-myc occur frequently in acquired immunodeficiency syndrome-associated lymphomas. *Blood*, 84, 883.

32. Gauwerky, C. E. and Croce, C. M. (1993) Chromosomal translocations in leukaemia. *Semin. Cancer Biol.*, 4, 333.

33. Bhatia, K., Huppi, K., Spangler, G., Siwarski, D., Iyer, R., and Magrath, I. (1993) Point mutations in the c-Myc transactivation domain are common in Burkitt's lymphoma and mouse plasmacytomas. *Nat. Genet.*, 5, 56.

34. Yano, T., Sander, C. A., Clark, H. M., Dolezal, M. V., Jaffe, E. S., and Raffeld, M. (1993) Clustered mutations in the second exon of the MYC gene in sporadic Burkitt's lymphoma. *Oncogene*, 8, 2741.

35. Clark, H. M., Yano, T., Otsuki, T., Jaffe, E. S., Shibata, D., and Raffeld, M. (1994) Mutations in the coding region of c-MYC in AIDS-associated and other aggressive lymphomas. *Cancer Res.*, 54, 3383.

36. Schwab, M. and Amler, L. C. (1990) Amplification of cellular oncogenes: a predictor of clinical outcome in human cancer. *Genes Chrom. Cancer*, 1, 181.

37. Barrios, C., Castresana, J. S., Ruiz, J., and Kreicbergs, A. (1994) Amplification of the c-myc proto-oncogene in soft tissue sarcomas. *Oncology*, 51, 13.

38. Berns, E. M., Klijn, J. G., van Stavern, I. L., Portengen, H., Noordegraff, E., and Foekens,

J. A. (1992) Prevalence of amplification of the oncogenes c-myc, HER2/neu, and int-2 in one thousand human breast tumours: correlation with steroid receptors. *Eur. J. Cancer,* 28, 697.

39. Johnson, B. E., Brennan, J. F., Ihde, D. C., and Gazdar, A. F. (1992) myc family DNA amplification in tumors and tumor cell lines from patients with small-cell lung cancer. *Monogr. Natl. Cancer Inst.,* 13, 39.

40. Schwab, M. (1990) Oncogene amplification in neoplastic development and progression of human cancers. *Crit. Rev. Oncog.,* 2, 35.

41. Fuller, G. N. and Bigner, S. H. (1992) Amplified cellular oncogenes in neoplasms of the human central nervous system. *Mutat. Res.,* 276, 299.

42. Evan, G. I. and Littlewood, T. D. (1993) The role of c-myc in cell growth. *Curr. Opin. Genet. Dev.,* 3, 44.

43. Roussel, M. F., Cleveland, J. L., Shurtleff, S. A., and Sherr, C. J. (1991) Myc rescue of a mutant CSF1 receptor impaired in mitogenic signalling. *Nature,* 353, 361.

44. Eilers, M., Schirm, S., and Bishop, J. M. (1991) The MYC protein activates transcription of the alpha-prothymosin gene. *EMBO J.,* 10, 133.

45. Dang, C. V., Barrett, J., Villa-Garcia, M., Resar, L. M., Kato, G. J., and Fearon, E. R. (1991) Intracellular leucine zipper interactions suggest c-Myc hetero-oligomerization. *Mol. Cell. Biol.,* 11, 954.

46. Littlewood, T. D., Amati, B., Land, H., and Evan, G. I. (1992) Max and c-Myc/Max DNA-binding activities in cell extracts. *Oncogene,* 7, 1783.

47. Amati, B. and Land, H. (1994) Myc-Max-Mad: a transcription factor network controlling cell cycle progression, differentiation and death. *Curr. Opin. Genet. Dev.,* 4, 102.

48. Blackwood, E. M. and Eisenman, R. N. (1991) Max: a helix-loop-helix zipper protein that forms a sequence-specific DNA-binding complex with Myc. *Science,* 251, 1211.

49. Prendergast, G. C., Lawe, D., and Ziff, E. B. (1991) Association of Myn, the murine homolog of max, with c-Myc stimulates methylation-sensitive DNA binding and ras cotransformation. *Cell,* 65, 395.

50. Amati, B., Dalton, S., Brooks, M. W., Littlewood, T. D., Evan, G. I., and Land, H. (1992) Transcriptional activation by the human c-Myc oncoprotein in yeast requires interaction with Max. *Nature,* 359, 423.

51. Reddy, C. D., Dasgupta, P., Saikumar, P., Dudek, H., Rauscher, F., and Reddy, E. P. (1992) Mutational analysis of Max: role of basic, helix-loop-helix/leucine zipper domains in DNA binding, dimerization and regulation of Myc-mediated transcriptional activation. *Oncogene,* 7, 2085.

52. Blackwell, T. K., Huang, J., Ma, A., Kretzner, L., Alt, F. W., Eisenman, R. N., *et al.* (1993) Binding of myc proteins to canonical and noncanonical DNA sequences. *Mol. Cell. Biol.,* 13, 5216.

53. Ayer, D. E., Kretzner, L., and Eisenman, R. N. (1993) Mad: a heterodimeric partner for Max that antagonizes Myc transcriptional activity. *Cell,* 72, 211.

54. Zervos, A. S., Gyuris, J., and Brent, R. (1993) Mxi1, a protein that specifically interacts with Max to bind Myc-Max recognition sites. *Cell,* 72, 223.

55. Larsson, L. G., Pettersson, M., Oberg, F., Nilsson, K., and Luscher, B. (1994) Expression of mad, mxi1, max and c-myc during induced differentiation of hematopoietic cells: opposite regulation of mad and c-myc. *Oncogene,* 9, 1247.

56. Ayer, D. E. and Eisenman, R. N. (1993) A switch from Myc:Max to Mad:Max heterocomplexes accompanies monocyte/macrophage differentiation. *Genes Dev.,* 7, 2110.

57. Ayer, D. E., Lawrence, Q. A., and Eisenman, R. N. (1995) Mad-Max transcriptional repression is mediated by ternary complex formation with mammalian homologs of yeast repressor Sin3. *Cell*, 80, 767.

58. Schreiber-Agus, N., Chin, L., Chen, K., Torres, R., Rao, G., Guida, P., *et al.* (1995) An amino-terminal domain of Mxi1 mediates anti-myc oncogenic activity and interacts with a homolog of the yeast transcriptional repressor SIN3. *Cell*, 80, 777.

59. Gupta, S., Seth, A., and Davis, R. J. (1993) Transactivation of gene expression by Myc is inhibited by mutation at the phosphorylation sites Thr-58 and Ser-62. *Proc. Natl. Acad. Sci. USA*, 90, 3216.

60. Lutterbach, B. and Hann, S. R. (1994) Hierarchical phosphorylation at N-terminal transformation-sensitive sites in c-Myc protein is regulated by mitogens and in mitosis. *Mol. Cell. Biol.*, 14, 5510.

61. Berberich, S. J. and Cole, M. D. (1992) Casein kinase II inhibits the DNA-binding activity of Max homodimers but not Myc/Max heterodimers. *Genes Dev.*, 6, 166.

62. Bousset, K., Henriksson, M., Luscher-Firzlaff, J. M., Litchfield, D. W., and Luscher, B. (1993) Identification of casein kinase II phosphorylation sites in Max: effects on DNA-binding kinetics of Max homo- and Myc/Max heterodimers. *Oncogene*, 8, 3211.

63. Rustgi, A. K., Dyson, N., and Bernards, R. (1991) Amino-terminal domains of c-myc and N-myc proteins mediate binding to the retinoblastoma gene product. *Nature*, 352, 541.

64. Beijersbergen, R. L., Hijmans, E. M., Zhu, L., and Bernards, R. (1994) Interaction of c-Myc with the pRb-related protein p107 results in inhibition of c-Myc-mediated transactivation. *EMBO J.*, 13, 4080.

65. Adnane, J. and Robbins, P. D. (1995) The retinoblastoma susceptibility gene product regulates Myc-mediated transcription. *Oncogene*, 10, 381.

66. Gu, W., Bhatia, K., Magrath, I. T., Dang, C. V., and Dalla-Favera, R. (1994) Binding and suppression of the Myc transcriptional activation domain by p107. *Science*, 264, 251.

67. Hateboer, G., Timmers, H. T., Rustgi, A. K., Billaud, M., van't Veer, L. J., and Bernards, R. (1993) TATA-binding protein and the retinoblastoma gene product bind to overlapping epitopes on c-Myc and adenovirus E1A protein. *Proc. Natl. Acad. Sci. USA*, 90, 8489.

68. Roy, A. L., Carruthers, C., Gutjahr, T., and Roeder, R. G. (1994) Direct role for Myc in transcription initiation mediated by interactions with TFII-I. *Nature*, 365, 359.

69. Shrivastava, A., Saleque, S., Kalpana, G. V., Artandi, S., Goff, S. P., and Calame, K. (1993) Inhibition of transcriptional regulator Yin-Yang-1 by association with c-Myc. *Science*, 262, 1889.

70. Sherr, C. J. and Roberts, J. M. (1995) Inhibitors of mammalian G1 cyclin-dependent kinases. *Genes Dev.*, **9**, 1149.

71. Philipp, A., Schneider, A., Vasrik, I., Finke, K., Xiong, Y., Beach, D., *et al.* (1994) Repression of cyclin D1: a novel function of MYC. *Mol. Cell. Biol.*, 14, 4032.

72. Hermeking, H. and Eick, D. (1994) Mediation of c-Myc-induced apoptosis by p53. *Science*, 265, 2091.

73. Packham, G. and Cleveland, J. L. (1994) Ornithine decarboxylase is a mediator of c-Myc-induced apoptosis. *Mol. Cell. Biol.*, 14, 5741.

74. Gaubatz, S., Meichle, A., and Eilers, M. (1994) An E-box element localized in the first intron mediates regulation of the prothymosin alpha gene by c-myc. *Mol. Cell. Biol.*, 14, 3853.

75. Benvenisty, N., Leder, A., Kuo, A., and Leder, P. (1992) An embryonically expressed gene is a target for c-Myc regulation via the c-Myc-binding sequence. *Genes Dev.*, 6, 2513.

76. Bello-Fernandez, C., Packham, G., and Cleveland, J. L. (1993) The ornithine decarboxylase gene is a transcriptional target of c-Myc. *Proc. Natl. Acad. Sci. USA*, 90, 7804.

77. Reisman, D., Elkind, N. B., Roy, B., Beamon, J., and Rotter, V. (1993) c-Myc transactivates the p53 promoter through a required downstream CACGTG motif. *Cell Growth Diff.*, 4, 57.

78. Jansen-Durr, P., Meichle, A, Steiner, P., Pagano, M., Finke, K., Botz, J., *et al.* (1993) Differential modulation of cyclin gene expression by MYC. *Proc. Natl. Acad. Sci. USA*, 90, 3685.

79. Li, L. H., Nerlov, C., Prendergast, G., MacGregor, D., and Ziff, E. B. (1994) c-Myc represses transcription in vivo by a novel mechanism dependent on the initiator element and Myc box II. *EMBO J.*, 13, 4070.

80. Reddy, E. P. (1988) The myb oncogene. In *The oncogene handbook* (ed. E. P. Reddy, A. M. Skalka, and T. Curran), p. 327. Elsevier Science Publishers, Amsterdam.

81. Luscher, B. and Eisenman, R. N. (1990) New light on Myc and Myb. Part II. Myb. *Genes Dev.*, 4, 2235.

82. Ogata, K., Morikawa, S., Nakamura, H., Sekikawa, A., Inoue, T., Kanai, H., *et al.* (1994) Solution structure of a specific DNA complex of the Myb DNA-binding domain with cooperative recognition helices. *Cell*, 79, 639.

83. Patel, G., Kreider, B., Rovera, G., and Reddy, E. P. (1993) v-myb blocks granulocyte colony-stimulating factor-induced myeloid cell differentiation but not proliferation. *Mol. Cell. Biol.*, 13, 2269.

84. Cuddihy, A. E., Brents, L. A., Aziz, N., Bender, T. P., and Kuehl, W. M. (1993) Only the DNA binding and transactivation domains of c-Myb are required to block terminal differentiation of murine erythroleukemia cells. *Mol. Cell. Biol.*, 13, 3505.

85. Press, R. D., Reddy, E. P., and Ewert, D. L. (1994) Overexpression of C-terminally but not N-terminally truncated Myb induces fibrosarcomas: a novel nonhematopoietic target cell for the myb oncogene. *Mol. Cell. Biol.*, 14, 2278.

86. Barletta, C., Pelicci, P. G., Kenyon, L. C., Smith, S. D., and Dalla-Favera, R. (1987) Relationship between the c-myb locus and the 6q-chromosomal aberration in leukemias and lymphomas. *Science*, 235, 1064.

87. Dasgupta, P., Linnenbach, A. J., Giaccia, A. J., Stamato, T. D., and Reddy, E. P. (1989) Molecular cloning of the breakpoint region on chromosome 6 in cutaneous malignant melanoma: evidence for deletion in the c-myb locus and translocation of a segment of chromosome 12. *Oncogene*, 4, 1201.

88. Park, J. G. and Reddy, E. P. (1992) Large-scale molecular mapping of human c-myb locus: c-myb proto-oncogene is not involved in 6q- abnormalities of lymphoid tumors. *Oncogene*, 7, 1603.

89. Toth, C. R., Hostutler, R. F., Baldwin, A. S., and Bender, T. P. (1995) Members of the nuclear factor κB family transactivate the murine *c-myb* gene. *J. Biol. Chem.*, 270, 7661.

90. Dasgupta, P. and Reddy, E. P. (1989) Identification of alternatively spliced transcripts for human c-myb: molecular cloning and sequence analysis of human c-myb exon 9A sequences. *Oncogene*, 4, 1419.

91. Shen-Ong, G. L., Luscher, B., and Eisenman, R. N. (1989) A second c-myb protein is translated from an alternatively spliced mRNA expressed from normal and 5'-disrupted myb loci. *Mol. Cell. Biol.*, 9, 5456.

92. Weber, B. L., Westin, E. H., and Clarke, M. F. (1990) Differentiation of mouse ery-throleukemia cells enhanced by alternatively spliced c-myb mRNA. *Science*, 249, 1291.

93. Nomura, T., Sakai, N., Sarai, A., Sudo, T., Kanei-Ishii, C., Ramsay, R. G. *et al.* (1993) Negative autoregulation of c-Myb activity by homodimer formation through the leucine zipper. *J. Biol. Chem.*, 268, 21914.

94. Vorbrueggen, G., Kalkbrenner, F., Guehmann, S., and Moelling, K. (1994) The car-boxyterminus of human c-myb protein stimulates activated transcription in trans. *Nucleic Acids Res.*, 22, 2466.

95. Favier, D. and Gonda, T. J. (1994) Detection of proteins that bind to the leucine zipper motif of c-Myb. *Oncogene*, 9, 305.

96. Luscher, B., Christenson, E., Litchfield, D. W., Krebs, E. G., and Eisenman, R. N. (1990) Myb DNA binding inhibited by phosphorylation at a site deleted during oncogenic activation. *Nature*, 344, 517.

97. Myrset, A. H., Bostad, A., Jamin, N., Lirsac, P. N., Toma, F., and Gabrielsen, O. S. (1993) DNA and redox state induced conformational changes in the DNA-binding domain of the Myb oncoprotein. *EMBO J.*, 12, 4625.

98. Ness, S. A., Marknell, A., and Graf, T. (1989) The v-myb oncogene product binds to and activates the promyelocyte-specific mim-1 gene. *Cell*, 59, 1115.

99. Aurigemma, R. E., Blair, D. G., and Ruscetti, S. K. (1992) Transactivation of erythroid transcription factor GATA-1 by a myb-ets-containing retrovirus. *J. Virol.*, 66, 3056.

100. Ku, D. H., Wen, S. C., Engelhard, A., Nicolaides, N. C., Lipson, K. E., Marino, T. A., *et al.* (1993) c-myb transactivates cdc2 expression via Myb binding sites in the 5′-flanking region of the human cdc2 gene [published erratum appears in *J. Biol. Chem.* 1993 268, 13010]. *J. Biol. Chem.*, 268, 2255.

101. Siu, G., Wurster, A. L., Lipsick, J. S., and Hedrick, S. M. (1992) Expression of the CD4 gene requires a Myb transcription factor. *Mol. Cell. Biol.*, 12, 1592.

102. Melotti, P. and Calabretta, B. (1994) Ets-2 and c-Myb act independently in regulating expression of the hematopoietic stem cell antigen CD34. *J. Biol. Chem.*, 269, 25303.

103. Dasgupta, P., Reddy, C. D., Saikumar, P., and Reddy, E. P. (1992) The cellular proto-oncogene product Myb acts as transcriptional activator of the long terminal repeat of human T-lymphotropic virus type I. *J. Virol.*, 66, 270.

104. Foos, G., Natour, S., and Klempnauer, K. H. (1993) TATA-box dependent transactiva-tion of the human HSP70 promoter by Myb proteins. *Oncogene*, 8, 1775.

105. Cogswell, J. P., Cogswell, P. C., Kuehl, W. M., Cuddihy, A. M., Bender, T. M., Engelke, U., *et al.* (1993) Mechanism of c-myc regulation by c-Myb in different cell lineages. *Mol. Cell. Biol.*, 13, 2858.

106. Introna, M., Luchetti, M., Castellano, M., Arsura, M., and Golay, J. (1994) The myb oncogene family of transcription factors: potent regulators of hematopoietic cell prolif-eration and differentiation. *Semin. Cancer Biol.*, 5, 113.

107. Mettus, R. V., Litvin, J., Wali, A., Toscani, A., Latham, K., Hatton, K., *et al.* (1994) Murine A-myb: evidence for differential splicing and tissue-specific expression. *Onco-gene*, 9, 3077.

108. Mizuguchi, G., Nakagoshi, H., Nagase, T., Nomura, N., Date, T., Ueno, Y., *et al.* (1990) DNA binding activity and transcriptional activator function of the human B-myb pro-tein compared with c-MYB. *J. Biol. Chem.*, 265, 9280.

109. Watson, R. J., Robinson, C., and Lam, E. W. (1993) Transcription regulation by murine B-myb is distinct from that by c-myb. *Nucleic Acids Res.*, 21, 267.

110. Lam, E. W., Morris, J. D., Davies, R., Crook, T., Watson, R. J., and Vousden, K. H. (1994) HPV 16 E7 oncoprotein deregulates B-myb expression: correlation with targeting of p107/E2F complexes. *EMBO J.*, 13, 871.

111. Seth, A., Ascione, R., Fisher, R. J., Mavrothalassitis, G. J., Bhat, N. K., and Papas, T. S. (1992) The ets gene family. *Cell Growth Diff.*, 3, 327.

112. Mavrothalassitis, G., Fisher, R. J., Smyth, F., Watson, D. K., and Papas, T. S. (1994) Structural inferences of the ETS1 DNA-binding domain determined by mutational analysis. *Oncogene*, 9, 425.

113. Donaldson, L. W., Petersen, J. M., Graves, B. J., and McIntosh, L. P. (1994) Secondary structure of the ETS domain places murine Ets-1 in the superfamily of winged helix-turn-helix DNA-binding proteins. *Biochemistry*, 33, 13509.

114. Lim, F., Kraut, N., Framptom, J., and Graf, T. (1992) DNA binding by c-Ets-1, but not v-Ets, is repressed by an intramolecular mechanism. *EMBO J.*, 11, 643.

115. Wang, C. Y., Petryniak, B., Ho, I. C., Thompson, C. B., and Leiden, J. M. (1992) Evolutionarily conserved Ets family members display distinct DNA binding specificities [published erratum appears in *J. Exp. Med.* 1993 178, 1133]. *J. Exp. Med.*, 175, 1391.

116. Wotton, D., Ghysdael, J., Wang, S., Speck, N. A., and Owen, M. J. (1994) Cooperative binding of Ets-1 and core binding factor to DNA. *Mol. Cell. Biol.*, 14, 840.

117. Treisman, R. (1994) Ternary complex factors: growth factor regulated transcriptional activators. *Curr. Opin. Genet. Dev.*, 4, 96.

118. Pongubala, J. M., Nagulapalli, S., Klemsz, M. J., McKercher, S. R., Maki, R. A., and Atchison, M. L. (1992) PU.1 recruits a second nuclear factor to a site important for immunoglobulin kappa 3′ enhancer activity. *Mol. Cell. Biol.*, 12, 368.

119. Clark, N. M., Smith, M. J., Hilfinger, J. M., and Markovitz, D. M. (1993) Activation of the human T-cell leukemia virus type I enhancer is mediated by binding sites for Elf-1 and the pets factor. *J. Virol.*, 67, 5522.

120. La Marco, K., Thompson, C. C., Byers, B. P., Walton, E. M., and McKnight, S. L. (1991) Identification of Ets- and notch-related subunits in GA binding protein. *Science*, 253, 789.

121. Wasylyk, C., Maira, S. M., Sobieszczuk, P., and Wasylyk, B. (1994) Reversion of Ras transformed cells by Ets transdominant mutants. *Oncogene*, 9, 3665.

122. Metz, T. and Graf, T. (1991) Fusion of the nuclear oncoproteins v-Myb and v-Ets is required for the leukemogenicity of E26 virus. *Cell*, 66, 95.

123. Kraut, N., Frampton, J., McNagny, K. M., and Graf, T. (1994) A functional Ets DNA-binding domain is required to maintain multipotency of hematopoietic progenitors transformed by Myb-Ets. *Genes Dev.*, 8, 33.

124. Kraut, N., Frampton, J., and Graf, T. (1995) Rem-1, a putative direct target gene of the Myb-Ets fusion oncoprotein in haematopoietic progenitors, is a member of the recoverin family. *Oncogene*, 10, 1027.

125. Ben-David, Y. and Bernstein, A. (1991) Friend virus-induced erythroleukemia and the multistage nature of cancer. *Cell*, 66, 831.

126. Delattre, O., Zucman, J., Plougastel, B., Desmaze, C., Melot, T., Peter, M., *et al.* (1992) Gene fusion with an ETS DNA-binding domain caused by chromosome translocation in human tumours. *Nature*, 359, 162.

127. Sorensen, P. H., Lessnick, S. L., Lopez-Terrada, D., Liu, X. F., Triche, T. J., and Denny, C. T. (1994) A second Ewing's sarcoma translocation, t(21; 22), fuses the EWS gene to another ETS-family transcription factor, ERG. *Nat. Genet.*, 6, 146.

128. Jeon, I.-S., Davis, J. N., Braun, B. S., Sublett, J. E., Roussel, M. F., Denny, C. T., *et al.* (1995) A varian Ewing's sarcoma translocation (7;22) fuses the EWS genes to the ETS gene ETV1. *Oncogene,* 10, 1229.

129. Ichikawa, H., Shimizu, K., Hayashi, Y., and Ohki, M. (1994) An RNA-binding protein gene, TLS/FUS, is fused to ERG in human myeloid leukemia with t(16;21) chromosomal translocation. *Cancer Res.,* 54, 2865.

130. Crozat, A., Aman, P., Mandahl, N., and Ron, D. (1993) Fusion of CHOP to a novel RNA-binding protein in human myxoid liposarcoma. *Nature,* 363, 640.

131. Bailly, R. A., Bosselut, R., Zucman, J., Cormier, F., Delattre, O., Roussel, M., *et al.* (1994) DNA-binding and transcriptional activation properties of the EWS-FLI-1 fusion protein resulting from the t(11; 22) translocation in Ewing sarcoma. *Mol. Cell. Biol.,* 14, 3230.

132. Zinszner, H., Albalat, R., and Ron, D. (1994) A novel effector domain from the RNA-binding protein TLS or EWS is required for oncogenic transformation by CHOP. *Genes Dev.,* 8, 2513.

133. May, W. A., Gishizky, M. L., Lessnick, S. L., Lunsford, L. B., Lewis, B. C., Delattre, O., *et al.* (1993) Ewing sarcoma 11; 22 translocation produces a chimeric transcription factor that requires the DNA-binding domain encoded by FLI1 for transformation. *Proc. Natl. Acad. Sci. USA,* 90, 5752.

134. Zucman, J., Delattre, O., Desmaze, C., Epstein, A. L., Stenman, G., Speleman, F., *et al.* (1993) EWS and ATF-1 gene fusion induced by t(12; 22) translocation in malignant melanoma of soft parts. *Nat. Genet.,* 4, 341.

135. Ladanyi, M. and Gerald, W. (1994) Fusion of the EWS and WT1 genes in the desmoplastic small round cell tumor. *Cancer Res.,* 54, 2837.

136. Golub, T. R., Barker, G. F., Lovett, M., and Gilliland, D. G. (1994) Fusion of PDGF receptor beta to a novel ets-like gene, tel, in chronic myelomonocytic leukemia with t(5; 12) chromosomal translocation. *Cell,* 77, 307.

137. Papadopoulos, P., Ridge, S. A., Boucher, C. A., Stocking, C., and Wiedmann, L. M. (1995) The novel activation of ABL by fusion to an ets-related gene, TEL. *Cancer Res.,* 55, 34.

138. Buijs, A., Sherr, S., van Baal, S., van Bezouw, S., van der Plas, D., van Kessel, A. G., *et al.* (1995) Translocation (12;22) (p13;q11) in myeloproliferative disorders results in fusion of the ETS-like TEL gene on 12p13 to the MN1 gene on 22q11. *Oncogene,* 10, 1511.

139. Roussel, M. F., Davis, J. N., Cleveland, J. L., Ghysdael, J., and Hiebert, S. W. (1994) Dual control of myc expression through a single DNA binding site targeted by ets family proteins and E2F-1. *Oncogene,* 9, 405.

140. Nakagoshi, H., Kanei-Ishii, C., Sawazaki, T., Mizuguchi, G., and Ishii, S. (1992) Transcriptional activation of the c-myc gene by the c-myb and B-myb gene products. *Oncogene,* 7, 1233.

141. Zobel, A., Kalkbrenner, F., Vorbrueggen, G., and Moelling, K. (1992) Transactivation of the human c-myc gene by c-Myb. *Biochem. Biophys. Res. Commun.,* 186, 715.

142. Nicolaides, N. C., Correa, I., Casadevall, C., Travali, S., Soprano, K. J., and Calabretta, B. (1992) The Jun family members, c-Jun and JunD, transactivate the human c-myb promoter via an Ap1-like element. *J. Biol. Chem.,* 267, 19665.

143. Adams, J. M., Harris, A. W., Pinkert, C. A., Corcoran, L. M., Alexander, W. S., Cory, S., *et al.* (1985) The c-myc oncogene driven by immunoglobulin enhancers induces lymphoid malignancy in transgenic mice. *Nature,* 318, 533.

144. Schmidt, E. V., Pattengale, P. K., Weir, L., and Leder, P. (1988) Transgenic mice bearing

the human c-myc gene activated by an immunoglobulin enhancer: a pre-B-cell lymphoma model. *Proc. Natl. Acad. Sci. USA*, 85, 6047.

145. Suda, Y., Aizawa, S., Hirai, S., Inoue, T., Furuta, Y., Suzuki, M., *et al.* (1987) Driven by the same Ig enhancer and SV40 T promoter ras induced lung adenomatous tumors, myc induced pre-B cell lymphomas and SV40 large T gene a variety of tumors in transgenic mice. *EMBO J.*, 6, 4055.

146. Dildrop, R., Ma, A., Ximmerman, K.,Hsu, E., Tesfaye, A., De Pinho, R., *et al.* (1989) IgH enhancer-mediated deregulation of N-myc gene expression in transgenic mice: generation of lymphoid neoplasias that lack c-myc expression. *EMBO J.*, 8, 1121.

147. Moroy, T., Fisher, P., Guidos, C., Ma, A., Zimmerman, K., Tesfaye, A., *et al.*, (1990) IgH enhancer deregulated expression of L-myc: abnormal T lymphocyte development and T cell lymphomagenesis. *EMBO J.*, 9, 3659.

148. Tsujimoto, Y., Jaffe, E., Cossman, J., Gorham, J., Nowell, P. C., and Croce, C. M. (1985) Clustering of breakpoints on chromosome 11 in human B-cell neoplasms with the t(11; 14) chromosome translocation. *Nature*, 315, 340.

149. Lovec, H., Grzeschiczek, A., Kowalski, M. B., and Moroy, T. (1994) Cyclin D1/bcl-1 cooperates with myc genes in the generation of B-cell lymphoma in transgenic mice. *EMBO J.*, 13, 3487.

150. Johnson, R. S., Spiegelman, B. M., and Papaioannou, V. (1992) Pleiotropic effects of a null mutation in the c-fos proto-oncogene. *Cell*, 71, 577.

151. Wang, Z. Q., Ovitt, C., Grigoriadis, A. E., Mohle-Steinlein, U., Ruther, U., and Wagner, E. F. (1992) Bone and haematopoietic defects in mice lacking c-fos. *Nature*, 360, 741.

152. Hu, E., Mueller, E., Oliviero, S., Papaioannou, V. E., Johnson, R., and Spiegelman, B. M. (1994) Targeted disruption of the c-fos gene demonstrates c-fos-dependent and -independent pathways for gene expression stimulated by growth factors or oncogenes. *EMBO J.*, 13, 3094.

153. Jain, J., Nalefski, E. A., McCaffrey, P. G., Johnson, R. S., Spiegelman, B. M., Papaioannou, V., *et al.* (1994) Normal peripheral T-cell function in c-Fos-deficient mice. *Mol. Cell. Biol.*, 14, 1566.

154. Johnson, R. S., van Lingen, B., Papaioannou, V. E., and Spiegelman, B. M. (1993) A null mutation at the c-jun locus causes embryonic lethality and retarded cell growth in culture. *Genes Dev.*, 7, 1309.

155. Davis, A. C., Wims, M., Spotts, G. D., Hann, S. R., and Bradley, A. (1993) A null c-myc mutation causes lethality before 10.5 days of gestation in homozygotes and reduced fertility in heterozygous female mice. *Genes Dev.*, 7, 671.

156. Charron, J., Malynn, B. A., Fisher, P., Stewart, V., Jeannotte, L., Goff, S. P., *et al.* (1992) Embryonic lethality in mice homozygous for a targeted disruption of the N-myc gene. *Genes Dev.*, 6, 2248.

157. Sawai, S., Shimono, A., Hanaoka, K., and Kondoh, H. (1991) Embryonic lethality resulting from disruption of both N-myc alleles in mouse zygotes. *New Biol.*, 3, 861.

158. Chambers, C. A. (1994) TKO'ed: lox, stock and barrel. *Bioessays*, 16, 865.

159. Moens, C. B., Auerbach, A. B., Conlon, R. A., Joyner, A. L., and Rossant, J. (1992) A targeted mutation reveals a role for N-myc in branching morphogenesis in the embryonic mouse lung. *Genes Dev.*, 6, 691.

160. Moens, C. B., Stanton, B. R., Parada, L. F., and Rossant, J. (1993) Defects in heart and lung development in compound heterozygotes for two different targeted mutations at the N-myc locus. *Development*, 119, 485.

161. Chatton, B., Bocco, J. L., Goetz, J., Gaire, M., Lutz, Y., and Kedinger, C. (1994) Jun and Fos heterodimerize with ATFa, a member of the ATF/CREB family and modulate its transcriptional activity. *Oncogene*, 9, 375.

162. Hai, T. and Curran, T. (1991) Cross-family dimerization of transcription factors Fos/Jun and ATF/CREB alters DNA binding specificity. *Proc. Natl. Acad. Sci. USA*, 88, 3720.

163. Chevray, P. M. and Nathans, D. (1992) Protein interaction cloning in yeast: identification of mammalian proteins that react with the leucine zipper of Jun. *Proc. Natl. Acad. Sci. USA*, 89, 5789.

164. Kerppola, T. K. and Curran, T. (1994) Maf and Nrl can bind to AP-1 sites and form heterodimers with Fos and Jun. *Oncogene*, 9, 675.

165. Kataoka, K., Fujiwara, K. T., Noda, M., and Nishizawa, M. (1994) MafB, a new Maf family transcription activator that can associate with Maf and Fos but not with Jun. *Mol. Cell. Biol.*, 14, 7581.

166. Kataoka, K., Igarashi, K., Itoh, K., Fujiwara, K. T., Noda, M., Yamamoto, M., *et al.* (1995) Small Maf proteins heterodimerize with Fos and may act as competitive repressors of the NF-E2 transcription factor. *Mol. Cell. Biol.*, 15, 2180.

167. Hsu, W., Kerppola, T. K., Chen, P. L., Curran, T., and Chen-Kiang, S. (1994) Fos and Jun repress transcription activation by NF-IL6 through association at the basic zipper region. *Mol. Cell. Biol.*, 14, 268.

168. Blanar, M. A. and Rutter, W. J. (1992) Interaction cloning: identification of a helix-loop-helix zipper protein that interacts with c-Fos. *Science*, 256, 1014.

169. Monteclaro, F. S. and Vogt, P. K. (1993) A Jun-binding protein related to a putative tumor suppressor. *Proc. Natl. Acad. Sci. USA*, 90, 6726.

170. Jain, J., McCaffrey, P. G., Milner, Z., Kerppola, T. K., Lambert, J. N., Verdine, G. L. *et al.* (1993) The T-cell transcription factor NFATp is a substrate for calcineurin and interacts with Fos and Jun. *Nature*, 365, 352.

171. Kerppola, T. K., Luk, D., and Curran, T. (1993) Fos is a preferential target of glucocorticoid receptor inhibition of AP-1 activity *in vitro*. *Mol. Cell. Biol.*, 13, 3782.

172. Stein, B., Baldwin, A., Jr., Ballard, D. W., Greene, W. C., Angel, P., and Herrlich, P. (1993) Cross-coupling of the NF-kappa B p65 and Fos/Jun transcription factors produces potentiated biological function. *EMBO J.*, 12, 3879.

173. Ransone, L. J., Kerr, L. D., Schmitt, M. J., Wamsley, P., and Verma, I. M. (1993) The bZIP domains of Fos and Jun mediate a physical association with the TATA box-binding protein. *Gene Expr.*, 3, 37.
174. Metz, R., Bannister, A. J., Sutherland, J. A., Hagemeier, C., O'Rourke, E. C., Cook, A., *et al.* (1994) c-Fos-induced activation of a TATA-box-containing promoter involves direct contact with TATA-box-binding protein. *Mol. Cell. Biol.*, 14, 6021.
175. Bengal, E., Ransone, L., Scharfmann, R., Dwarki, V. J., Tapscott, S. J., Weintraub, H., *et al.* (1992) Functional antagonism between c-Jun and MyoD proteins: a direct physical association. *Cell*, 68, 507.

Part II

TUMOUR SUPPRESSORS AND CELL CYCLE CONTROL

7 | Mammalian cell cycle control

JONATHON PINES

1. Introduction

A proliferating cell must co-ordinate DNA replication and chromosomal separation to ensure that the genome is replicated completely, and that a single copy is correctly inherited by each daughter cell. The cell cycle is the co-ordinated series of events that achieves these aims. Our current understanding of the basic mechanism underlying the cell cycle is that many of the key events are initiated by a family of conserved serine/threonine protein kinases, the cyclin-dependent kinases (CDKs), that are activated by the cyclin family of proteins. In turn, the cyclin–CDK complexes are modulated by other protein kinases or phosphatases, and by binding specific inhibitor proteins. The tremendous variety of ways in which CDK activity can be regulated allows the cell cycle to respond both to external growth signals (positive or negative), and to internal signals generated by preceding events in the cell cycle. Moreover, the uncontrolled proliferation of some cancer cells can be ascribed to defects in the cyclin–CDK machinery. This review will outline the components and principles which we currently believe to control the cell cycle in proliferating mammalian cells.

2. Controlpoints and checkpoints

2.1 Controlpoints

By convention, the somatic cell cycle is divided into four phases: DNA replication (S phase) and chromosome separation (M phase) are separated by gap phases (G1 and G2). During the gap phases the cell prepares for either DNA synthesis or mitosis by transcribing and synthesizing components of the replication or mitotic machinery. In many embryonic cell cycles, where these components are stockpiled in the egg, there are no G1 or G2 phases (reviewed in ref. 1). The decision to begin the next stage in the cell cycle is carefully regulated at what I will call controlpoints (Fig. 1), in particular:

- the commitment to another round of DNA replication
- the initiation of DNA replication
- the initiation of mitosis

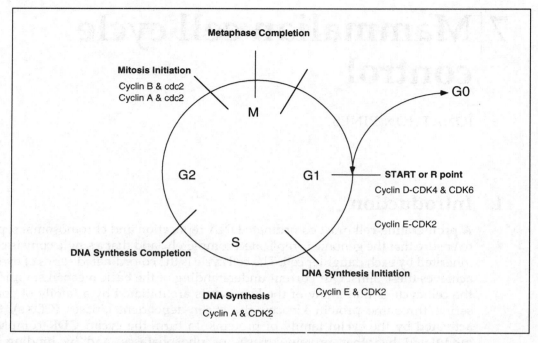

Fig. 1 The main control points in the mammalian cell cycle. The four phases of the cell cycle—G1, S, G2, and M—are illustrated, along with the cyclin–CDK complexes most directly correlated with their control.

The effectors of many of the cell cycle controlpoints are the cyclin-dependent kinases (CDKs) (2, 3). CDKs are activated by binding a member of the cyclin family (4, 5), whose synthesis is cell cycle-dependent. In the mammalian cell cycle, particular CDKs have been implicated in the control of specific control points (Fig. 1), and the cell cycle can be envisaged as a succession of different cyclin–CDK activities. Once the decision to commit to another round of DNA replication and mitosis has been made, these waves of CDK kinase activity succeed one another in an almost cell autonomous fashion.

2.2 Checkpoints

In between controlpoints the cell is able to respond to adverse conditions by arresting the cell cycle at various 'checkpoints' (6). Under normal conditions, checkpoints are silent, but specific signals activate them and stop the cell cycle, often through modulating specific cyclin–CDK complexes (Fig. 2). For example, DNA damage is able to arrest cells before S phase and before mitosis, such that either the damage is repaired, or the cell undergoes apoptosis. This prevents DNA mutations from being replicated, and damaged DNA from interfering with the separation of sister chromatids in mitosis. Another important checkpoint is activated when chromosomes are incorrectly aligned in metaphase, causing cells to stay in metaphase until the chromosomes

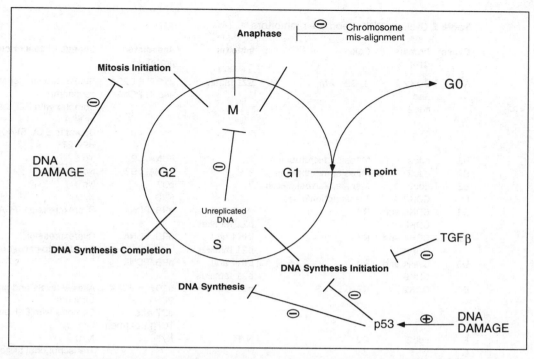

Fig. 2 Checkpoints. The points at which various factors, such as DNA damage, are able to arrest the cell cycle are shown.

are correctly configured. However, one of the hallmarks of cancer cells is their genetic instability; chromosomes are often rearranged or even lost when cells divide, and this indicates that some checkpoints must be inoperative (reviewed in ref. 7). Cancer cells must have lost, or be able to ignore, those checkpoints that normally prevent the replication of damaged DNA, and those checkpoints that normally prevent cells from carrying out mitosis with misaligned or imbalanced chromosomes. The molecular basis for these changes is in part due to the differences in the regulation and composition of the cyclin–CDK complexes.

2.3 The cyclin–CDK motif

2.3.1 CDK regulation by cyclin and CAK

Different cyclin–CDK complexes drive the cell through most of the major cell cycle control points. In the mammalian cell cycle some CDKs have more clearly defined roles than others (reviewed in ref. 8; see Table 1). Thus cdc2 is the primary mitotic kinase, CDK2 is required for the G1–S transition and S phase itself, CDK4 and CDK6 are probably involved at the restriction point (R, see below), and CDK7 appears to have dual roles; as a CDK activating kinase (CAK, see below), and as part of the TFIIH

Table 1 Cyclins, CDKs, and their inhibitors

Cyclin	Primary CDK	Role	Inhibitor	Associated proteins[a]	Change in cancer cells
A-	CDK2 and cdc2	S, G2 → M	p21 family	p107 + E2F-1 and 4, PCNA	Stabilization in hepatocellular carcinoma Complex with E2F disrupted by E1A Bound to E1A, SV40 T Ag, HPV E7
B1-	cdc2	Mitosis, microtubules	?	PCNA, p9?	No
B2	cdc2	Mitosis, membranes	?	PCNA, p9?	No
B3	cdc2	Mitosis, karyoskeleton	?	p9?	No
C-	CDK8	Transcription?		N/D	N/D
D1	CDK4 and CDK6	R?	INK4 and p21 families	pRB, PCNA	Overexpression (*PRAD1, BCL1*)
D2	CDK4 and CDK6	R?	INK4 and p21 families	pRB, PCNA	Overexpression (*Vin-1* proto-oncogene)
D3	CDK4 and CDK6	R?	INK4 and p21 families	pRB, PCNA	
E-	CDK2	R?, G1 → S	p21 family	p107 + E2F-4, PCNA p27 after TGFβ treatment	Altered levels and protein in tumours Complex with E2F disrupted by E1A
F	cdc2	G2	N/D	N/D	N/D
G	?	?			Transcriptional target of p53
H	CDK7	CAK, TFIIH	N/D	N/D	N/D

[a] PCNA not bound to cyclin–CDK complexes in most cancer cells.

transcription factor complex. In principle, the protein kinase activity of all CDKs can be controlled in the same ways; by cyclin synthesis, cyclin binding, cyclin destruction, by phosphorylation, and by binding inhibitors. What follows is a brief overview of the ways in which cyclin–CDK complexes are regulated (Fig. 3). For more detailed reviews see (9, 10).

CDKs must bind a cyclin to be active, and almost all the CDKs are present in constant, excess amounts over the cyclins throughout the cell cycle. This means that CDK activity can be regulated by controlling the amount of its partner cyclin. To this end, mammalian cyclin genes are transcribed in a cell cycle-dependent fashion, and some cyclins are also degraded at specific points in the cell cycle.

The changes wrought in the structure of a CDK when it binds a cyclin have recently been determined through a comparison of the crystal structure of monomeric CDK2 (11) with CDK2 in a complex with cyclin A (12). In sum, cyclin changes the conformation in which ATP is bound, and moves a domain of CDK2—the T loop—away from a position blocking access to the catalytic cleft. However, for some cyclin–CDK complexes, this only generates a partially active kinase (13, 14). Full activity is conferred when a conserved threonine residue in the T loop is phosphorylated (15,

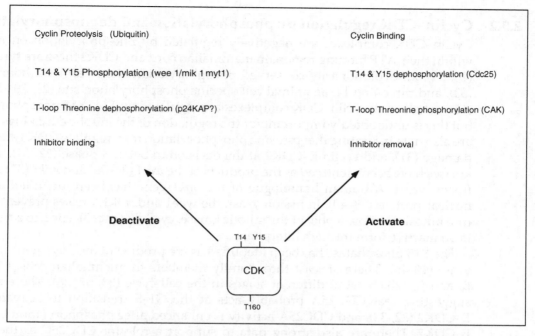

Fig. 3 CDK regulation. The mechanisms by which cyclin-dependent kinases can be turned on and off are illustrated.

16). This residue is specifically phosphorylated by a CDK activating kinase, or CAK (17). A potential CAK has recently been purified as a cyclin–CDK complex, between cyclin H (18–20) and CDK7 (21–23). CAK could therefore be subject to cell cycle regulation, although thus far CAK activity appears to be constant throughout the cell cycle.

An unexpected development has been the isolation of CDK7–cyclin H as part of the TFIIH transcription factor complex (24, 25). TFIIH is part of the basal transcription machinery, and also required for DNA repair. The TFIIH–associated kinase has been implicated as (one of) the kinase responsible for phosphorylating the carboxy terminal domain (CTD) of RNA polymerase II, which correlates with the release of RNA polymerase from the transcription initiation complex. Therefore, either cyclin H–CDK7 performs two functions in the cell—potentially linking DNA repair and transcription to other cell cycle events—or there is another CAK still to be isolated.

The phosphatase that dephosphorylates the T loop threonine—usually once the cyclin partner has been degraded—has not been unambiguously identified. However, there are data to suggest that it is p24$^{\text{Cdi1/KAP}}$ (T. Hunter, personal communication) a dual specificity phosphatase that was first isolated in a yeast two-hybrid screen with cdc2 (26, 27).

2.3.2 Cyclin–CDK regulation by phosphorylation and dephosphorylation

Cyclin–CDK complexes are negatively regulated by phosphorylation on residues within their ATP binding region. In mammalian cdc2 and CDK2 these are tyrosine 15 (28, 29), an evolutionarily conserved phosphorylation site in all cdc2 homologues (30), and threonine 14, an animal cell-specific phosphorylation site (28, 29). It is not clear whether all cyclin–CDK complexes are regulated by T14/Y15 phosphorylation, but this is undoubtedly important for the regulation of the mitotic cdc2 kinase. There are also data indicating that tyrosine phosphorylation may regulate CDK4 after DNA damage (31), and cyclin E–CDK2 at the decision to begin S phase (32, 33). The Y15 kinases have been identified as the products of the *wee1* (34–36) and *mik1* (37) genes in fission yeast. A human homologue of the *mik1* gene has been identified and is a nuclear protein (38–40). In fission yeast, the wee1 and mik1 kinases prevent premature mitosis to allow a pool of the mitotic kinase, cyclin B (cdc13)–cdc2, to accumulate in an inactive form through interphase.

The Y15 phosphatase has been identified as the product of the *cdc25* gene in fission yeast (41–46). There at least three family members in mammalian cells, CDC25A, B, and C, which act at different stages in the cell cycle (33, 37, 38). There are data suggesting that CDC25A probably acts at the G1–S transition to activate cyclin E–CDK2 (32, 33), and CDC25A activity is enhanced after phosphorylation by cyclin E–CDK2. There are also strong data to support a role for CDC25C as the crucial phosphatase that activates cyclin B–cdc2 at the G2–M transition and CDC25C activity is enhanced by phosphorylation by cyclin B–cd2 (reviewed in Ref. 49).

2.3.3 Regulation by CDK inhibitors

The most recently identified manner of regulating cyclin–CDK complexes is by specific inhibitor proteins. In mammalian cells there are at least two classes of these inhibitors. One class, the INK4 proteins (50–53), bind the monomeric form of CDK4 and CDK6, the partners of the D-type cyclins. The INK4 proteins are mostly comprised of repeated ankyrin motifs and include p15 (52), p16 (50), p18, and p19 (51, 53), one of which, p16, has been implicated as an important tumour suppressor (54, 55 and Chapter 10). The other class of inhibitors include p21 (56–60), p27 (61, 62), and p57 (63, 64), which have significant homology to one another in their amino termini and are able to bind a variety of cyclin–CDK complexes. These inhibitors only bind to cyclin–CDKs once they form a complex, and more than one molecule of the inhibitor is required to inhibit the kinase activity (65). This means that cyclin–CDK complexes can retain kinase activity when bound to a single inhibitor molecule, so that the inhibitors could have an additional role, such as targeting the complex to other molecules.

2.3.4 Regulation by cyclin proteolysis

An important aspect of a cyclin is its cell cycle-regulated destruction, which consequently inactivates its partner CDK and contributes to the irreversibility of progress from one phase of the cell cycle to the next. Recent studies have shown that, at heart, the cell cycle is based on alternating phases of ubiquitin-mediated proteolysis involving the destruction of both cyclins and CDK inhibitors (66, 67). Ubiquitin-mediated proteolysis requires a ubiquitin conjugating enzyme (UBC), often in partnership with a ubiquitin ligase, to transfer ubiquitin to the substrate. Once ubiquitinated, the substrate is degraded by the 26S proteosome (reviewed in ref. 68). In terms of their destruction there are broadly two classes of cyclins; those that are constitutively unstable and degraded throughout the cell cycle, for example cyclins D and E, and those that are degraded only at a specific point in the cell cycle, such as cyclins A and B.

The D- and E-type cyclins are short-lived proteins ($t_{1/2} \sim 20$ min) (69–71), which means that their levels are primarily determined by the rate of their transcription. D- and E-type cyclin instability is conferred by the carboxy terminal third of the protein which is rich in 'PEST' sequences. In budding yeast, the instability of the G1 phase cyclins is in large part conferred by PEST regions (72, 73), and these cyclins are degraded by the ubiquitin pathway (74), so that a similar mechanism is likely to prevail for the mammalian D- and E-type cyclins.

The A- and B-type cyclins are stable throughout most of interphase but are rapidly degraded once cells enter mitosis (4, 75, 76). This property is dependent on a partially conserved ten amino acid region in the amino terminus, called the destruction box (77). Cyclins are recognized by a specific ubiquitin ligase (78, 79), but usually only when bound to a CDK (80, 81). Some of the components of the ubiquitin ligase have recently been identified and are conserved between budding yeast and humans. These are the products of the *S. cerevisiae* genes *CDC16*, *CDC23*, and *CDC27*, which form part of a large multiprotein complex, variously called the 'anaphase promoting complex' (APC) or the 'cyclosome' (78, 79, 82, 83). In budding yeast, the mitotic cyclins are subsequently degraded via a specific 26S protease (84, 85). The APC is diffusely distributed in the nucleus and associated with the centrosome during interphase, but at mitosis it is strongly associated with the mitotic apparatus (83)—as indeed is one of its substrates, the cyclin B–cdc2 complex (86–88). Furthermore, there are strong indications that the APC is itself indirectly activated through cyclin B1–cdc2 kinase activity (78, 89). In effect the B-type cyclins trigger their own destruction, as well as the destruction of the A-type cyclins and as yet unidentified proteins that link the sister chromatids (90; and see below).

2.3.5 Cyclin–CDK deregulation in cancer cells

In cancer cells, controlpoints and checkpoints could be deregulated or ablated if a positive CDK regulator (e.g. a cyclin) is overexpressed or a negative regulator is removed. Examples of both conditions are found in tumours. Some tumours over-express certain cyclins, especially the D-type cyclins, whereas other tumours have lost inhibitor proteins. Cell cycle regulation is also essential to alternative cell fates such as differentiation, senescence, and meiosis. Thus some cell cycle regulators have important roles in, for example, differentiation, which could be relevant to their involvement in oncogenesis.

3. The cell cycle is regulated by a succession of control-points and checkpoints

3.1 The restriction point, R

In G1 phase, the mammalian cell commits itself to a round of DNA replication and mitosis, rather than to the alternative fates of quiescence or differentiation—which usually involve withdrawal from the cell cycle. It is also in G1 phase that growth is coupled to proliferation. Thus the point(s) in G1 phase at which the decision is made to begin the mitotic cell cycle is the one at which most external influences impinge upon the cell cycle, and not surprisingly, the components involved in regulating this decision are those most closely implicated in cancer.

The time when a cell becomes committed to proliferate is called the restriction point (R) in mammalian cells (91). However, R is rather an amorphous entity, defined as the point after which cells no longer need serum to continue on into S phase. By comparison, the point at which a yeast cell commits itself to another round of DNA replication is much more clearly defined. This controlpoint is called START, and it is where a yeast cell arrests in the presence of mating pheromone, or in the absence of sufficient nutrients. The regulators of START have been identified by genetic analysis; mutations in several cell cycle regulators—notably the principle CDK (*cdc2* in fission yeast and *CDC28* in budding yeast)—will arrest the cell at START (92, 93). Thus, by analogy with START, it has been postulated that R is regulated by cyclin–CDK complexes. This analogy is strengthened by the original observations on the restriction point which imply that a short-lived protein (94), such as a D- or E-type cyclin, is required to pass through R.

3.1.1 Specific transcription factors required to begin DNA synthesis

In budding yeast, START is mainly controlled by the interplay between cyclin–CDK complexes and specific transcription factors (reviewed in ref. 95). The most important of these transcription factors are SBF and MBF, which are activated through phosphorylation by the G1 cyclin–CDC28 complexes at START (96–98). SBF and MBF are responsible for transcribing the genes required for DNA synthesis, such as DNA polymerase and ribonucleotide reductase, and the CLB5 and CLB6 cyclins that are also involved in S phase (99, 100). To continue the analogy between START and R, the mammalian transcription factor most closely implicated in the stimulation of DNA synthesis genes is E2F (reviewed in ref. 101 and Chapter 8). However, the components of E2F show very limited homology to the components of SBF and MBF (102), so that it is possible that the true mammalian homologues of SBF and MBF remain to be discovered. The canonical E2F binding site is found in many genes required for DNA synthesis, such as DNA polymerase α, thymidine kinase, and ribonucleotide reductase, as well as cyclins E and A which appear to be necessary for S phase (reviewed in ref. 101). Furthermore, E2F is able to induce transcription from these genes when artificially expressed in quiescent cells (103).

The DNA binding activity defined as E2F can be any of several different heterodimers between a member of the E2F family (five known members) and one of the DP family (three known members) (reviewed in ref. 102 and Chapter 8). The differences between DP1, 2, and 3 are unclear; thus far DP1 has been shown to be present in all E2F activities in the mammalian cell cycle (104). The E2F components vary in their properties, in particular in their ability to bind members of the retinoblastoma (RB) tumour suppressor family that are implicated as transcriptional repressors (reviewed in ref. 105 and Chapter 8). pRB is one of three cloned proteins, pRB, p107, and p130, that bear significant homology to each other in a region called the 'pocket'. (reviewed in ref. 106). This region is targeted by certain viral proteins, including the SV40 T antigen, adenovirus E1A proteins, and the E7 protein of papilloma virus, and is also the region involved in binding E2F and certain cyclins (reviewed in ref. 107). It has been shown that E2F-1, -2, and -3 are all able to bind to pRB (108–112), but not p107 or p130, whereas E2F-4 (113, 114) and E2F-5 bind p107 and p130, but not pRB (115–117).

There is a rather complicated pattern of E2F binding activities that varies in a cell cycle-dependent manner. In quiescent cells, the predominant E2F DNA binding activity is associated with p130 and composed of E2F-4 and E2F-5 (113–117). When cells are serum stimulated, p130 is replaced by p107, and these complexes also contain cyclin E in G1 phase (118), and cyclin A in S and G2 phase (118–120). Thus, the E2F-4 and E2F-5 family members correlate with the re-entry of the cell from quiescence to proliferation (113, 114, 116).

Once serum stimulated cells enter G1 phase, pRB-associated E2F also appears (121–123)—largely composed of E2F-1, whose transcription begins after serum stimulation (124). This implicates E2F-1 in the transcription of genes required for DNA synthesis, and in support of this overexpressing E2F-1 is sufficient to drive a significant fraction (20%) of transfected cells into S phase (125). However, E2F-1 alone is not sufficient for a physiological S phase because the cells go on to die by apoptosis.

Thus distinct E2F transcription factor complexes are likely to control the transcription of different sets of genes, from those required to re-enter the proliferation cycle to those required for DNA synthesis. It is likely that different E2F family members confer specificity in binding to promoters and that regulation by different pocket proteins and cyclins co-ordinates transcription with the cell cycle.

3.1.2 D-type cyclin–CDKs are correlated with passage through R

In yeast, START is clearly regulated by G1 cyclin–CDK complexes (96, 97, 126). In budding yeast, one G1 cyclin (CLN3) also plays an important role at START in integrating growth control—i.e. cell size—with proliferation (72, 127). However, because of its ill-defined nature, transition through R has thus far only been correlated with the appearance of certain cyclin–CDK complexes. In particular, these are the cyclin D–CDK4/CDK6, and the cyclin E– CDK2 complexes (reviewed in ref. 128). Overproducing either D-type cyclins or cyclin E moderately shortens G1 phase in mammalian cells (129–131), whereas overproducing both D- and E-type cyclins significantly shortens G1 phase (132). This suggests that the two types of cyclin regulate different aspects of G1 phase, and because D-type cyclin kinase activities appear earlier than cyclin E kinase activity, they are more closely correlated with R.

There are three known D-type cyclins, D1, D2, and D3, which display some tissue specificity, and potentially redundancy (69, 133–136). Most cells contain cyclin D3 and either D1 or D2 but not all three. The D-type cyclins act as a read-out of the presence of growth factors because, in the absence of serum, D-type cyclin transcription stops and therefore the proteins rapidly disappear. Indeed, one of the ways in which cyclin D1 was first isolated was in a differential screen for mRNAs up-regulated four to six hours after the readdition of CSF-1 to quiescent macrophages (69). The D-type cyclins have several properties that set them apart from other mammalian cyclins (cyclins A, B1, B2, and E). The D-type cyclins alone have an L–X–C–X–E motif such that they are able to bind directly to pRB (137, 138). Their two main CDK partners, CDK4 (138) and CDK6 (141) only bind to D-type cyclins whereas, for example, CDK2 is able to bind to cyclin D (141), cyclin A (142, 143), or cyclin E (71). CDK4 and CDK6 in turn are uniquely bound by the INK4 family of inhibitor proteins, p15, p16, p18, and p19 (50–53).

3.1.3 D-type cyclins are commonly overexpressed in cancer

Of all cyclins, the D-type cyclins are the most strongly implicated as proto-oncogenes. Human cyclin D1 maps to chromosome 11q13 and was originally identified as the *PRAD1* or *BCL1* proto-concogene (133, 134). Cyclin D1 (PRAD1) is overexpressed in parathyroid adenomas because of a chromosomal inversion, inv (11)(p15;q13), such that it comes under the control of regulatory elements of the parathyroid hormone gene on 11p15 (133). The overexpression of cyclin D1 probably results in a purely proliferative lesion because the tumours are benign and non-invasive. In mantel cell lymphomas (centrocytic lymphomas) cyclin D1 expression is brought under the influence of the immunoglobulin heavy chain enhancer by a chromosomal translocation at the BCL1 breakpoint, t(11;14)(q13;q32) (134 and Chapter 1). The cyclin D1 locus is also amplified and overexpressed in a wide variety of tumours including breast cancer, oesophageal carcinoma, and squamous cell carcinoma. In mice, both the cyclin D1 and the cyclin D2 loci are the sites of integration of murine leukaemia virus (144, 145). Cyclin D1 is able to co-operate with RAS (146), a defective E1A protein (147), and MYC (148) in cellular transformation assays or for lymphomagenesis in transgenic mice. Furthermore, transgenic mice overexpressing cyclin D1 from the MMTV promoter develop mammary carcinomas at a substantially increased frequency (149). Lymphoid cells appear to be particularly susceptible to transformation by deregulated D-type cyclins, and in this regard it is very interesting to note that the lymphotropic Herpes virus saimiri encodes a cyclin homologue (150) that is able to bind and activate CDK6, the primary D-type cyclin partner in lymphoid cells.

Human cyclin D3, the *CCND3* gene (151, 152), maps to chromosome 6p21 but has not yet been identified as a proto-oncogene.

3.1.3 The INK4 family of inhibitors are potential tumour suppressors

Cyclin D–CDK complexes are negatively regulated by the INK4 family of inhibitors, and the prediction that this family of inhibitors would be down-regulated in cancer cells has proved to be the case. The p16^{INK4A} protein is very commonly lost in tumours and transformed cell lines (54, 55, 153). Although some of the changes in p16[INK4A] in culture appear to be a secondary consequence of establishing cell lines, nevertheless p16[INK4A] is a good candidate for one of the familial melanoma genes. Furthermore, in cell lines which retain p16[INK4A] the protein is mutated such that it is unable to inhibit cyclin D1–CDK kinase activity (154), and p16 is unable to inhibit growth in cells without a functional retinoblastoma protein (155, 156). The emerging picture is that cancer cells deregulate D-type cyclin function by removing or inactivating either pRB or p16.

The other INK4 family members have not been found to be as commonly mutated in cancer. p15[INK4B] appears to be on one pathway through which some cells arrest in response to TGFβ. For example p15 mRNA and protein levels are induced more that 30-fold when HaCaT cells are exposed to TGFβ (52).

3.1.4 D-type cyclins are regulators of the retinoblastoma protein

The significance of D-type cyclin deregulation in oncogenesis is underlined by their interaction with pRB. A specific role for the D-type cyclins in the regulation of pRB is indicated by data indicating that pRB-positive cells are prevented from entering S phase when anti-cyclin D1 antibodies are microinjected in G1 phase. In contrast, pRB-negative cells are insensitive to these antibodies, suggesting that in the absence of pRB, cyclin D1 function is dispensable (157).

Yet the role of D-type cyclins in the mitotic cell cycle is still undefined. pRB has been proposed as the principle regulator of the G1–S transition, with the D-type cyclins acting to neutralize pRB by phosphorylation and to allow the cell to begin S phase (reviewed in ref. 158 and Chapter 8). In support of this, pRB is underphosphorylated in G1 phase, progressively phosphorylated in mid–late G1 phase, and remains hyper-phosphorylated in S and G2 phases (159,–161). Cyclins D1, E, A, but also B1, are able to phosphorylate pRB *in vitro* on sites that are phosphorylated in vivo (162–164). The hypophosphorylated form of pRB is able to bind a large number of proteins, such as E2F, that are not bound by hyperphosphorylated pRB. A significant difference between hypo- and hyperphosphorylated pRB is also suggested by the observation that transforming antigens target only the underphosphorylated from of pRB. These studies have led to the proposal that the phosphorylation of pRB releases sequestered factors required for DNA replication at the G1 to S transition (reviewed in ref. 106).

However, there are problems with this model, principally that neither pRB nor individual D-type cyclins are essential to the control of the initiation of DNA replication. Cells without pRB are able to regulate the G1–S transition correctly during proliferation, such that the $RB^{-/-}$ mouse is able to develop as far as day 13 before dying, after numerous cell divisions and substantial differentiation (165, 166). Rather than regulating basic cell division, the lack of pRB appears to be important for specific differentiation pathways, primarily in the development of the liver, in haematopoiesis, and in some neuronal development (165, 166). In addition, pRB phosphorylation does not correlate exactly with the G1–S transition; there is a significant proportion of pRB that remains underphosphorylated as cells traverse S phase. Moreover, the G1 arrest caused by transient transfection of pRB into pRB-negative cells is reversed much more efficiently by A- and B-type cyclin–CDKs than by D-type cyclin–CDKs (163).

In a similar fashion to their proposed regulation of pRB, D-type cyclins have also been correlated with regulation of p107. In 3T3 cells, phosphorylated p107 is unable to bind to E2F-4, cyclin D1 levels and p107 phosphorylation increase at the same time after serum stimulation, and a dominant negative CDK4 will prevent the phosphorylation of p107 (167). These studies, combined with data showing that p107 can sequester and inhibit cyclins E and A (168), have led to the suggestion that the D-type cyclins activate E2F-4 transcription in G1 phase, after which E2F-4 is turned off by association with p107–cyclin E in late G1 phase, and p107–cyclin A in S and G2 phases (168).

3.1.5 The decision to proliferate or differentiate or senesce

Evidence is accumulating to support a primary role for pRB and the D-type cyclins in signal transduction to the cell cycle machinery, as part of the integration of signals (at R) when the decision is made whether to proliferate, or to differentiate, or to senesce (Fig. 4). The instability of the D-type cyclins and their growth factor-dependent transcription means that they act as an accurate read-out of the presence or absence of growth factors in the environment. If they are involved in signal transduction, D-type cyclin synthesis might also be sensitive to differentiation as well as growth factors. In support of this, D-type cyclins have a profound inhibitory effect on differentiation.

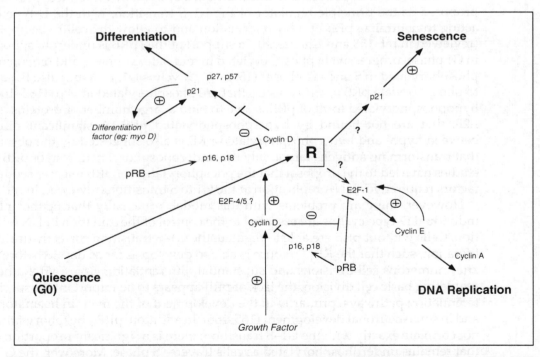

Fig. 4 Cell fate decisions. The various cell fate alternatives, quiescence, differentiation, senescence, and proliferation are shown. The hypothesis is made that the fate is decided upon at R and the various cell cycle components that have been implicated in the different decisions are shown.

The clearest evidence for this comes from studies on 32D myeloid cells (169). These cells normally express cyclins D2 and D3 in a growth factor-dependent manner, and proliferate in culture until G-CSF is added, which induces them to differentiate. When the cells are transfected with either cyclin D2 or D3 under a constitutive promoter, the cells are unable to differentiate in the presence of G-CSF; they continue to proliferate until they die. Constitutive expression of cyclin D1 has no effect on their differentiation, nor does expression of cyclin D2 and D3 mutants that are unable to bind RB (169). Thus deregulating the D-type cyclins might prevent differentiation, one of the conditions that predisposes a cell to transformation (170).

4. The G1–S checkpoint

4.1 p53 and p21

Once a cell has made the decision to proliferate, rather than to senesce or differentiate, it is vital that only undamaged DNA is replicated, because if DNA damage is substantial, its replication can lead to chromosome loss or rearrangement. Thus, there is a major checkpoint in late G1 phase that is activated by damaged DNA. At this checkpoint, cells are prevented from entering S phase, although there is some debate over whether cells are able to repair their DNA and go on to enter S phase (171) or whether they are permanently arrested in a state resembling senescence (172). This checkpoint requires wild-type p53 (171, 172). Thus p53 may enhance the genetic stability of the cell by preventing cells from replicating damaged DNA, and this may be one of the reasons why it functions as a tumour suppressor (see Chapter 9).

One of the important effectors of the p53-dependent G1 arrest is the cyclin-dependent kinase inhibitor p21$^{CIP1/WAF1}$. p21 seems to be a general inhibitor of almost all cyclin–CDK complexes, including cyclin D–CDK4, cyclin E–CDK2, and cyclin A–CDK2. It is much less effective at inhibiting cyclin B–cdc2 (56, 58, 173). The p21 gene has a p53 consensus site in its promoter, and is a transcriptional target of wild-type p53 (57 and Chapter 9). When p53 is activated by DNA damage, the amount of p21 increases substantially and probably arrests the cell cycle by inhibiting cyclin D– and cyclin E–CDK complexes (57, 174). Mutant p53 is unable to activate p21 transcription, and this may be one reason why the G1–S checkpoint is defective in many tumour cells. It may also explain why very much less p21 is bound to cyclin–CDK complexes in transformed cells (173).

However, there are data showing that phosphorylation of the Y15 equivalent of CDK4 is also important to this checkpoint. After DNA damage, cyclin D–CDK4 becomes phosphorylated on tyrosine and mutating this residue to phenylalanine prevents cells from arresting in G1 (31). This is in apparent conflict to the inhibitory effect of p21, which should still have been expressed in these cells.

The p21 protein can be divided into two domains. The amino terminus of the protein binds and inhibits cyclin–CDK complexes (175) and more than one molecule of p21 is required to inhibit one cyclin–CDK complex (65). This has led to the suggestion that p21 could act as a threshold to inhibit cyclin–CDK activity until the cyclin–CDK complexes have accumulated above the level of p21 (176, 177). Alternatively, p21 might function as part of an active cyclin–CDK complex and, indeed, most cyclin–CDK complexes in non-transformed cells contain p21. One idea is that p21 could target a cyclin–CDK complex within the cell and some credence to this is given by the observation that the carboxy terminus of p21 binds to PCNA, the auxillary subunit of DNA polymerase δ (175, 178).

4.2 p21 is involved in senescence and differentiation

Increased p21 levels are not simply associated with the activation of wild-type p53. One of the ways in which p21 was isolated was because of its increased abundance in senescent cells (60). This may be germane to the argument over whether the p53-mediated G1 arrest point is reversible or resembles senescence. Similarly, several terminally differentiated cell types also have large amounts of p21, and *in situ* hybridization studies show that p21 is associated in particular with developing muscle. Indeed, MYO D and p21 form a potential positive feedback loop in differentiating muscle cells (179). Thus p21 appears to be an effector of cell cycle arrest under a variety of conditions.

4.3 The p21 family includes p27 and p57

There are at least two other cyclin–CDK inhibitors in the p21 family, p27[KIP1] and p57[KIP2], all related by their amino terminal sequences that are responsible for inhibiting cyclin–CDK complexes (62, 180 and reviewed in ref. 177). Like p21, p27 is able to arrest cells in response to a checkpoint. In this case, p27 is closely associated with cell cycle arrest in response to contact inhibition, or in some cells to TGFβ (180). However, unlike p21, transcription is not responsible for the increase in active p27. Rather, p27 is present in a latent form in the cytoplasm through association with a heat labile repressor (180, 181), and is unmasked by TGFβ treatment or cell–cell contact, and by cAMP treatment of macrophages (182). Tumour cells are often unresponsive to contact inhibition and a reason for this may be found in the level or form of p27 in these cells.

Once unmasked, p27 binds and inhibits the cyclin E–CDK2 complex, although in proliferating cells most p27 is bound to cyclin D–CDK4/6 complexes (62), which could therefore be the heat labile repressor (183). p27 may inhibit cyclin D–CDK4 through preventing the phosphorylation of the T loop threonine residue in CDK4 (T172) by CAK (182). Increasing the amount of p27 (cAMP treatment of macrophages) or decreasing the amount of CDK4 (TFGβ treatment) would both block cells in G1 phase (177). Conversely, in T lymphocytes, IL-2 treatment depresses p27 levels, whilst antigen stimulation increases cyclin D2 and D3 synthesis, causing T cells to proliferate (184).

p27 is closely related in its amino and carboxy terminal sequences to p57, but p57 has in addition one large proline-rich and one acidic domain in the middle of the protein. p57 also maps to 11p15, a chromosomal region that is implicated in many tumours (64). Like p27, p57 is able to inhibit cyclin D-, cyclin E-, and cyclin A-associated kinases, and does not require pRB or wild-type p53 to induce G1 arrest when transfected into tissue culture cells.

In a similar manner to p21, *in situ* hybridization data link p27 with differentiation, in particular in muscle and nervous tissue, and p57 is present in a restricted set of the same tissues as p27 (63, 64).

Recently, it has been shown that the pRB-related protein p107 appears to be able to inhibit cyclin A–CDK2 activity in an analogous fashion to p21/p27/p57. Furthermore, p107, p21, and p27 share a small region of homology and bind to cyclin–CDKs in a mutually exclusive fashion (168). Thus, it has been proposed that p107 functions as an inhibitor of cyclin–CDK activity as well as to target cyclin–CDK complexes to E2F.

5. The G1 to S controlpoint

5.1 Cyclin E–CDK2

The clearest evidence points to cyclin E as the primary regulator of the initiation of S phase, and comes from studies on *Drosophila* that are mutant in cyclin E. In these flies, cells arrest in G1 phase when the maternal supply of cyclin E is exhausted, and these cells can then be made to undergo another round of DNA replication by the ectopic expression of cyclin E (185, 186). Interestingly, the cells undergo endo-reduplication when cyclin E is expressed in the absence of the mitotic cyclins (186).

A homologue of the mammalian E2F transcription factor has been isolated from *Drosophila* and one of its target genes is cyclin E (187, 188). Furthermore, ectopically expressed cyclin E is able to overcome the cell cycle arrest caused by a defective E2F gene (187). Thus it appears that cyclin E is one of the major limiting downstream targets of E2F in the initiation of S phase. Conversely, E2F is unable to rescue a defect in cyclin E, so that cyclin E-associated kinase activity must be required for more than just the activation of E2F (187).

The cyclin E gene looks to be an evolutionarily conserved target for E2F because mammalian cyclin E (and cyclin A) synthesis is strongly stimulated by ectopic E2F-1 (103). In mammalian cells, cyclin E–CDK2 interacts with E2F complexes in late G1 phase through binding to p107 (118). However, the amount of E2F bound to cyclin E–CDK2 is small, and the effect of cyclin E–CDK2 on E2F activity is unclear. Given the feedback between E2F and cyclin E in *Drosophila*, mammalian cyclin E–CDK2 could stimulate E2F activity at the G1–S transition, but there are little data to confirm this.

Further evidence for a requirement for cyclin E–CDK2 to initiate S phase is that in *Xenopus* egg extracts, almost all the CDK2 is bound to cyclin E, and DNA synthesis is blocked when CDK2 is depleted (189, 190). Similarly anti-CDK2 antibodies (191) or a dominant negative form of CDK2 (192) will inhibit the initiation of DNA replication in mammalian cells, blocking cells in G1 phase, at which point CDK2 is primarily bound to cyclin E (71, 193).

In mammalian cells in tissue culture, G1 phase is slightly shortened when cyclin E is overexpressed (132), which is indirect evidence that cyclin E could be rate limiting for the G1–S decision point. However, it is not clear whether the activity of cyclin E–CDK2 is mainly regulated by the amount of cyclin and inhibitor proteins (61, 62, 180, 193) or whether phosphorylation of Y15/T14 is also a significant factor. The CDC25A phosphatase does appear to be necessary for the entry into S phase, and it can be activated by phosphorylation (32, 33). *In vitro*, CDC25A is a very good substrate for cyclin E–CDK2 (33), but whether it is activated by cyclin E–CDK2 *in vivo* has not been confirmed. Similarly, the substrate for CDC25A has not been defined but, given the high degree of specificity exhibited by these phosphatases for the inhibitory T14 and Y15 sites on a CDK, the best candidate is cyclin E–CDK2. Thus, it is possible that there is a positive feedback loop between the cyclin–CDK2 complexes and CDC25A at the initiation of S phase, in the same manner as for cyclin B–cdc2 and CDC25C at mitosis (47). There are also recent data to suggest that CDC25A associates with RAF (see Chapter 5) and that when overexpressed, CDC25A is able to co-operate with activated RAS in transforming cells (194). However, the significance of this to the regulation of S phase is not immediately apparent.

5.2 Cyclin A–CDK2

In contrast to both *Drosophila* and *Xenopus*, there are data indicating that in mammalian cells cyclin A may also be required for DNA replication. Both antisense cyclin A mRNA and cyclin A antibody microinjection experiments prevent, or dramatically decrease, DNA replication in tissue culture cells (195–197). Cyclin A also co-localizes with mammalian origins of replication (198, 199) but a SV40 T antigen-depdendent *in vitro* system does not need cyclin A to replicate DNA (200). This suggests that if cyclin A-associated kinase activity is required, then it might only be needed for origin unwinding/initiation and not elongation. However, contrasting data using *Xenopus* extracts suggest that cyclin A could be needed for the switch between initiation and elongation (190). One difference between cyclin A in mammalian cells compared with *Xenopus* embryos is that in the embryos cyclin A only associates with cdc2 (201), whereas in mammalian cells it binds both CDK2 and cdc2. Moreover, cyclin A–CDK2 predominates in S phase whereas cyclin A–cdc2 appears later in G2 phase (196). Thus it is possible that cyclin A has taken on an additional role in mammalian DNA replication through its association with CDK2. Furthermore, after *Xenopus* gastrulation, the adult form of cyclin A begins to be transcribed and this associates with CDK2 (201), although it has not been determined whether this complex is required for DNA replication in adult frog cells.

5.2.1 Cyclin A and cancer

Cyclin A has also been implicated in cancer. One of the ways in which human cyclin A was identified was as the site of integration of a hepatitis B virus in a hepatocellular carcinoma (202). The integration was into the first intron of the gene generating a fusion protein between the pre-S protein of HBV and cyclin A, removing the amino terminal region of cyclin A including the destruction box (203). However, it is still not clear whether this event was the cause of the carcinoma, nor whether the critical change was in generating a non-degradable form of cyclin A.

Cyclin A has been linked to cancer in a second manner, by its identification as one of the targets of DNA tumour virus transforming antigens. Cyclin A is one of the proteins that form a complex with adenovirus E1A (204), and is also associated with SV40 T antigen (205) and HPV E7 protein (206), in each case with its CDK2 partner. Again it is not certain why cyclin A–CDK2 is targeted by these antigens, but it may be in order to deregulate E2F. Cyclin A directly binds with E2F-1, -2, and -3 (207), and also forms a complex with E2F-4 and -5 (118–120) through binding to the spacer region of p107 (208 and Chapter 8). As mentioned above, the E2F transcription factors appear to be responsible for transcribing S phase genes, and there are data indicating that cyclin A is able to phosphorylate E2F-1 to prevent it binding DNA (207).

The prevailing hypothesis is that cyclin A negatively regulates E2F once cells have entered S phase, to shut down the genes encoding components of the replication machinery and help to ensure that there is only one round of DNA replication per cell cycle. Thus, viral antigens may target cyclin A in order to block cells in a state permissive for DNA replication. This theory requires that cyclin A bound to the viral proteins is still able to perform the actions necessary for DNA replication indicated by the antisense and antibody injection experiments mentioned above.

6. DNA replication

6.1 Proteins bound to origins of replication differ before and after firing

The initiation of DNA replication is one of the most important and carefully regulated controlpoints in the cell cycle. It is very important that cells should replicate each and every part of the genome once, but only once, per cell cycle. The mechanism by which the cell distinguishes between replicated and unreplicated DNA is not clear, but there are data to connect it with the state of the origins of replication and with which cyclin–CDK complexes are present in the cell.

In vivo and *in vitro* footprinting of yeast origins of replication have shown that origins are constitutively bound throughout the cell cycle by a multiprotein complex called the origin replication complex, ORC (209, 210), and some replication proteins, such as RPA, assemble on the chromosome scaffold at the end of mitosis (211). The ORC footprint differs between replication origins in G1 phase, when they are competent to initiate DNA synthesis but have not yet fired, compared with S and G2 phase once they have initiated DNA replication (212, 213). This indicates that pre-replication complexes assemble on origins in G1 phase, which differ by one or more components compared with origins that have initiated DNA replication. One of the yeast proteins that may be unique to pre-replication origins is the product of the *CDC6* gene, which interacts with ORC and becomes very unstable when cells enter S phase (212). The fission yeast homologue of *CDC6* is *cdc18*, which has itself been implicated in the proper regulation of S phase (214). In the absence of *cdc18*, fission yeast cells will enter prematurely into mitosis without replicating their DNA (214), suggesting that *cdc18* is part of the mechanism that generates a negative signal to prevent mitosis while DNA replication is in progress (see below).

6.2 Cyclin–CDK complexes define pre- and post-replicated cell states

The fission yeast cell appears to be able to tell which phase of the cell cycle it is in by which cyclin–CDK complex is present in the cell. A specific mutation in the G2/mitosis specific B-type cyclin, cdc13, makes it thermolabile. When cells with this allele of *cdc13* are raised to the restrictive temperature, they degrade cdc13 and re-replicate their DNA without undergoing mitosis (215). The cell has apparently been fooled into believing it is back in G1 phase through the loss of cdc13. Similarly, cells with a thermolabile cdc2 protein re-replicate their DNA after being raised to the restrictive temperature (216), perhaps because cdc2 is newly synthesized as the G1 phase form. Fission yeast cells also re-replicate their DNA if the rum1 protein is overexpressed (217). The rum1 protein inhibits the cdc13–cdc2 complex, so that overexpressing rum1 would prevent the appearance of any mitotic cyclin–cdc2 activity, which may be functionally equivalent to degrading cdc13. Conversely, deleting *rum1* causes fission yeast cells to begin mitosis before START without replicating their DNA (217), so (that) it appears that pre-START rum1 is required to prevent cyclin B–cdc2 mitosis-inducing activity. Once DNA synthesis has begun, mitosis is inhibited by the presence of replication complexes (see below).

6.3 Licensing factor

Studies with *Xenopus* cell-free extracts cells have shown that nuclei can also be induced to re-replicate DNA without an intervening mitosis if the nuclear membrane is artificially disrupted (218, 219). These observations led to the 'licensing factor' model of DNA replication which postulates that there is (are) a factor(s) required for replication that is unable to cross the nuclear membrane, and is inactivated once DNA is replicated (218). This factor can only gain access to the DNA when the nuclear membrane breaks down at mitosis. A partial purification from *Xenopus* extracts of the proteins required to cause re-replication identified components of the MCM family (220–222) (mini-chromosome maintenance genes), proteins that are well conserved between yeast and animals cells. However, the MCM proteins are able to cross an intact nuclear membrane, so that the original licensing factor remains unidentified.

DNA can also be re-replicated if G2 nuclei are treated with protein kinase inhibitors such as 6-dimethyl amino purine (6-DMAP) (223) or staurosporin (224). Thus, a recent synthesis of the licensing factor model and observations on cyclin–CDK complexes in yeast has proposed that the G2-specific cyclin–CDK complexes, cyclins A and B in animals cells, may directly, or indirectly, block re-replication by preventing the assembly of pre-replication complexes (225). This would inhibit the initiation of DNA replication but not DNA elongation. Pre-replication complexes would normally be able to assemble and origins become competent to initiate DNA replication when cyclins A and B are degraded at mitosis. However, this effect could be mimicked artificially by inactivating the cyclin–CDK complexes with protein kinase inhibitors, or in some way by permeabilizing the nuclear membrane (225).

This model is consistent with data from experiments on *Drosophila*. Cells in developing *Drosophila* embryos that are mutant in cyclin A all arrest in G2 phase once the maternal store of cyclin A is exhausted (226), whereas cells from embryos that lack cyclin E arrest in G1 phase (185). A pulse of cyclin E from a transgene will drive cells through another round of S phase and mitosis but, in the absence of cyclin A, cells are unable to enter mitosis and instead go through a round of re-replication. One possible conclusion from this is that cyclin A is required to prevent re-replication (186). This correlates with the presence of cyclin E and absence of cyclins A and B in wild-type cells that naturally re-replicate their DNA (185, 186), where cyclin E negatively regulates its own expression (186).

6.4 An S phase checkpoint involving p21 and PCNA?

The p53–p21 pathway theoretically provides a means to arrest cells after UV damage while they are replicating DNA (Chapter 9). This is because p21 is able to bind and inhibit PCNA, which is required for leading strand synthesis in DNA replication (200). The carboxy terminus of p21 inhibits PCNA *in vitro* (175, 178), and blocks DNA replication in an *in vitro* SV40 T antigen-dependent replication system (227), without the mediation of cyclin–CDK complexes. Furthermore, DNA excision repair, which requires PCNA, is not sensitive to p21 inhibition (228), so that cells could repair their DNA while DNA replication is blocked. However, it has not yet been clearly demonstrated whether p21 ever acts through inhibiting PCNA *in vivo*. On the one hand, tissue culture cells are arrested when transfected with either the amino or the carboxyl half of p21 (229, 230). Conversely, in *Xenopus* egg extracts, exogenous p21 inhibits DNA replication exclusively through inhibiting cyclin–CDKs, such that replication is restored by the addition of cyclin E or cyclin A kinase (190, 231).

7. G2 phase: rad and hus checkpoints and the G2 to M controlpoint

7.1 Unreplicated DNA inhibits mitosis through Y15 phosphorylation on cdc2

Remarkably, studies on the budding and fission yeast cell cycles have shown that when a cell commits itself to DNA replication it simultaneously commits itself to mitosis, such that mitosis is only prevented by ongoing DNA replication. There are three fission yeast genes which are needed for DNA replication to begin, and are also needed to prevent mitosis before the DNA has been replicated. These include the

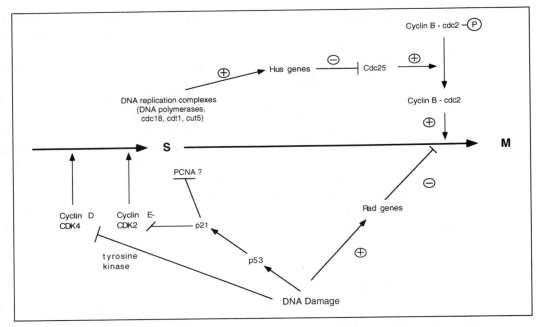

Fig. 5 The rad and hus checkpoints. The negative effect of DNA damage and unreplicated DNA on the entry into mitosis, and the components involved as identified by genetic analysis, are shown.

products of the *cdc18* (214), *cdt1* (232), and *cut5* (233, 234) genes. Components of the DNA replication machinery, such as DNA polymerase α and ε (235, 236), are also thought to help to generate the mitosis-inhibiting signal, which will therefore only disappear when the last replication complex disassembles upon completion of DNA synthesis. Some of the genes (the *hus* genes) in the pathway coupling the signal to the mitotic machinery have been defined by genetic analysis (237, 238). This pathway prevents the dephosphorylation of Y15 on cdc2, such that mutating Y15 in fission yeast cdc2 renders the yeast insensitive to the replication state of the DNA when they initiate mitosis (238, 239). Before yeast have committed themselves to DNA replication/mitosis, i.e. before START, mitosis is inhibited by a mechanism that is independent of cdc2 Y15 phosphorylation. One component is the rum1 inhibitor protein (217), and another is that cyclin B and cdc2 are prevented from forming a complex (240).

Studies on *Xenopus* egg extracts have also shown that unreplicated DNA will prevent cells from initiating mitosis (241). There are data indicating that the arrest is effected by inhibiting the dephosphorylation of Y15 in cdc2, and/or by a titratable inhibitor protein (242). This inhibitor might be one of the p21 family but because none of these is very effective in inhibiting cyclin B–cdc2 *in vitro*, there could be a specific mitotic kinase inhibitor still to be identified. Such an inhibitor could be related to fission yeast p13^{suc1}, the first cyclin–CDK binding protein (243) to be identified, which is a conserved and essential gene. p13^{suc1} will inhibit the G2–M transition when added to *Xenopus* extracts (244), but its role in the cell cycle is still an enigma.

Both transformed and non-transformed mammalian cell lines arrest in S phase with DNA synthesis inhibitors and are therefore responsive to the replication state of the DNA. However, the tsBN2 temperature-sensitive cell line will begin mitosis with unreplicated DNA at the non-permissive temperature (245, 246). This has a defect in the RCC1 protein, which is a GTP exchange factor (247, 248) for the RAN/TC4 G protein required for nuclear import (249). At the non-permissive temperature, RCC1 is degraded and cyclin B–cdc2 is subsequently activated by CDC25C when the cells prematurely initiate mitosis (245, 246). The components downstream of RCC1 and RAN/TC4 have not been identified, but it is likely that premature mitosis is due to an interruption in the inhibitory signal generated by unreplicated DNA. Premature mitosis is also the consequence of adding the phosphatase 1 and 2A inhibitor okadaic acid (250) to hamster cells, which appears to inhibit the phosphatase(s) that usually keeps CDC25C inactive until mitosis (251). Thus CDC25C may be one of the targets of the inhibitory signal generated by unreplicated DNA in mammalian cells.

7.2 Damaged DNA inhibits mitosis, but not directly through cdc2

There is clearly a G2 phase checkpoint responsive to DNA damage after DNA replication. This checkpoint has been studied in most detail in yeast. In budding yeast, one of the crucial players involved is the product of the RAD9 gene (252). Indeed, studies on RAD9 generated the concept of the checkpoint itself (6). The RAD9 gene is not essential to cell growth under normal conditions, however, when cells are irradiated with γ-rays RAD9 mutants are unable to arrest in G2 phase to repair their DNA. Thus γ-irradiated RAD9 mutant cells initiate mitosis with damaged DNA which is normally a lethal event (252, 253). The RAD9 checkpoint pathway inhibits mitosis by a mechanism that does not directly act on CDC28, the major CDK in budding yeast. Similarly, the damaged DNA checkpoint pathway in fission yeast does not act through phosphorylating and inhibiting cdc2 (254, 255). Although there is some overlap between the genes involved in inhibiting mitosis in the presence of unreplicated DNA and of damaged DNA in fission and budding yeasts, some genes are unique to each pathway (238, 256–258) (Fig. 5).

Transformed and non-transformed mammalian cells differ in their ability to arrest in G2 after DNA damage (259), but given the lack of genetic analysis, it has proved difficult to determine whether the arrest is effected directly by modulating the cyclin–CDK complexes. Radiation or chemical damage to DNA arrests cells in G2 phase with cdc2 phosphorylated on Y15 (259, 260), but this may not be a direct effect. Radiation or chemical damage to DNA causes cyclin B1 mRNA (261) but not cyclin A (262) to be down-regulated in G2 phase, and this is at the level of mRNA stability (263). Cyclin B1 protein levels have also been proposed to decrease (261). Decreasing the amount of cyclin B1 would contribute to a G2 phase arrest by preventing cyclin B1–cdc2 complexes from reaching the (putative) threshold amount required to enter mitosis.

8. The G2 to M controlpoint

8.1 The antagonism between wee1/mik1 and cdc25

Mitosis is initiated by the activation of the pool of cyclin B–cdc2 complexes that have accumulated through G2 phase. An analysis of *Drosophila* embryos that have a mutation in cyclin A shows that cyclin A plays an essential role in initiating mitosis but its exact role has not been defined (264). Cyclin A–CDK complexes are likely to be involved in the initiation of spindle assembly, because in *Xenopus* cell-free extracts cyclin A–CDK kinase activity causes centrosomes to nucleate arrays of microtubules (265, 266). Similarly, cyclin F is also active in G2 phase and although its substrates have not been identified, antisense data suggest that cyclin F is also required for entry into M phase (267).

There are a number of different cyclin B–cdc2 complexes in mammalian cells and these appear to act both as upstream activators of other mitotic kinases, and as 'workhorse' kinases (268) that phosphorylate a number of cytoskeletal components in order to reorganize the cellular architecture at mitosis. For a more detailed discussion of the mitotic substrates of cyclin B–cdc2 kinases see (10, 268, 269). In the context of oncogenesis, it is relevant to mention that two non-receptor tyrosine kinases, c-ABL and c-SRC (see Chapter 4), are substrates for the cyclin B–cdc2 kinase in mitosis. Phosphorylation by cyclin B–cdc2 appears to abolish the DNA binding activity of c-ABL (270), whereas it increases the kinase activity of c-SRC (271).

One of the primary controls on cyclin B–cdc2 kinase activity is through the phosphorylation and dephosphorylation of T14 and Y15 of cdc2 (reviewed in ref. 49). Mutating either of these sites to non-phosphorylatable residues partially deregulates mitosis when the mutant cdc2 is introduced into tissue culture cells or in frog egg extracts (28, 29). If both residues are mutated the cell is unable to prevent the activation of cdc2 kinase and appears to enter mitosis prematurely.

The T14 kinase has been only partially characterized but interestingly it is membrane associated (272) and may therefore be especially important in the regulation of cyclin B2–cdc2 (see below). Tyrosine 15 is phosphorylated by the wee1 and mik1 kinases, maintaining cyclin B–cdc2 in an inactive state (reviewed in ref. 49). At mitosis, wee1/mik1 kinase activity is down-regulated through wee1/mik1 phosphorylation by at least two protein kinases, one of which is encoded by the *nim*1 gene in fission yeast (273–276). At the same time, the T14 and Y15 phosphatase, CDC25C, is activated by phosphorylation. Subsequently a positive feedback loop is set-up between active cyclin B–cdc2 and CDC25C (47). However, the identity of the kinase that initially activates CDC25C at mitosis is still unknown. The kinase may be one of the MPM2 kinases (277), because activated CDC25C is recognized by the MPM2 monoclonal antibody (278)—which binds a mitosis-specific phosphorylation epitope found on a variety of proteins phosphorylated at mitosis (279). Two MPM2 kinases have been partially characterized and are clearly distinct from the CDK family (277). The weaker of the two kinases is a member of the MAP kinase family (see Chapter 5).

8.1.1 Localization and translocation

Mammalian cells have two types of cyclin B; cyclin B1 (280) and cyclin B2 (281). There may be other B-type cyclins in human cells because nematodes, *Drosophila*, and chicken (282) cells all have a cyclin B3, frogs have five types of B cyclin (Mike Howell and Tim Hunt, personal communication), and nine B-type cyclin loci were mapped onto the mouse genome (283), although some of these loci are likely to be pseudo-genes. The different cyclin B–cdc2 complexes are activated and inactivated at the same time in the cell cycle but they differ in their cellular localization which may give us clues to their likely role in mitosis.

Cyclin B3 is a nuclear protein (282) and so could be involved in reorganizing the karyoskeleton, for example in lamin disassembly or in chromosome condensation. The nuclear lamins are the most thoroughly defined substrates for cyclin B–cdc2, and phosphorylation has been shown to promote lamina disassembly (284–287). Histone H1 is a good substrate for most cyclin–CDK complexes (288, 289) and is routinely used for CDK assays *in vitro*. However, it is unclear whether this phosphorylation contributes to chromosome condensation or not. A better candidate for the kinase involved in chromosome condensation is the product of the NIMA gene in the filamentous fungus *Aspergillus nidulans* (290). NIMA is a very unstable protein that is stabilized by phosphorylation at mitosis, in all likelihood by cyclin B–cdc2 kinase activity (291); artificially stabilized NIMA will cause chromosome condensation if it is mis-expressed at any stage in the cell cycle (292). As yet, no mammalian homologue of NIMA has been isolated, but the *Aspergillus* protein will produce chromosome condensation independently of cdc2 kinase activity in human cells (293), so that it is likely that its role has been conserved in evolution.

Human cyclin B2 is a cytoplasmic protein that is almost exclusively associated with the Golgi apparatus (294). It is therefore likely that cyclin B2 is involved in the disassembly of the Golgi apparatus and inhibition of membrane traffic that occurs at mitosis (295–297), and which can be reconstituted *in vitro* by mitotic cyclin–cdc2 kinase (297, 298). Cyclin B2 remains associated with membrane vesicles throughout metaphase, before being degraded along with the other B-type cyclins when cells begin anaphase (294).

In contrast, in interphase, human cyclin B1 is associated with microtubules (86, 299) and in particular with MAP4 (300), but at mitosis it translocates into the nucleus before nuclear envelope breakdown (86). There are also data to suggest that CDC25C undergoes a similar translocation event at the same time (39). Thus, cyclin B1 may also be able to act as the lamin kinase. During metaphase, cyclin B1 strongly associates with the mitotic apparatus, a feature that is conserved in evolution because fission yeast cdc13 also binds to the spindle and spindle poles (301). *In vitro* studies show that cyclin B–cdc2 kinase activity changes the dynamic instability of microtubules and inhibits their nucleation at centrosomes (267, 268, 302). This is the behaviour that microtubules exhibit at mitosis, so that it is likely that cyclin B1–cdc2 is involved in the reorganization of the microtubule network into the spindle.

9. The metaphase–anaphase checkpoint

9.1 A phosphorylation epitope unique to misaligned chromosomes

The physical connection between the spindle and cyclin B1–cdc2 complexes is probably integral to the control of cyclin degradation and thus to the metaphase–anaphase checkpoint.

Normally, once chromosomes are correctly paired on the metaphase plate, cyclin B is degraded and the cells enter anaphase. When chromosomes are incorrectly aligned in metaphase, or the spindle is incorrectly formed, a checkpoint is activated and cells stay in metaphase until the error is removed. This is through the inhibition (or non-activation) of the proteolysis machinery responsible for degrading the proteins that link sister chromatids and for degrading cyclin B (but not A) (90). High cyclin B–cdc2 kinase activity maintains the spindle, and because sister chromatids are still linked together, the cell will remain in metaphase (90, 303).

A cell senses errors in the spindle through a lack of tension in the spindle micro-tubules. Only when all the microtubules are under equal tension will the cell begin anaphase (304–306). Exactly how the force is measured is not known, although it appears to be sensed by the kinetochores (306, 307), but the inhibitory signal gener-ated may have been identified. A monoclonal antibody raised to a phosphorylation epitope has been found to label kinetochores that are misaligned more strongly than those on chromosomes equidistant between spindle poles (306, 308). This suggests that a kinetochore protein is dephosphorylated once chromosomes are properly aligned on the metaphase plate. Moreover, even one incorrectly aligned kinetochore would generate a positive signal to inhibit anaphase via its phosphorylated compo-nent, explaining why cells are able to arrest in metaphase even if only one chromo-some is delayed in reaching the metaphase plate (Fig. 6; and reviewed in ref. 309). The kinase responsible for phosphorylating the unidentified kinetochore component in metaphase may be a member of the MAP kinase family, because the metaphase arrest checkpoint can be reconstituted in frog egg extracts by the addition of MAP kinase (310).

9.2 MOS and CSF

The role of MAP kinase in maintaining cells in metaphase may be relevant to the identification of the product of the proto-oncogene c-MOS as cytostatic factor (CSF) in meiosis (311, 312). CSF is an activity able to arrest cells in metaphase (313) and is normally generated specifically in meiosis in order to arrest oocytes in metaphase II before fertilization. c-MOS protein is normally only present in germ cells, and has CSF activity when injected into oocytes or cleaving embryos (311, 312, 314). MOS is required to prevent DNA replication between the first and second meiotic division in frog oocytes, (315), and if MOS is ablated in mouse oocytes they are unable to arrest in

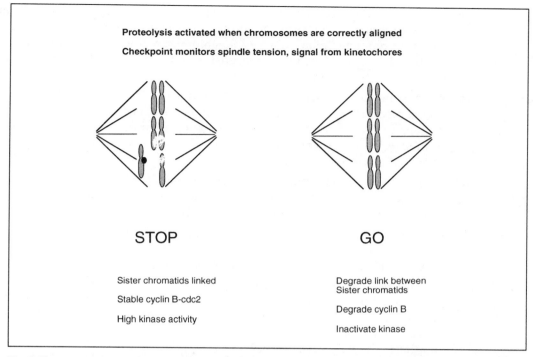

Fig. 6 The metaphase–anaphase checkpoint. The presence of even one misaligned kinetochore is able to inhibit the entry into anaphase. The misaligned kinetochore (black dot) is recognized by a phospho-epitope specific monoclonal and generates an inhibitory signal that only disappears once all the chromosomes are correctly aligned.

metaphase II (316, 317). c-MOS is a serine threonine kinase that acts as a MAP kinase kinase (318), the equivalent of RAF in signal transduction pathways (Chapter 5). Thus MOS might promote metaphase arrest by activating the MAP kinase responsible for the metaphase–anaphase checkpoint.

The role of MOS as a MAP kinase kinase during meiosis (318, 319), may explain why it is able to transform somatic cells. MOS normally disappears immediately after fertilization, so that its expression in somatic cells might aberrantly stimulate the MAP kinase pathway, mimicking the effect of growth factors. An alternative model is that when the M phase promoting properties of MOS are superimposed on the somatic cell cycle, this perturbs the normal morphology of cells and increases genetic instability by compromising interphase and mitotic checkpoint controls (320, 321).

10. Drug targets

Our understanding of the mechanics of cell cycle control continues to increase rapidly. With the identification of cell cycle components deregulated in transformed compared with non-transformed cells comes the possibility of new targets for anti-cancer therapy. A number of approaches suggest themselves.

(a) We may be able to reconstitute checkpoints lost in transformed cells and thus arrest tumour cell growth, or induce apoptosis when the cell recognizes the genomic damage it has already sustained. In this respect, the alterations in cyclin–CDK complexes in many transformed cells, such as the absence of p21 or PCNA, are obvious targets for drug development.

(b) We may be able to take advantage of the lack of checkpoints in transformed cells, that may leave them vulnerable to therapy tolerated by normal cells. This is one of the factors in current radiation treatment and chemotherapy, because some transformed cells are unable to arrest in G2 phase and so enter mitosis with the damaged DNA, which is a lethal event.

(c) We may be able to inhibit positive regulators of proliferation in tumour cells, for example the cyclin D–CDK4/CDK6 complexes. In this case, inhibitors could be substrate analogues or mimics of the INK4 family.

(d) We may be able to alter the decision made at various control points to prevent the cell from proliferating. For example, at R we may be able to induce the cell to differentiate, or to senesce, or to undergo apoptosis.

(e) We may be able to identify defects in the components of the cell cycle machinery in tumour cells that act at particular controlpoints, and thus specifically inhibit proliferation in these cells. For example, cells could be prevented from initiating DNA replication (cyclin E–CDK2), or mitosis (cyclin B–cdc2 or CDC25C), or anaphase (the APC/cyclosome).

Note added in proof

Since this review was written, the cdc2 threonine 14 membrane-associated kinase has been isolated as an integral membrane protein and named myt1 (Mueller, P. R., Coleman, T. R., Kumagai, A., and Dunphy, W. G. 1995. Myt1: a membrane-associated inhibitory kinase that phosphorylates cdc2 on both threonine-14 and tyrosine-15. *Science*, **270**, 86–90). In addition, one of the kinases that activates Cdc25C in frogs has been identified as the *polo* homologue, Plx1 (Kumagai, A., and Dunphy, W. G. 1996. Purification and molecular cloning of Plx1, a Cdc25-regulatory kinase from Xenopus egg extracts. *Science*, **273**, 1377–80.)

References

1. Murray, A. and Hunt, T. (1993) *The cell cycle: an introduction.* W. H. Freeman and Co., New York.
2. Meyerson, M., Faha, B., Su, L. K., Harlow, E., and Tsai, L. H. (1991) The cyclin-dependent kinase family. *Cold Spring Harbor Symp. Quant. Biol.*, **56**, 177.
3. Pines, J. and Hunter, T. (1991) Cyclin-dependent kinases: a new cell cycle motif? *Trends Cell. Biol.*, **1**, 117.
4. Evans, T., Rosenthal, E. T., Youngblom, J., Distel, D., and Hunt, T. (1983) Cyclin: A protein specified by maternal mRNA in sea urchin eggs that is destroyed at each cleavage division. *Cell*, **33**, 389.

5. Hunt, T. (1991) Cyclins and their partners: from a simple idea to complicated reality. *Semin. Cell Biol.*, **2**, 213.

6. Hartwell, L. H. and Weinert, T. A. (1989) Checkpoints: controls that ensure the order of cell cycle events. *Science*, **246**, 629.

7. Hartwell, L. H. and Kastan, M. B. (1994) Cell Cycle Control and Cancer. *Science*, **266**, 1821.

8. Pines, J. and Hunter, T. (1995) Cyclin-dependent kinases: an embarrassment of riches? In *Cell cycle control* (ed. Hutchison and Glover), p. 144. IRL Press, Oxford.

9. Morgan, D. O. (1995) Principles of CDK regulation. *Nature*, **374**, 131.

10. Pines, J. (1995) Cyclins and cyclin-dependent kinases: a biochemical view. *Biochem. J.*, **308**, 697.

11. De Bondt, H. L., Rosenblatt, J., Jancarik, J., Jones, H. D., Morgan, D. O., and Kim, S.-H. (1993) Crystal structure of human CDK2: implications for the regulation of cyclin-dependent kinases by phosphorylation and cyclin binding. *Nature*, **363**, 595.

12. Jeffrey, P. D., Russo, A. A., Polyak, K., Gibbs, E., Hurwitz, J., Massague, J., et al. (1995) Structure of a cyclin A-CDK2 complex. *Nature*, **376**, 313.

13. Connell, C. L., Solomon, M. J., Wei, N., and Harper, J. W. (1993) Phosphorylation independent activation of human cyclin-dependent kinase 2 by cyclin A *in vitro. Mol. Biol. Cell*, **4**, 79.

14. Desai, D., Wessling, H. C., Fisher, R. P., and Morgan, D. O. (1995) Effects of Phosphorylation by CAK on Cyclin Binding by CDC2 and CDK2. *Mol. Cell. Biol.*, **15**, 345.

15. Ducommun, B., Brambilla, P., Félix, M.-A., Franza, B. R., Jr, Karsenti, E., and Draetta, G. (1991) cdc2 phosphorylation is required for its interaction with cyclin. *EMBO J.*, **10**, 3311.

16. Gould, K. L., Moreno, S., Owen, D. J., Sazer, S., and Nurse, P. (1991) Phosphorylation at Thr167 is required for *Schizosaccharomyces pombe* p34[cdc2] function. *EMBO J.*, **10**, 3297.

17. Solomon, M. J., Lee, T., and Kirschner, M. W. (1992) Role of phosphorylation in p34cdc2 activation: identification of an activating kinase. *Mol. Biol. Cell*, **3**, 13.

18. Fisher, R. P. and Morgan, D. O. (1994) A novel cyclin associates with MO15/CDK7 to form the CDK-activating kinase. *Cell*, **78**, 713.

19. Makela, T. P., Tassan, J.-P., Nigg, E. A., Frutiger, S., Hughes, G. J., and Weinberg, R. A. (1994) A cyclin associated with the CDK-activating kinase MO15. *Nature*, **371**, 254.

20. Tassan, J.-P., Schultz, S. J., Bartek, J., and Nigg, E. A. (1994) Cell cycle analysis of the activity, subcellular localization and subunit composition of human CAK (CDK-activating kinase). *J. Cell. Biol.*, **127**, 467.

21. Fesquet, D., Labbe, J. C., Derancourt, J., Capony, J. P., Galas, S., Girard, F., et al. (1993) The MO15 gene encodes the catalytic subunit of a protein kinase that activates cdc2 and other cyclin-dependent kinases (CDKs) through phosphorylation of Thr161 and its homologues. *EMBO J.*, **12**, 3111.

22. Poon, R. Y. C., Yamashita, K., Adaczewski, J., Hunt, T., and Shuttleworth, J. (1993) The cdc2-related protein p40[MO15] is the catalytic subunit of a protein kinase that can activate p33[cdk2] and p34[cdc2]. *EMBO J.*, **12**, 3123.

23. Solomon, M. J., Harper, J. W., and Shuttleworth, J. (1993) CAK, the p34[cdc2] activating kinase, contains a protein identical or closely related to p40[MO15]. *EMBO J.*, **12**, 3133.

24. Feaver, W. J., Svejstrup, J. Q., Henry, N. L., and Kornberg, R. D. (1994) Relationship of CDK-Activating Kinase and RNA Polymerase II CTD Kinase TFIIH/TFIIK. *Cell*, **79**, 1103.

25. Roy, R., Adamczewski, J. P., Seroz, T., Vermeulen, W., Tassan, J.-P., Schaeffer, L., et al.

(1994) The MO15 Cell Cycle Kinase Is Associated with the TFIIH Transcription-DNA Repair Factor. *Cell*, **79**, 1093.

26. Gyuris, J. E. G., Chertkov, H., and Brent, R. (1993) Cdi1, a human G1 and S phase protein phosphatase that associates with Cdk2. *Cell*, **75**, 791.

27. Hannon, G., Casso, D., and Beach, D. (1994) KAP: A dual specificity phosphatase that interacts with cyclin-dependent kinases. *Proc. Natl. Acad. Sci. USA*, **91**, 1731.

28. Krek, W. and Nigg, E. A. (1991) Mutations of p34cdc2 phosphorylation sites induce premature mitotic events in HeLa cells: evidence for a double block to p34cdc2 kinase activation in vertebrates. *EMBO J.*, **10**, 3331.

29. Norbury, C., Blow, J., and Nurse, P. (1991) Regulatory phosphorylation of the p34^{cdc2} protein kinase in vertebrates. *EMBO J.*, **10**, 3321.

30. Gould, K. L. and Nurse, P. (1989) Tyrosine phosphorylation of the fission yeast *cdc2*$^+$ protein kinase regulates entry into mitosis. *Nature*, **342**, 39.

31. Terada, Y., Tatsuka, M., Jinno, S., and Okayama, H. (1995) Requirement for tyrosine phosphorylation of Cdk4 in G1 arrest induced by ultraviolet irradiation. *Nature*, **376**, 358.

32. Jinno, S., Suto, K., Nagata, A., Igarashi, M., Kanaoka, Y., Nojima, H., *et al.* (1994) Cdc25A is a novel phosphatase functioning early in the cell cycle. *EMBO J.*, **13**, 1549.

33. Hoffmann, I., Draetta, G., and Karsenti, E. (1994) Activation of the phosphatase activity of human cdc25A by a cdk2-cyclin E dependent phosphorylation at the G_1/S transition. *EMBO J.*, **13**, 4302.

34. Russell, P. and Nurse, P. (1987) Negative regulation of mitosis by wee1+, a gene encoding a protein kinase homolog. *Cell*, **49**, 559.

35. Featherstone, C. and Russell, P. (1991) Fission yeast p107wee1 mitotic inhibitor is a tyrosine/serine kinase. *Nature*, **349**, 808.

36. Parker, L. L., Atherton-Fessler, S., Lee, M. S., Ogg, S., Falk, J. L., Swenson, K. I., *et al.* (1991) Cyclin promotes the tyrosine phosphorylation of p34cdc2 in a wee1+ dependent manner. *EMBO J.*, **10**, 1255.

37. Lundgren, K., Walworth, N., Booher, R., Dembski, M., and Beach, D. (1991) mik1 and wee1 cooperate in the inhibitory tyrosine phosphorylation of cdc2. *Cell*, **64**, 1111.

38. Parker, L. L. and Piwnica-Worms, H. (1992) Inactivation of the p34cdc2-cyclin B complex by the human WEE1 tyrosine kinase. *Science*, **257**, 1955.

39. Heald, R., McLoughlin, M., and McKeon, F. (1993) Human Wee1 maintains mitotic timing by protecting the Nucleus from cytoplasmically activated Cdc2 kinase. *Cell*, **74**, 463.

40. McGowan, C. H. and Russell, P. (1993) Human Wee1 kinase inhibits cell division by phosphorylating p34cdc2 exclusively on Tyr15. *EMBO J.*, **12**, 75.

41. Russell, P. and Nurse, P. (1986) cdc25+ functions as an inducer in the mitotic control of fission yeast. *Cell*, **45**, 145.

42. Dunphy, W. G. and Kumagai, A. (1991) The cdc25 protein contains an intrinsic phosphatase activity. *Cell*, **67**, 189.

43. Girard, F., Strausfeld, U., Cavadore, J. C., Russell, P., Fernandez, A., and Lamb, N. J. (1992) cdc25 is a nuclear protein expressed constitutively throughout the cell cycle in nontransformed mammalian cells. *J. Cell. Biol.*, **118**, 785.

44. Gautier, J., Solomon, M. J., Booher, R. N., Bazan, J. F., and Kirschner, M. W. (1991) cdc25 is a specific tyrosine phosphatase that directly activates p34^{cdc2}. *Cell*, **67**, 197.

45. Strausfeld, U., Labbé, J. C., Fesquet, D., Cavadore, J. C., Picard, A., Sadhu, K., *et al.*

(1991) Dephosphorylation and activation of a p34cdc2/cyclin B complex *in vitro* by human cdc25 protein. *Nature*, **351**, 242.

46. Millar, J. B., Blevitt, J., Gerace, L., Sadhu, K., Featherstone, C., and Russell, P. (1991) p55CDC25 is a nuclear protein required for the initiation of mitosis in human cells. *Proc. Natl. Acad. Sci. USA*, **88**, 10500.

47. Hoffmann, I., Clarke, P. R., Marcote, M. J., Karsenti, E., and Draetta, G. (1993) Phosphorylation and activation of human cdc25-C by cdc2–cyclin B and its involvement in the self-amplification of MPF at mitosis. *EMBO J.*, **12**, 53.

48. Galaktionov, K. and Beach, D. (1991) Specific activation of cdc25 tyrosine phosphatases by B-type cyclins: evidence for multiple roles of mitotic cyclins. *Cell*, **67**, 1181.

49. Dunphy, W. G. (1994) The decision to enter mitosis. *Trends Cell Biol.*, **4**, 202.

50. Serrano, M., Hannon, G. J., and Beach, D. (1993) A new regulatory motif in cell cycle control causing specific inhibition of cyclin D/CDK4. *Nature*, **366**, 704.

51. Guan, K.-L., Jenkins, C. W., Li, Y., Nichols, M. A., Wu, X., O'Keefe, C. L., et al. (1994) Growth suppression by p18, a p16$^{INK4/MTS1}$-and p14$^{INK4B/MTS2}$-related CDK6 inhibitor, correlates with wild-type pRb function. *Genes Dev.*, **8**, 2939.

52. Hannon, G. and Beach, D. (1994) p15^{INK4B} is a potential effector of TGF-β-induced cell cycle arrest. *Nature*, **371**, 257.

53. Hirai, H., Roussel, M. F., Kato, J., Ashmun, R. A., and Sherr, C. J. (1995) Novel INK4 proteins, p19 and p18, are specific inhibitors of cyclin D-dependent kinases CDK4 and CDK6. *Mol. Cell. Biol.*, **15**, 2672.

54. Kamb, A., Gruis, N. A., Weaver-Feldhaus, J., Liu, Q., Harshman, K., Tavtigian, S. V., et al. (1994) A cell cycle regulator potentially involved in genesis of many tumor types. *Science*, **264**, 436.

55. Nobori, T., Miura, K., Wu, D. J., Lois, A., Takabayashi, K., and Carson, D. A. (1994) Deletions of the cyclin-dependent kinase-4 inhibitor gene in multiple human cancers. *Nature*, **368**, 753.

56. Xiong, Y., Hannon, G. J., Zhang, H., Casso, D., Kobayashi, R., and Beach, D. (1993) p21 is a universal inhibitor of cyclin kinases. *Nature*, **366**, 701.

57. El-Deiry, W. S., Tokino, T., Velculesco, V. E., Levy, D. B., Parsons, R., Trent, J. M., et al. (1993) WAF1, a potential mediator of p53 tumor suppression. *Cell*, **75**, 817.

58. Harper, J. W., Adami, G. R., Wei, N., Keyomarsi, K., and Elledge, S. J. (1993) The p21 Cdk-interacting protein Cip1 is a potent inhibitor of G1 cyclin-dependent kinases. *Cell*, **75**, 805.

59. Gu, Y., Turck, C. W., and Morgan, D. O. (1993) Inhibition of CDK2 activity *in vivo* by an associated 20K regulatory subunit. *Nature*, **366**, 707.

60. Noda, A., Ning, Y., Venable, S. F., Pereira-Smith, O. M., and Smith, J. R. (1994) Cloning of senescent cell-derived inhibitors of DNA synthesis using an expression screen. *Exp. Cell Res.*, **211**, 90.

61. Polyak, K., Lee, M.-H., Erdjument-Bromage, H., Koff, A., Roberts, J. M., Tempst, P., et al. (1994) Cloning of p27Kip1, a cyclin-dependent kinase inhibitor and a potential mediator of extracellular antimitogenic signals. *Cell*, **78**, 59.

62. Toyoshima, H. and Hunter, T. (1994) p27, a novel inhibitor of G1 cyclin-Cdk protein kinase activity, is related to p21. *Cell*, **78**, 67.

63. Lee, M. H., Reynisdóttir, I., and Massagué, J. (1995) Cloning of p57^{Kip2}, a cyclin-dependent kinase inhibitor with unique domain structure and tissue distribution. *Genes Dev.*, **9**, 639.

64. Matsuoka, S., Edwards, M., Bai, C., Parker, S., Zhang, P., Baldini, A., *et al.* (1995) p57[KIP2], a structurally distinct member of the p21[CIP1] cdk inhibitor family, is a candidate tumor suppressor gene. *Genes Dev.*, **9**, 650.

65. Zhang, H., Hannon, G. J., and Beach, D. (1994) p21-containing cyclin kinases exist in both active and inactive states. *Genes Dev.*, **8**, 1750.

66. Amon, A., Irniger, S., and Nasmyth, K. (1994) Closing the Cell Cycle Circle in Yeast: G2 Cyclin Proteolysis Initiated at Mitosis Persists until the Activation of G1 Cyclins in the Next Cycle. *Cell*, **77**, 1037.

67. Schwob, E., Böhm, T., Mendenhall, M. D., and Nasmyth, K. (1994) The B-type cyclin kinase inhibitor p40[SIC1] controls the G1/S transition in *Saccharomyces cerevisiae*. *Cell*, **79**, 233.

68. Ciechanover, A. (1994) The ubiquitin-proteasome proteolytic pathway. *Cell*, **79**, 13.

69. Matsushime, H., Roussel, M. F., Ashmun, R. A., and Sherr, C. J. (1991) Colony-Stimulating Factor 1 regulates novel cyclins during the G1 phase of the cell cycle. *Cell*, **65**, 701.

70. Koff, A., Cross, F., Fisher, A., Schumacher, J., Phillipe, M., and Roberts, J. M. (1991) Cyclin E, a new class of human cyclin that can activate the p34cdc2/CDC28 kinase. *Cell*, **66**, 1217.

71. Dulic, V., Lees, E., and Reed, S. I. (1992) Association of human cyclin E with a periodic G1-S phase protein kinase. *Science*, **257**, 1958.

72. Cross, F. (1988) DAF1, a mutant gene affecting size control, pheremone arrest and cell cycle kinetics of *S. cerevisiae*. *Mol. Cell. Biol.*, **8**, 4675.

73. Wittenberg, C., Sugimoto, K., and Reed, S. I. (1990) G1-specific cyclins of *S. cerevisiae*: cell cycle periodicity, regulation by mating pheromone, and association with the p34CDC28 protein kinase. *Cell*, **62**, 225.

74. Deshaies, R. J., Chau, V., and Kirschner, M. (1995) Ubiquitination of the G_1 cyclin Cln2p by a Cdc34p-dependent pathway. *EMBO J.*, **14**, 303.

75. Standart, N., Minshull, J., Pines, J., and Hunt, T. (1987) Cyclin synthesis, modification and destruction during meiotic maturation of the starfish oocyte. *Dev. Biol.*, **124**, 248.

76. Hunt, T., Luca, F. C., and Ruderman, J. V. (1992) The requirements for protein synthesis and degradation, and the control of destruction of cyclins A and B in the meiotic and mitotic cell cycles of the clam embryo. *J. Cell. Biol.*, **116**, 707.

77. Glotzer, M., Murray, A. W., and Kirschner, M. W. (1991) Cyclin is degraded by the ubiquitin pathway. *Nature*, **349**, 132.

78. Hershko, A., Ganoth, D., Sudakin, V., Dahan, A., Cohen, L. H., Luca, F. C., *et al.* (1994) Components of a system that ligates cyclin to ubiquitin and their regulation by the protein kinase cdc2. *J. Biol. Chem.*, **269**, 4940.

79. King, R. W., Peters, J.-M., Tugendreich, S., Rolfe, M., Hieter, P., and Kirschner, M. W. (1995) A 20S complex containing CDC27 and CDC16 catalyzes the mitosis-specific conjugation of ubiquitin to cyclin B. *Cell*, **81**, 279.

80. Stewart, E., Kobayashi, H., Harrison, D., and Hunt, T. (1994) Destruction of Xenopus cyclins A and B2, but not B1, requires binding to p34cdc2. *EMBO J.*, **13**, 584.

81. Van der Velden, H. M. W. and Lohka, M. J. (1994) Cell cycle-regulated degradation of *Xenopus* cyclin B2 requires binding to p34[cdc2]. *Mol. Biol. Cell*, **5**, 713.

82. Irniger, S., Piatti, S., Michaelis, C., and Nasmyth, K. (1995) Genes involved in sister chromatid separation are needed for B-type cyclin proteolysis in budding yeast. *Cell*, **81**, 269.

83. Tugendreich, S., Tomkiel, J., Earnshaw, W., and Hieter, P. (1995) CDC27Hs colocalizes

with CDC16Hs to the centrosome and mitotic spindle and is essential for the metaphase to anaphase transition. *Cell*, **81**, 261.

84. Ghislain, M., Udvardy, A., and Mann, C. (1993) *S. cerevisiae* 26S protease mutants arrest cell division in G2/metaphase. *Nature*, **366**, 358.

85. Gordon, C., McGurk, G., Dillon, P., Rosen, C., and Hastie, N. D. (1993) Defective mitosis due to a mutation in the gene for a fission yeast 26S protease subunit. *Nature*, **366**, 355.

86. Pines, J. and Hunter, T. (1991) Human cyclins A and B are differentially located in the cell and undergo cell cycle dependent nuclear transport. *J. Cell Biol.*, **115**, 1.

87. Gallant, P. and Nigg, E. A. (1992) Cyclin B2 undergoes cell cycle-dependent nuclear translocation and, when expressed as a non-destructible mutant, causes mitotic arrest in HeLa cells. *J. Cell Biol.*, **117**, 213.

88. Ookata, K., Hisanaga, S., Okano, T., Tachibana, K., and Kishimoto, T. (1992) Relocation and distinct subcellular localization of p34cdc2-cyclin B complex at meiosis reinitiation in starfish oocytes. *EMBO J.*, **11**, 1763.

89. Luca, F. C., Shibuya, E. K., Dohrmann, C. E., and Ruderman, J. V. (1991) Both cyclin A delta 60 and B delta 97 are stable and arrest cells in M-phase, but only cyclin B delta 97 turns on cyclin destruction. *EMBO J.*, **10**, 4311.

90. Holloway, S. L., Glotzer, M., King, R. W., and Murray, A. W. (1993) Anaphase is initiated by proteolysis rather than by the inactivation of Maturation-Promoting factor. *Cell*, **73**, 1393.

91. Pardee, A. B. (1989) G1 events and regulation of cell proliferation. *Science*, **246**, 603.

92. Hartwell, L. H. (1978) Cell division from a genetic perspective. *J. Cell Biol.*, **77**, 627.

93. Nurse, P. and Bisset, Y. (1981) Gene required in G1 for commitment to cell cycle and in G2 for control of mitosis in fission yeast. *Nature*, **292**, 558.

94. Croy, R. G. and Pardee, A. B. (1983) Enhanced synthesis and stabilization of Mr 68,000 protein in transformed BALB/c-3T3 cells: Candidate for restriction point control of cell growth. *Proc. Natl. Acad. Sci. USA*, **80**, 4699.

95. Koch, C. and Nasmyth, K. (1994) Cell cycle regulated transcription in yeast. *Curr. Opin. Cell Biol.*, **6**, 451.

96. Cross, F. R. and Tinkelenberg, A. H. (1991) A potential positive feedback loop controlling CLN1 and CLN2 gene expression at the start of the yeast cell cycle. *Cell*, **65**, 875.

97. Dirick, L. and Nasmyth, K. (1991) Positive feedback in the activation of G1 cyclins in yeast. *Nature*, **351**, 754.

98. Moll, T., Tebb, G., Surana, U., Robitsch, H., and Nasmyth, K. (1991) The role of phosphorylation and the CDC28 protein kinase in cell cycle-regulated nuclear import of the *S. cerevisiae* transcription factor SWI5. *Cell*, **66**, 743.

99. Epstein, C. B. and Cross, F. (1992) Clb5: a novel B cyclin from budding yeast with a role in S phase. *Genes Dev.*, **6**, 1695.

100. Schwob, E. and Nasmyth, K. (1993) CLB5 and CLB6, a new pair of B cyclins involved in DNA replication in *Saccharomyces cervisiae*. *Genes Dev.*, **7**, 1160.

101. Nevins, J. R. (1992) E2F: a link between the Rb tumor suppressor protein and viral oncoproteins. *Science*, **258**, 424.

102. La Thangue, N. (1994) DP and E2F proteins: components of a heterodimeric transcription factor implicated in cell cycle control. *Curr. Opin. Cell Biol.*, **6**, 443.

103. DeGregori, J., Kowalik, T., and Nevins, J. R. (1995) Cellular targets for activation by the E2F1 transcription factor include DNA synthesis- and G1/S-regulatory genes. *Mol. Cell. Biol.*, **15**, 4215.

104. Girling, R., Partridge, J. F., Bandara, L. R., Burden, N., Totty, N. F., Hsuan, J. J., *et al.* (1993) A new component of the transcription factor DRTF1/E2F. *Nature*, **362**, 83.

105. Kouzarides, T. (1995) Transcriptional control by the retinoblastoma protein. *Semin. Cancer Biol.*, **6**, 91.

106. Whyte, P. (1995) The retinoblastoma protein and its relatives. *Semin. Cancer Biol.*, **6**, 83.

107. Livingston, D. M., Kaelin, W., Chittenden, T., Qin, X. (1993) Structural and functional contributions to the G1 blocking action of the retinoblastoma protein, *Br. J. Cancer*, **68**, 264.

108. Bagchi, S., Weinmann, R., and Raychaudhuri, P. (1991) The retinoblastoma protein copurifies with E2F-I, an E1A-regulated inhibitor of the transcription factor E2F. *Cell*, **65**, 1063.

109. Bandara, L. R., Buck, V. M., Zamanian, M., Johnston, L. H., and La-Thangue, N. B. (1993) Functional synergy between DP-1 and E2F-1 in the cell cycle-regulating transcription factor DRTF1/E2F. *EMBO J.*, **12**, 4317.

110. Ivey, H. M., Conroy, R., Huber, H. E., Goodhart, P. J., Oliff, A., and Heimbrook, D. C. (1993) Cloning and characterization of E2F-2, a novel protein with the biochemical properties of transcription factor E2F. *Mol. Cell. Biol.*, **13**, 7802.

111. Shan, B., Zhu, X., Chen, P. L., Durfee, T., Yang, Y., Sharp, D., *et al.* (1992) Molecular cloning of cellular genes encoding retinoblastoma-associated proteins: identification of a gene with properties of the transcription factor E2F. *Mol. Cell. Biol.*, **12**, 5620.

112. Lees, J. A., Saito, M., Vidal, M., Valentine, M., Look, T., Harlow, E., *et al.* (1993) The retinoblastoma protein binds to a family of E2F transcription factors. *Mol. Cell. Biol.*, **13**, 7813.

113. Beijersbergen, R. L., Kerkhoven, R. M., Zhu, L., Carlée, L., Voorhoeve, P. M., and Bernards, R. (1994) E2F-4, a new member of the E2F gene family, has oncogenic activity and associates with p107 in vivo. *Genes Dev.*, **8**, 2680.

114. Ginsberg, D., Vairo, G., Chittenden, T., Xiao, Z.-X., Xu, G., Wydner, K. L., *et al.* (1994) E2F-4, a new member of the E2F transcription factor family, interacts with p107. *Genes Dev.*, **8**, 2665.

115. Hijmans, E. M., Voorhoeve, P. M., Beijersbergen, R. L., van't Veer, L. J., and Bernards, R. (1995) E2F-5, a new E2F family member that interacts with p130 *in vivo*. *Mol. Cell. Biol.*, **15**, 3082.

116. Sardet, C., Vidal, M., Cobrinik, D., Geng, Y., Onufryk, C., Chen, A., *et al.* (1995) E2F-4 and E2F-5, two members of the E2F family, are expressed in the early phases of the cell cycle. *Proc. Natl. Acad. Sci. USA*, **92**, 2403.

117. Vairo, G., Livingston, D. M., and Ginsberg, D. (1995) Functional interaction between E2F-4 and p130: evidence for distinct mechanisms underlying growth suppression by different retinoblastoma protein family members. *Genes Dev.*, **9**, 869.

118. Lees, E., Faha, B., Dulic, V., Reed, S. I., and Harlow, E. (1992) Cyclin E/cdk2 and cyclin A/cdk2 kinases associate with p107 and E2F in a temporally distinct manner. *Genes Dev.*, **6**, 1874.

119. Mudryj, M., Devoto, S. H., Hiebert, S., Hunter, T., Pines, J., and Nevins, J. R. (1991) Cell cycle regulation of the E2F transcription factor involves an interaction with cyclin A. *Cell*, **65**, 1243.

120. Devoto, S. H., Mudryj, M., Pines, J., Hunter, T., and Nevins, J. R. (1992) A cyclin A-protein kinase complex possesses sequence-specific DNA binding activity: p33^{cdk2} is a component of the E2F-cyclin A complex. *Cell*, **68**, 167.

121. Chellappan, S. P., Hiebert, S., Mudryj, M., Horowitz, J. M., and Nevins, J. R. (1991) The E2F transcription factor is a cellular target for the RP protein. *Cell*, **65**, 1053.

122. Helin, K., Harlow, E., and Fattaey, A. (1993) Inhibition of E2F-1 Transactivation by Direct Binding of the Retinoblastoma Protein. *Mol. Cell. Biol.*, **13**, 6501.

123. Shirodkar, S., Ewen, M., DeCaprio, J. A., Morgan, J., Livingston, D. M., and Chittenden, T. (1992) The transcription factor E2F interacts with the retinoblastoma product and a p107-cyclin A complex in a cell cycle-regulated manner. *Cell*, **68**, 157.

124. Johnson, D. G., Ohtani, K., and Nevins, J. R. (1994) Autoregulatory control of *E2F1* expression in response to positive and negative regulators of cell cycle progression. *Genes Dev.*, **8**, 1514.

125. Johnson, D. G., Schwarz, J. K., Cress, W. D., and Nevins, J. R. (1993) Expression of transcription factor E2F1 induces quiescent cells to enter S phase. *Nature*, **365**, 349.

126. Richardson, H. E., Wittenberg, C., Cross, F., and Reed, S. I. (1989) An essential G1 function for cyclin-like proteins in yeast. *Cell*, **59**, 1127.

127. Tyers, M., Tokiwa, G., Nash, R., and Futcher, B. (1992) The Cln3-Cdc28 kinase complex of *S. cerevisiae* is regulated by proteolysis and phosphorylation. *EMBO J.*, **11**, 1773.

128. Sherr, C. J. (1993) Mammalian G1 cyclins. *Cell*, **73**, 1059.

129. Ohtsubo, M. and Roberts, J. M. (1993) Cyclin-dependent regulation of G1 in mammalian fibroblasts. *Science*, **259**, 1908.

130. Quelle, D. E., Ashmun, R. A., Shutleff, S. A., Kato, J., Bar-Sagi, D., Roussel, M. F., *et al.* (1993) Overexpression of mouse D-type cyclins accelerates G_1 phase in rodent fibroblasts. *Genes Dev.*, **7**, 1559.

131. Resnitzky, D., Gossen, M., Bujard, H., and Reed, S. I. (1994) Acceleration of the G1/S Phase Transition by Expression of Cyclins D1 and E with an Inducible System. *Mol. Cell. Biol.*, **14**, 1669.

132. Resnitzky, D. and Reed, S. I. (1995) Different roles for cyclins D1 and E in regulation of the G1-to-S transition. *Mol. Cell. Biol.*, **15**, 3463.

133. Motokura, T., Bloom, T., Kim, H. G., Jüppner, H., Ruderman, J. V., Kronenberg, H. M., *et al.* (1991) A novel cyclin encoded by a bcl-linked candidate oncogene. *Nature*, **350**, 512.

134. Withers, D. A., Harvey, R. C., Faust, J. B., Melnyk, O., Carey, K., and Meeker, T. C. (1991) Characterization of a candidate bcl-1 gene. *Mol. Cell. Biol.*, **11**, 4846.

135. Motokura, T., Keyomarsi, K., Kronenberg, H. M., and Arnold, A. (1992) Cloning and characterization of human cyclin D3, a cDNA closely related in sequence to the PRAD1/cyclin D1 proto-oncogene. *J. Biol. Chem.*, **267**, 20412.

136. Xiong, Y., Connolly, T., Futcher, B., and Beach, D. (1991) Human D-type cyclin. *Cell*, **65**, 691.

137. Dowdy, S. F., Hinds, P. W., Louie, K., Reed, S. I., Arnold, A., and Weinberg, R. A. (1993) Physical interaction of the retinoblastoma protein with human D cyclins. *Cell*, **73**, 499.

138. Kato, J.-Y., Matsuoka, M., Strom, D. K., and Sherr, C. J. (1994) Regulation of cyclin D-dependent kinase 4 (cdk4) by cdk-activating enzyme. *Mol. Cell. Biol.*, **14**, 2713.

139. Bates, S., Bonetta, L., MacAllan, D., Parry, D., Holder, A., Dickson, C., *et al.* (1994) CDK6 (PLSTIRE) and CDK4 (PSK-J3) are a distinct subset of the cyclin-dependent kinases that associate with cyclin D1. *Oncogene*, **9**, 71.

140. Meyerson, M. and Harlow, E. (1994) Identification of G1 kinase activity for cdk6, a novel cyclin D partner. *Mol. Cell. Biol.*, **14**, 2077.

141. Xiong, Y., Xhang, H., and Beach, D. (1992) D type cyclins associate with multiple protein kinases and the DNA replication and repair factor PCNA. *Cell*, **71**, 504.

142. Elledge, S. J. and Spottswood, M. R. (1991) A new human p34 protein kinase, CDK2, identified by complementation of a cdc28 mutation in *Saccharomyces cerevisiae*, is a homolog of Xenopus Eg1. *EMBO J.*, **10**, 2653.

143. Tsai, L.-H., Harlow, E., and Meyerson, M. (1991) Isolation of the human cdk2 gene that encodes the cyclin A and adenovirus E1A-associated p33 kinase *Nature*, **353**, 174.

144. Lammie, G. A., Smith, R., Silver, J., Brookes, S., Dickson, C., and Peters, G. (1992) Proviral insertions near cyclin D1 in mouse lymphomas: a parallel for BCL1 translocations in human B-cell neoplasms. *Oncogene*, **7**, 2381.

145. Hanna, Z., Jankowski, M., Tremblay, P., Jiang, X., Milatovich, A., Francke, U., *et al.* (1993) The Vin-1 gene, identified by provirus insertional mutagenesis, is the cyclin D2. *Oncogene*, **8**, 1661.

146. Lovec, H., Sewing, A., Lucibello, F., Müller, R., and Möröy, T. (1994) Oncogenic activity of cyclin D1 revealed through cooperation with Ha-ras: link between cell cycle control and malignant transformation. *Oncogene*, **9**, 323.

147. Hinds, P. W., Dowdy, S. F., Eaton, E. N., Arnold, A., and Weinberg, R. A. (1994) Function of a human cyclin gene as an oncogene. *Proc. Natl. Acad. Sci. USA*, **91**, 709.

148. Bodrug, S., Warner, B., Bath, M., Lindeman, G., Harris, A., and Adams, J. (1994) Cyclin D1 transgene impedes lymphocyte maturation and collaborates in lymphomagenesis with the *myc* gene. *EMBO J.*, **13**, 2124.

149. Wang, T. C., Cardiff, R. D., Zukerberg, L., Lees, E., Arnold, A., and Schmidt, E. V. (1994) Mammary hyperplasia and carcinoma in MMTV-cyclin D1 transgenic mice. *Nature*, **369**, 669.

150. Nicholas, J., Cameron, K. R., and Honess, R. W. (1992) Herpesvirus saimiri encodes homologues of G protein-coupled receptors and cyclins. *Nature*, **355**, 362.

151. Motokura, T., Yi, H. F., Kronenberg, H. M., McBride, O. W., and Arnold, A. (1992) Assignment of the human cyclin D3 gene (CCND3) to chromosome 6p–q13. *Cytogenet. Cell Genet.*, **61**, 5.

152. Xiong, Y., Menninger, J., Beach, D., and Ward, D. C. (1992) Molecular cloning and chromosomal mapping of CCND genes encoding human D-type cyclins. *Genomics*, **13**, 575.

153. Spruck III, C. H., Gonzales-Zuleta, M., Shibata, A., Simoneau, A. R., Lin, M.-F., Gonzales, F., *et al.* (1994) p16 gene in uncultured tumours. *Nature*, **370**, 183.

154. Koh, J., Enders, G. H., Dynlacht, B. D., and Harlow, E. (1995) Tumour-derived p16 alleles encoding proteins defective in cell cycle inhibition. *Nature*, **375**, 506.

155. Lukas, J., Parry, D., Aagaard, L., Mann, D. J., Bartkova, J., Strauss, M., *et al.* (1995) Retinoblastoma protein-dependent cell cycle inhibition by the tumour suppressor p16. *Nature*, **375**, 503.

156. Medema, R. H., Herrera, R. E., Lam, F., and Weinberg, R. A. (1995) Growth suppression by p16[INK4A] requires functional retinoblastoma protein. *Proc. Natl. Acad. Sci. USA*, **92**, 6289.

157. Lukas, J., Pagano, M., Staskova, Z., Draetta, G., and Bartek, J. (1994) Cyclin D1 protein oscillates and is essential for cell cycle progression in human tumour cell lines. *Oncogene*, **9**, 707.

158. Weinberg, R. A. (1995) The retinoblastoma protein and cell cycle control. *Cell*, **81**, 323.

159. Furukawa, Y., DeCaprio, J. A., Freedman, A., Kanakura, Y., Nakamura, M., Ernst, T. J.,

et al. (1990) Expression and state of phosphorylation of the retinoblastoma susceptibility gene product in cycling and noncycling human hematopoietic cells. *Proc. Natl. Acad. Sci. USA*, **87**, 2770.

160. DeCapiro, J. A., Ludlow, J. W., Lynch, D., Furukawa, Y., Griffin, J., Piwnica-Worms, H., *et al.* (1989) The product of the retinoblastoma susceptibility gene has the properties of a cell cycle regulatory element. *Cell*, **58**, 1085.

161. DeCapiro, J. A., Furukawa, Y., Ajchenbaum, F., Griffin, J. D., and Livingston, D. M. (1992) The retinoblastoma-susceptibility gene product becomes phosphorylated in multiple stages during cell cycle entry and progression. *Proc. Natl. Acad. Sci. USA*, **89**, 1795.

162. Lees, J. A., Buchkovich, K. J., Marshak, D. R., Anderson, C. W., and Harlow, E. (1991) The retinoblastoma protein is phosphorylated on multiple sites by human cdc2. *EMBO J.*, **10**, 4279.

163. Hinds, P. W., Mittnacht, S., Dulic, V., Arnold, A., Reed, S. I., and Weinberg, R. A. (1992) Regulation of retinoblastoma protein functions by ectopic expression of human cyclins. *Cell*, **70**, 993.

164. Ewen, M. E., Sluss, H. K., Sherr, C. J., Matsushime, H., Kato, J.-y., and Livingstone, D. M. (1993) Functional interactions of the retinoblastoma protein with the mammalian D-type cyclins. *Cell*, **73**, 487.

165. Lee, E. Y., Chang, C. Y., Hu, N., Yang, Y. C., Lai, C. C., Herrup, K. *et al.* (1992) Mice deficent for Rb are nonviable and show defects in neurogenesis and haematopoiesis. *Nature*, **359**, 288.

166. Jacks, T., Faxeli, A., Schmitt, E. M., Bronson, R. T., Goodell, M. A., and Weinberg, R. A. (1992) Effects of an Rb mutation in the mouse. *Nature*, **359**, 295.

167. Beijersbergen, R. L., Carlée, L., Kerkhoven, R. M., and Bernards, R. (1995) Regulation of the retinoblastoma protein-regulated p107 by G1 cyclin complexes. *Genes Dev.*, **9**, 1340.

168. Zhu, L., Harlow, E., and Dynlacht, B. D. (1995) p107 uses a p21Cip1-related domain to bind cyclin/Cdk2 and regulate interactions with E2F. *Genes Dev.*, **9**, 1740.

169. Kato, J. and Sherr, C. J. (1993) Inhibition of granulocyte differentiation by G1 cyclins D2 and D3 but not D1. *Proc. Natl. Acad. Sci. USA*, **90**, 11513.

170. Hunter, T. (1991) Cooperation between oncogenes. *Cell*, **64**, 249.

171. Duli'c, V., Kaufmann, W. K., Wilson, S. J., Tisty, T. D., Lees, E., Harper, W. J., *et al.* (1994) p53-dependent inhibition of cyclin-dependent kinase activities in human fibroblasts during radiation-induced G1 arrest. *Cell*, **76**, 1013.

172. Di Leonardo, A., Linke, S. P., Clarkin, K., and Wahl, G. M. (1994) DNA damage triggers a prolonged p53-dependent G1 arrest and long term induction of Cip1 in normal human fibroblasts. *Genes Dev.*, **8**, 2540.

173. Xiong, Y., Zhang, H., and Beach, D. (1993) Subunit rearrangement of the cyclin-dependent kinases is associated with cellular transformation. *Genes Dev.*, **7**, 1572.

174. El-Deiry, W. S., Harper, J. W., O'Connor, P. M., Velculescu, V. E., Canman, C. E., Jackman, J., *et al.* (1994) WAF1/CIP1 is induced in p53-mediated G1 arrest and apoptosis. *Cancer Res.*, **54**, 1169.

175. Chen, J., Jackson, P. K., Kirschner, M. W., and Dutta, A. (1995) Separate domains of p21 involved in the inhibition of cdk kinase and PCNA. *Nature*, **374**, 386.

176. Nasmyth, K. and Hunt, T. (1993) Cell cycle. Dams and sluices. *Nature*, **366**, 634.

177. Sherr, C. J. and Roberts, J. M. (1995) Inhibitors of mammalian cyclin-dependent kinases. *Genes Dev.*, **9**, 1149.

178. Warbrick, E., Lane, D. P., Glover, D. M., and Cox, L. S. (1995) A small peptide inhibitor of DNA replication defines the site of interaction between the cyclin-dependent kinase inhibitor p21^{WAF1} and proliferating cell nuclear antigen. *Curr. Biol.*, **5**, 275.

179. Parker, S. B., Eichele, G., Zhang, P., Rawls, A., Sands, A. T., Bradley, A., *et al.* (1995) p53-independent expression of p21^{Cip1} in muscle and other terminally differentiating cells. *Science*, **267**, 1024.

180. Polyak, K., Kato, J.-y., Solomon, M., Sherr, C. J., Massague, J., Roberts, J. M., *et al.* (1994) p27^{Kip1} and cyclin D-CDK4, interacting regulators of CDK2, link TGF-B and contact inhibition to cell cycle arrest. *Genes Dev.*, **8**, 9.

181. Slingerland, J. M., Hengst, L., Pan, C.-H., Alexander, D., Stampfer, M., and Reed, S. I. (1994) A novel inhibitor of cyclin-Cdk activity detected in transforming growth factor b-arrested epithelial cells. *Mol. Cell. Biol.*, **14**, 3683.

182. Kato, J.-y., Matsuoka, M., Polyak, K., Massagué, J., and Sherr, C. J. (1994) Cyclin AMP-induced G1 phase arrest mediated by an inhibitor (p27^{KIP1}), of cyclin-dependent kinase 4 activation. *Cell*, **79**, 487.

183. Peters, G. (1994) Stifled by inhibitions. *Nature*, **371**, 204.

184. Firpo, E., Koff, A., Solomon, M., and Roberts, J. (1994) Inactivation of a Cdk2 Inhibitor during Interleukin 2-Induced Proliferation of Human T Lymphocytes. *Mol. Cell. Biol.*, **14**, 4889.

185. Knoblich, J. A., Sauer, K., Jones, L., Richardson, H., Saint, R., and Lehner, C. F. (1994) Cyclin E controls S phase progression and its down-regulation during *Drosophila* embryogenesis is required for the arrest of cell proliferation. *Cell*, **77**, 107.

186. Sauer, K., Knoblich, J. A., Richardson, H., and Lehner, C. F. (1995) Distinct modes of cyclin E/cdc2c kinase regulation and S-phase control in mitotic and endoreduplication cycles of *Drosophila* embryogenesis. *Genes Dev.*, **9**, 1327.

187. Duronio, R. J. and O'Farrell, P. H. (1995) Developmental control of the G1 to S transition in *Drosophila*: cyclin E is a limiting downstream target of E2F. *Genes Dev.*, **9**, 1456.

188. Duronio, R. J., O'Farrell, P. H., Xie, J.-E., Brook, A., and Dyson, N. (1995) The transcription factor E2F is required for S phase during *Drosophila* embryogenesis. *Genes Dev.*, **9**, 1445.

189. Fang, F. and Newport, J. W. (1991) Evidence that the G1-S and G2-M Transitions are controlled by different cdc2 proteins in higher eukaryotes. *Cell*, **66**, 731.

190. Jackson, P. K., Chevalier, S., Philippe, M., and Kirschner, M. W. (1995) Early events in DNA replication require cyclin E and are blocked by p21^{CIP1}. *J. Cell Biol.*, **130**, 755.

191. Tsai, L.-H., Lees, E., Faha, B., Harlow, E., and Riabowol, K. (1993) The CDK2 kinase is required for the G1 to S transition in mammalian cells. *Oncogene*, **8**, 1593.

192. van den Heuvel, S. and Harlow, E. (1994) Distinct roles for cyclin-dependent kinases in cell cycle control. *Science*, **262**, 2050.

193. Koff, A., Ohtsuki, M., Polyak, K., Roberts, J. M., and Massague, J. (1993) Negative regulation of G1 in mammalian cells: inhibition of cyclin E-dependent kinase by TGF-beta. *Science*, **260**, 536.

194. Galaktionov, K., Jessus, C., and Beach, D. (1995) Raf1 interaction with Cdc25 phosphatase ties mitogeneic signal transduction to cell cycle activation. *Genes Dev.*, **9**, 1046.

195. Girard, F., Strausfeld, U., Fernandez, A., and Lamb, N. J. C. (1991) Cyclin A is required for the onset of DNA replication in mammalian fibroblasts. *Cell*, **67**, 1169.

196. Pagano, M., Pepperkok, R., Verde, F., Ansorge, W., and Draetta, G. (1992) Cyclin A is required at two points in the human cell cycle. *EMBO J.*, **11**, 961.

197. Zindy, F., Lamas, E., Chenivesse, X., Sobczak, J., Wang, J., Fesquet, D., *et al.* (1992) Cyclin A is required in S phase in normal epithelial cells. *Biochem. Biophys. Res. Commun.*, **182**, 1144.

198. Cardoso, M. C., Leonhardt, H., and Nadal-Ginard, B. (1993) Reversal of terminal differentiation and control of DNA replication: Cyclin A and Cdk2 specifically localize at subnuclear sites of DNA replication. *Cell*, **74**, 979.

199. Sobczak, T. J., Harper, F., Florentin, Y., Zindy, F., Brechot, C., and Puvion, E., (1993) Localization of cyclin A at the sites of cellular DNA replication. *Exp. Cell Res.*, **206**, 43.

200. Waga, S. and Stillman, B. (1994) Anatomy of a DNA replication fork revealed by reconstitution of SV40 DNA replication *in vitro*. *Nature*, **369**, 207.

201. Howe, J. A., Howell, M., Hunt, T., and Newport, J. W. (1995) Identification of a developmental timer regulating the stability of embryonic cyclin A and a new somatic A-type cyclin at gastrulation. *Genes Dev.*, **9**, 1164.

202. Wang, J., Chenivesse, X., Henglein, B., and Bréchot, C. (1990) Hepatitis B virus integration in a cyclin A gene in a hepatocellular carcinoma. *Nature*, **343**, 555.

203. Wang, J., Zindy, F., Chenivesse, X., Lamas, E., Henglein, B., and Brechot, C. (1992) Modification of cyclin A expression by hepatitis B virus DNA integration in a hepatocellular carcinoma. *Oncogene*, **7**, 1653.

204. Pines, J. and Hunter, T. (1990) Human cyclin A is adenovirus E1A-associated protein p60, and behaves differently from cyclin B. *Nature*, **346**, 760.

205. Adamczewski, J. P., Gannon, J. V., and Hunt, T. (1993) Simian virus 40 large T antigen associates with cyclin A and p33cdk2. *J. Virol.*, **67**, 6551.

206. Tommasino, M., Adamczewski, J. P., Carlotti, F., Barth, C. F., Manetti, R., Contorni, M., *et al.* (1993) HPV16 E7 protein associates with the protein kinase p33CDK2 and cyclin A. *Oncogene*, **8**, 195.

207. Krek, W., Ewen, M. E., Shirodkar, S., Arany, Z., Kaelin, W. G., and Livingstone, D. M. (1994) Negative regulation of the growth-promoting transcription factor E2F-1 by a stably bound cyclin A-dependent protein kinase. *Cell*, **78**, 161.

208. Ewen, M. E., Faha, B., Harlow, E., and Livingstone, D. M. (1992) Interaction of p107 with cyclin A independent of complex formation with viral oncoproteins. *Science*, **255**, 85.

209. Diffley, J. F. X. and Cocker, J. H. (1992) Protein-DNA interactions at a yeast replication origin. *Nature*, **357**, 169.

210. Bell, S. P. and Stillman, B. (1992) ATP-dependent recognition of eukaryotic origins of DNA replication by a multiprotein complex. *Nature*, **357**, 128.

211. Adachi, Y. and Laemmli, U. K. (1994) Study of the cell cycle-dependent assembly of the DNA pre-replication centres in *Xenopus* egg extracts. *EMBO J.*, **13**, 4153.

212. Liang, C., Weinreich, M. and Stillman, B. (1995) ORC and Cdc6p interact and determine the frequency of initiation of DNA replication in the genome. *Cell*, **81**, 667.

213. Rowley, A., Cocker, J. H., Harwood, J., and Diffley, J. F. X. (1995) Initiation complex assembly at budding yeast replication origins begins with the recognition of a bipartite sequence by limiting amounts of the initiator, ORC. *EMBO J.*, **14**, 2631.

214. Kelly, T. J., Martin, G. S., Forsburg, S. L., Stephen, R. J., Russo, A., and Nurse, P. (1993) The fission yeast cdc18$^+$ gene product couple S phase to START and Mitosis. *Cell*, **74**, 371.

215. Hayles, J., Fisher, D., Woollard, A., and Nurse, P. (1994) Temporal order of S phase and

Mitosis in fission yeast is determined by the state of the p34^{cdc2}-mitotic B cyclin complex. *Cell*, **78**, 813.

216. Broek, D., Barlett, R., Crawford, K., and Nurse, P. (1991) Involvement of p34cdc2 in establishing the dependency of S phase on mitosis. *Nature*, **349**, 388.

217. Moreno, S. and Nurse, P. (1994) Regulation of progression through the G1 phase of the cell cycle by the rum1 + gene. *Nature*, **367**, 236.

218. Blow, J. J. and Laskey, R. A. (1988) A role for the nuclear envelope in controlling DNA replication within the cell cycle. *Nature*, **332**, 546.

219. Leno, G. H., Downes, C. S., and Laskey, R. A. (1992) The nuclear membrane prevents replication of human G2 nuclei but not G1 nuclei in Xenopus egg extract. *Cell*, **69**, 151.

220. Kubota, Y., Mimura, S., Nishimoto, S.-i., Takisawa, H., and Nojima, H. (1995) Identification of the yeast MCM3-related protein as a component of Xenopus DNA replication licensing factor. *Cell*, **81**, 601.

221. Chong, J. P. J., Mahbubani, H. M., Khoo, C. Y., and Blow, J. J. (1995) Purification of an MCM-containing complex as a component of the DNA replication licensing system. *Nature*, **375**, 418.

222. Madine, M. A., Khoo, C.-Y., Mills, A. D., and Laskey, R. A. (1995) MCM3 complex required for cell cycle regulation of DNA replication in vertebrate cells. *Nature*, **375**, 421.

223. Blow, J. J. (1993) Preventing re-replication of DNA in a single cell cycle: Evidence for a replication licensing factor. *J. Cell. Biol.*, **122**, 993.

224. Usui, T., Yoshida, M., Abe, K., Osada, H., Isono, K., and Beppu, T. (1991) Uncoupled cell cycle without mitosis induced by a protein kinase inhibitor, K-252a. *J. Cell Biol.*, **115**, 1275.

225. Su, T. T., Follette, P. J., and O'Farrell, P. H. (1995) Qualifying for the license to replicate. *Cell*, **81**, 825.

226. Lehner, C. F. and O'Farrell, P. H. (1989) Expression and function of *Drosophila* cyclin A during embryonic cell cycle progression. *Cell*, **56**, 957.

227. Waga, S., Hannon, G. J., Beach, D., and Stillman, B. (1994) The p21 cyclin-dependent kinase inhibitor directly controls DNA replication via interaction with PCNA. *Nature*, **369**, 574.

228. Li, R., Waga, S., Hannon, G. J., Beach, D., and Stillman, B. (1994) Differential effects by the p21 CDK inhibitor on PCNA-dependent DNA replication and repair. *Nature*, **371**, 534.

229. Nakanishi, M., Robetorye, R. S., Adami, G. R., Pereira-Smith, O. M., and Smith, J. R. (1995) Identification of the active region of the DNA synthesis inhibitory gene p21$^{Sdi1/CIP1/WAF1}$. *EMBO J.*, **14**, 555.

230. Luo, Y., Hurwitz, J., and Massagué, J. (1995) Cell cycle inhibition mediated by functionally independent CDK and PCNA inhibitory domains in p21^{CIP1}. *Nature*, **375**, 159.

231. Strausfeld, U. P., Howell, M., Rempel, R., Maller, J. L., Hunt, T., and Blow, J. J. (1994) Cip 1 blocks the initiation of DNA replication in *Xenopus* extracts by inhibition of cyclin-dependent kinases. *Curr. Biol.*, **4**, 876.

232. Hofmann, J. and Beach, D. (1994) cdt1 is an essential target of the cdc 10/Sct1 transcription factor: requirement for DNA replication and inhibition of mitosis. *EMBO J.*, **13**, 425.

233. Saka, Y. and Yanagida, M. (1993) Fission yeast cut5$^+$, required for S phase onset and M phase restraint, is identical to the radiation-damage repair gene rad4$^+$. *Cell*, **74**, 383.

234. Saka, Y., Fantes, P., and Yanagida, M. (1994) Coupling of DNA replication and mitosis by fission yeast rad4/cut5. *J. Cell Sci.*, **18**, 57.

235. Murakami, H. and Okayama, H. (1995) A kinase from fission yeast responsible for blocking mitosis in S phase. *Nature*, **374**, 817.

236. Navas, T. A., Zheng, Z., and Elledge, S. J. (1995) DNA polymerase ε links the DNA replication machinery to the S phase checkpoint. *Cell*, **74**, 29.

237. Enoch, T. and Nurse, P. (1991) Coupling M phase and S phase: controls maintaining the dependence of mitosis on chromosome replication. *Cell*, **65**, 921.

238. Enoch, T., Carr, A. M., and Nurse, P. (1992) Fission yeast genes involved in coupling mitosis to completion of DNA replication. *Genes Dev.*, **6**, 2035.

239. Enoch, T. and Nurse, P. (1990) Mutation of fission yeast cell cycle control genes abolishes dependence of mitosis on DNA replication. *Cell*, **60**, 665.

240. Hayles, J. and Nurse, P. (1995) A pre-START checkpoint preventing mitosis in fission yeast acts independently of p34^{cdc2} tyrosine phosphorylation. *EMBO J.*, **14**, 2760.

241. Dasso, M. and Newport, J. W. (1990) Completion of DNA replication is monitored by a feedback system that controls the initiation of mitosis *in vitro*: studies in Xenopus. *Cell*, **61**, 811.

242. Kumagai, A. and Dunphy, W. G. (1995) Control of the cdc2/cyclin B complex in *Xenopus* egg extracts arrested at the G2/M checkpoint with DNA synthesis inhibitors. *Mol. Biol. Cell*, **6**, 199.

243. Brizuela, L., Draetta, G., and Beach, D. (1987) p13suc1 acts in the fission yeast cell division cycle as a component of the p34cdc2 protein kinase. *EMBO J.*, **6**, 3507.

244. Dunphy, W. and Newport, J. (1989) Fission yeast p13 blocks mitotic activation and tyrosine dephosphorylation of the Xenopus cdc2 protein kinase. *Cell*, **58**, 181.

245. Nishitani, H., Ohtsubo, M., Yamashita, K., Iida, H., Pines, J., Yasudo, H., *et al.* (1991) Loss of RCC1, a nuclear DNA-binding protein, uncouples the completion of DNA replication from the activation of cdc2 protein kinase and mitosis. *EMBO J.*, **10**, 1555.

246. Seki, T., Yamashita, K., Nishitani, H., Takagi, T., Russell, P., and Nishimoto, T. (1992) Chromosome condensation caused by loss of RCC1 function requires the cdc25C protein that is located in the cytoplasm. *Mol. Biol. Cell*, **3**, 1373.

247. Bischoff, F. R. and Ponstingl, H. (1991) Catalysis of guanine nucleotide exchange on Ran by the mitotic regulator RCC1. *Nature*, **354**, 80.

248. Bischoff, F. R. and Ponstingl, H. (1991) Mitotic regulator protein RCC1 is complexed with a nuclear ras-related polypeptide. *Proc. Natl. Acad. Sci. USA*, **88**, 10830.

249. Moore, M. S. and Blobel, G. (1993) The GTP-binding protein Ran/TC4 is required for protein import into the nucleus. *Nature*, **365**, 661.

250. Yamashita, K., Yasuda, H. Pines, J., Yasumoto, K., Nishitani, H., Ohtsubo, M., *et al.* (1991) Okadaic acid, a potent inhibitor of type 1 and type 2A protein phosphatases, activates cdc2/H1 kinase and transiently induces a premature mitosis-like state in BHK21 cells. *EMBO J.*, **9**, 4331.

251. Clarke, P. R., Hoffmann, I., Draetta, G., and Karsenti, E. (1993) Dephosphorylation of cdc25-C by a type-2A protein phosphatase: specific regulation during the cell cycle in Xenopus egg extracts. *Mol. Biol. Cell*, **4**, 397.

252. Weinert, T. A. and Hartwell, L. H. (1988) The RAD9 gene controls the cell cycle response to DNA damage in *Saccharomyces cerevisiae*. *Science*, **241**, 317.

253. Weinert, T. A. and Hartwell, L. H. (1990) Characterization of RAD9 of *Saccharomyces*

cerevisiae and evidence that its function acts posttranslationally in cell cycle arrest after DNA damage. *Mol. Cell. Biol.*, **10**, 6554.

254. Barbet, N. C. and Carr, A. M. (1993) Fission yeast wee1 protein kinase is not required for DNA damage-dependent mitotic arrest. *Nature*, **364**, 824.

255. Al-Khodairy, F., Fotou, E., Sheldrick, K., Griffiths, D., Lehmann, A., and Carr, A. (1994) Identification and Characterization of New Elements Involved in Checkpoint and Feedback Controls in fission Yeast. *Mol. Biol. Cell*, **5**, 147.

256. Weinert, T., Kiser, G., and Hartwell, L. (1994) Mitotic checkpoint genes in budding yeast and the dependence of mitosis on DNA replication and repair. *Genes Dev.*, **8**, 652.

257. Ford, J., Al-Khodairy, F., Fotou, E., Sheldrick, K., Griffiths, D., and Carr, A. (1994) 14-3-3 Protein Homologs Required for the DNA Damage Checkpoint in Fission Yeast. *Science*, **265**, 533.

258. Fenech, M., Carr, A. M., Murray, J., Watts, F. Z., and Lehman, A. R. (1991) Cloning and characterisation of the rad4 gene of schizosaccharomyces pombe—a gene showing short regions of sequence similarity to the human xrcc1 gene. *Nucleic Acids Res.*, **19**, 6737.

259. O'Connor, P. M., Ferris, D. K., White, G. A., Pines, J., Hunter, T., Longo, D. L., *et al.* (1992) Relationships between cdc2 kinase, DNA cross-linking, and cell cycle perturbations induced by nitrogen mustard. *Cell Growth Diff.*, **3**, 43.

260. Lock, R. B. (1992) Inhibition of p34cdc2 kinase activation, p34cdc2 tyrosine dephosphorylation, and mitotic progression in Chinese hamster ovary cells exposed to etoposide. *Cancer Res.*, **52**, 1817.

261. Muschel, R. J., Zhang, H. B., Iliakis, G., and McKenna, W. G. (1991) Cyclin B expression in HeLa cells during the G2 block induced by ionizing radiation. *Cancer Res.*, **51**, 5113.

262. O'Connor, P. M., Ferris, D. K., Pagano, M., Draetta, G., Pines, J., Hunter, T., *et al.* (1993) G2 delay induced by nitrogen mustard in human cells affects cyclin A/cdk2 and cyclin B1/cdc2-kinase complexes differently. *J. Biol. Chem.*, **268**, 8298.

263. Maity, A., McKenna, W. G., and Muschel, R. J. (1995) Evidence for post-transcriptional regulation of cyclin B1 mRNA in the cell cycle and following irradiation in HeLa cells. *EMBO J.*, **14**, 603.

264. Lehner, C. F. and O'Farrell, P. H. (1990) The roles of *Drosophila* cyclins A and B in mitotic control. *Cell*, **61**, 535.

265. Buendia, B., Draetta, G., and Karsenti, E. (1992) Regulation of the microtubule nucleating activity of centrosomes in Xenopus egg extracts: role of cyclin A-associated protein kinase. *J. Cell Biol.*, **116**, 1431.

266. Verde, F., Dogterom, M., Stelzer, E., Karsenti, E., and Leibler, S. (1992) Control of microtubule dynamics and length by cyclin A- and cyclin B-dependent kinases in Xenopus egg extracts. *J. Cell Biol.*, **118**, 1097.

267. Bai, C., Richman, R., and Elledge, S. J. (1994) Human cyclin F. *EMBO J.*, **13**, 6087.

268. Nigg, E. A. (1991) The substrates of the cdc2 kinase. *Semin. Cell Biol.*, **2**, 261.

269. Nigg, E. A. (1993) Cellular substrates of p34^{cdc2} and its companion cyclin-dependent kinases. *Trends Cell Biol.*, **3**, 296.

270. Kipreos, E. T. and Wang, J.-Y. (1992) Cell cycle-regulated binding of c-Abl tyrosine kinase to DNA. *Science*, **256**, 382.

271. Shenoy, S., Choi, J.-K., Bagrodia, S., Copeland, T. D., Maller, J. L., and Shalloway, D.

(1989) Purified maturation promoting factor phosphorylates pp60[c-src] at the sites phosphorylated during fibroblast mitosis. *Cell*, **57**, 763.

272. Kornbluth, S., Sebastian, B., Hunter, T., and Newport, J. (1994) Membrane localization of the kinase which phosphorylates p34cdc2 on threonine 14. *Mol. Biol. Cell*, **5**, 273.

273. Russell, P. and Nurse, P. (1987) The mitotic inducer nim1+ functions in a regulatory network of protein kinase homologs controlling the initiation of mitosis. *Cell*, **49**, 569.

274. Coleman, T. R., Tang, Z., and Dunphy, W. G. (1993) Negative regulation of the Wee1 protein kinase by direct action of the nim1/cdr1 mitotic inducer. *Cell*, **73**, 919.

275. Parker, L. L., Walter, S. A., Young, P. G., and Piwnica-Worms, H. (1993) Phosphorylation and inactivation of the mitotic inhibitor Wee1 by the nim1/cdr1 kinase. *Nature*, **363**, 736.

276. Wu, L. and Russell, P. (1993) Nim1 kinase promotes mitosis by inactivating wee1 tyrosine kinase. *Nature*, **363**, 738.

277. Kuang, J. and Ashorn, C. L. (1993) At least two kinases phosphorylate the MPM-2 epitope during Xenopus oocyte maturation. *J. Cell Biol.*, **123**, 859.

278. Kuang, J., Ashorn, C., Gonzales-Kuyvenhoven, M., and Penkala, J. (1994) cdc25 is one of the MPM-2 antigens involved in the activation of Maturation-promoting Factor. *Mol. Biol. Cell*, **5**, 135.

279. Davis, F., Tsao, T. Y., Fowler, S. K., and Rao, P. N. (1983) Monoclonal antibodies to mitotic cells. *Proc. Natl. Acad. Sci. USA*, **80**, 2926.

280. Pines, J. and Hunter, T. (1989) Isolation of a human cyclin cDNA: evidence for cyclin mRNA and protein regulation in the cell cycle and for interaction with p34[cdc2]. *Cell*, **58**, 833.

281. Lew, D. J., Dulic, V., and Reed, S. I. (1991) Isolation of three novel human cyclins by rescue of G1 cyclin (Cln) function in yeast. *Cell*, **66**, 1197.

282. Gallant, P. and Nigg, E. A. (1994) Identification of a novel vertebrate cyclin: cyclin B3 shares properties with both A- and B-type cyclins. *EMBO J.*, **13**, 595.

283. Lock, L. F., Pines, J., Hunter, T., Gilbert, D. J., Gopalan, G., Jenkins, N. A., *et al.* (1992) A single cyclin A gene and multiple cyclin B1-related sequences are dispersed in the mouse genome. *Genomics*, **13**, 415.

284. Peter, M., Nakagawa, J., Dorée, M., Labbé, J. C., and Nigg, E. A. (1990) *In vitro* disassembly of the nuclear lamina and M-phase specific phosphorylation of lamins by cdc2 kinase. *Cell*, **61**, 591.

285. Enoch, T., Peter, M., Nurse, P., and Nigg, E. A. (1991) p34cdc2 acts as a lamin kinase in fission yeast. *J. Cell Biol.*, **112**, 797.

286. Peter, M., Heitlinger, E., Haner, M., Aebi, U., and Nigg, E. A. (1991) Disassembly of *in vitro* formed lamin head-to-tail polymers by CDC2 kinase. *EMBO J.*, **10**, 1535.

287. Heald, R. and McKeon, F. (1990) Mutations of phosphorylation sites in lamin A that prevent nuclear lamina disassembly in mitosis. *Cell*, **61**, 579.

288. Langan, T. A., Zeilig, C. E., and Leichtling, B. (1980) Analysis of multiple site phosphorylation of H1 histone. In *Protein phosphorylation and bio-regulation* (ed. Thomas, Podesta, and Gordon). Karger, S., Basel,

289. Chambers, T. C. and Langan, T. A. (1990) Purification and characterization of growth-associated H1 histone kinase from Novikoff hepatoma cells. *J. Biol. Chem.*, **265**, 16940.

290. Osmani, A. H., McGuire, S. L., and Osmani, S.A. (1991) Parallel activation of the NIMA and p34cdc2 cell cycle-regulated protein kinases is required to initiate mitosis in *A. nidulans. Cell*, **67**, 283.

291. Ye, X. S., Xu, G., Pu, R. T., Fincher, R. R., McGuire, S. L., Osmani, A. H., *et al.* (1995) The NIMA protein kinase is hyperphosphorylated and activated downstream of p34cdc2-cyclin B: co-ordination of two mitosis promoting kinases. *EMBO J.*, **14**, 986.

292. O'Connell, M. J., Norbury, C., and Nurse, P. (1994) Premature chromatin condensation upon accumulation of NIMA. *EMBO J.*, **13**, 4926.

293. Luo, K. P. and Hunter, T. (1995) Evidence for a NIMA-like pathway in vertebrate cells. *Cell*, **81**, 413.

294. Jackman, M., Firth, M., and Pines, J. (1995) Human cyclins B1 and B2 are localised to strikingly different structures: B1 to microtubules, B2 primarily to the Golgi apparatus. *EMBO J.*, **14**, 1646.

295. Pypaert, M., Mundy, D., Souter, E., Labbe, J. C., and Warren, G. (1991) Mitotic cytosol inhibits invagination of coated pits in broken mitotic cells. *J. Cell Biol.*, **114**, 1159.

296. Stuart, R. A., Mackay, D., Adamczewski, J., and Warren, G. (1993) Inhibition of intra-Golgi transport in vitro by mitotic kinase. *J. Biol. Chem.*, **268**, 4050.

297. Woodman, P. G., Adamczewski, J. P., Hunt, T., and Warren, G. (1993) *In vitro* fusion of endocytic vesicles is inhibited by cyclin A-cdc2 kinase. *Mol. Biol. Cell*, **4**, 541.

298. Thomas, L., Clarke, P. R., Pagano, M., and Gruenberg, J. (1992) Inhibition of membrane fusion *in vitro* via cyclin B but not cyclin A [published erratum appears in *J. Biol. Chem.* 1992 Jul 5;267(19):13780]. *J. Biol. Chem.*, **267**, 6183.

299. Bailly, E., Pines, J., Hunter, T., and Bornens, M. (1992) Cytoplasmic accumulation of cyclin B1 in human cells: association with a detergent-resistant compartment and with the centrosome. *J. Cell Sci.*, **101**, 529.

300. Ookata, K., Hisanaga, S.-i., Bulinski, J. C., Murofushi, H., Aizawa, H., Itoh, T. J., *et al.* (1995) Cyclin B interaction with microtubule-associated protein 4 (MAP4) targets p34cdc2 kinase to microtubules and is a potential regulator of M-phase microtubule dynamics. *J. Cell Biol.*, **128**, 849.

301. Alfa, C. E., Ducommun, B., Beach, D., and Hyams, J. S. (1990) Distinct nuclear and spindle pole body populations of cyclin-cdc2 in fission yeast. *Nature*, **347**, 680.

302. Verde, F., Labbe, J. C., Doree, M., and Karsenti, E. (1990) Regulation of microtubule dynamics by cdc2 protein kinase in cell-free extracts of Xenopus eggs. *Nature*, **343**, 233.

303. Surana, U., Amon, A., Dowzer. C., McGrew, J., Byers, B., and Nasmyth, K. (1993) Destruction of the CDC28/CLB mitotic kinase is not required for the metaphase to anaphase transition in budding yeast. *EMBO J.*, **12**, 1969.

304. Rieder, C., Schultz, A., Cole, R., and Sluder, G. (1994) Anaphase onset in vertebrate somatic cells is controlled by a checkpoint that monitors sister kinetochore attachment to the spindle. *J. Cell Biol.*, **127**, 1301.

305. Li, X. and Nicklas, R. B. (1995) Mitotic forces control a cell-cycle checkpoint. *Nature*, **373**, 630.

306. Nicklas, R. B., Ward, S. C., and Gorbsky, G. J. (1995) Kinetochore chemistry is sensitive to tension and may link mitotic forces to a cell cycle checkpoint. *J. Cell Biol.*, **130**, 929.

307. Rieder, C. L., Cole, R. W., Khodjakov, A., and Sluder, G. (1995) The checkpoint delaying anaphase in response to chromosome monoorientation is mediated by an inhibitory signal produced by unattached kinetochores. *J. Cell Biol.*, **130**, 941.

308. Gorbsky, G. J. and Ricketts, W. A. (1993) Differential expression of a phosphoepitope at the kinetochores of moving chromosomes. *J. Cell Biol.*, **122**, 1311.

309. Murray, A. W. (1995) Tense spindles can relax [news; comment]. *Nature*, **373**, 560.

310. Minshull, J., Sun, H., Tonks, N. K., and Murray, A. W. (1994) A MAP Kinase-dependent spindle assembly checkpoint in Xenopus egg extracts. *Cell*, **79**, 475.

311. Sagata, N., Oskarsson, M., Copeland, T., Brumbaugh, J., and Vande Woude, G. F. (1988) Function of c-mos proto-oncogene product in meiotic maturation in Xenopus oocytes. *Nature*, **335**, 519.

312. Sagata, N., Daar, I., Oskarsson, M., Showalter, S. D., and Vande Woude, G. F. (1989) The product of the mos proto-oncogene as a candidate 'initiator' for oocyte maturation. *Science*, **245**, 643.

313. Masui, Y. and Markert, C. L. (1971) Cytoplasmic control of nuclear behavior during meiotic maturation of frog oocytes. *J. Exp. Zool.*, **17**, 129.

314. Daar, I., Paules, R. S., and Vande Woude, G. F. (1991) A characterization of cytostatic factor activity from Xenopus eggs and c-mos-transformed cells. *J. Cell Biol.*, **114**, 329.

315. Furuno, N., Nishizawa, M., Okazaki, K., Tanaka, H., Iwashita, J., Nakajo, N., *et al.* (1994) Suppression of DNA replication via Mos function during meiotic divisions in *Xenopus* oocytes. *EMBO J.*, **13**, 2399.

316. Colledge, W. H., Carlton, M. B., Udy, G. B., and Evans, M. J. (1994) Disruption of c-mos causes parthenogenetic development of unfertilized mouse eggs. *Nature*, **370**, 65.

317. Hashimoto, N., Watanabe, N., Furuta, Y., Tamemoto, H., Sagata, N., Yokoyama, M., *et al.* (1994) Parthenogenetic activation of oocytes in c-mos-deficient mice. *Nature*, **370**, 68.

318. Nebreda, A. R. and Hunt, T. (1993) The c-*mos* proto-oncogene protein kinase turns on and maintains the activity of MAP kinase, but not MPF, in cell-free extracts of *Xenopus* oocytes and eggs. *EMBO J.*, **12**, 1979.

319. Posada, J., Yew, N., Ahn, N. G., Vande Woude, G. F., and Cooper, J. A. (1993) Mos stimulates MAP kinase in *Xenopus* oocytes and activates a MAP kinase kinase *in vitro*. *Mol. Cell. Biol.*, **13**, 2546.

320. Yew, N., Strobel, M., and Vande Woude, G. F. (1993) Mos and the cell cycle: the molecular basis of the transformed phenotype. *Curr. Opin. Genet. Dev.*, **3**, 19.

321. Fukasawa, K. and Vande Woude, G. F. (1995) Mos overexpression in Swiss 3T3 cells induces meiotic-like alterations of the mitotic spindle. *Proc. Natl. Acad. Sci. USA*, **92**, 3430.

8 | The retinoblastoma gene product and its relatives

NICHOLAS B. LA THANGUE

1. Introduction

An overwhelming body of cancer research supports the idea that the integration of growth-promoting and growth-restraining pathways maintains the fidelity of the cell cycle (see Chapter 7). During the genesis of tumour cells, such pathways become aberrantly regulated, culminating in an absence of cell cycle control and uncontrolled proliferation. A key player in negative regulation of the cell cycle is the retinoblastoma tumour suppressor gene product (pRB), historically identified through studies on the rare recessive paediatric eye tumour, retinoblastoma, where predisposition to the hereditary form of the disease correlates with a loss of heterozygosity at chromosome 13q14 (1, 2). These studies, together with the recessive nature of the disease, suggests that inactivation of the *RB* gene is important in the generation of retinoblastoma, and implied a negative role for pRB in regulating proliferation. Subsequent molecular characterization of the *RB* gene indicated that the locus is invariably mutated in both hereditary and sporadic retinoblastoma as well as in a variety of other types of tumour (2, 3).

The pRB protein currently takes the central stage for those researchers with interests in the regulation of cellular proliferation and the mechanisms of tumorigenesis because it is now clear that pRB and its upstream and downstream effectors play a critical role in early cell cycle control. It is, arguably, the tumour suppressor gene product for which we have most information about its mechanism of action.

2. Cell cycle regulation of pRB

pRB is a 105 kDa protein believed to be constitutively expressed by most normal cycling cells in mammals (4–6). During cell cycle progression, the phosphorylation level of pRB is periodically regulated, being hypophosphorylated during the early cell cycle and acquiring greater levels of phosphorylation as cells progress into S phase and begin DNA synthesis (7–9). Introducing vectors which express wild-type pRB into tumour cells carrying a mutated endogenous *RB* allele causes cell cycle arrest towards S phase, implying that a principal physiological role of pRB is to regulate the transition from G1 into S phase (10; and see Chapter 7). Since a characteristic of the early cell cycle form of pRB is a low level of phosphorylation, it is believed that this hypophosphorylated form of pRB is active in negative growth control, and that increasing the degree of phosphorylation overcomes this growth-regulating capacity.

Considerable progress has been made in understanding the nature of the efferent signalling proteins which mediate and control the phosphorylation of pRB (Fig. 1). Members of the cyclin-dependent kinase (CDK) family of proteins together with a regulatory cyclin partner (see Chapter 7) appear to be critical regulators of pRB. When cells enter the cycle, the D-type cyclins and cyclin E are temporally induced as cells approach S phase (11, 12). The D-type cyclins (D1, D2, and D3) can be induced by mitogens as cells leave quiescence and form complexes with predominantly one of two CDK subunits, CDK4 or CDK6 (13–16). *In vitro*, the cyclin D–CDK4 and cyclin D–CDK6 kinase complexes preferentially phosphorylate pRB, as opposed to other good CDK substrates, such as histone H1 (17), supporting a physiological role in pRB phosphorylation. In addition, the D-type cyclins contain a short protein motif in their amino terminal region which enables them to associate with pRB (17–19), a feature which may influence their capacity to efficiently phosphorylate pRB. This same motif is present in certain viral oncoproteins which bind pRB (see later).

Cyclin D1 is endowed with proto-oncogenic activity (20–24), and when expressed at high levels can shorten the length of time cells spend in G1 (25). It is an attractive possibility that these effects are exerted through the phosphorylation of pRB and

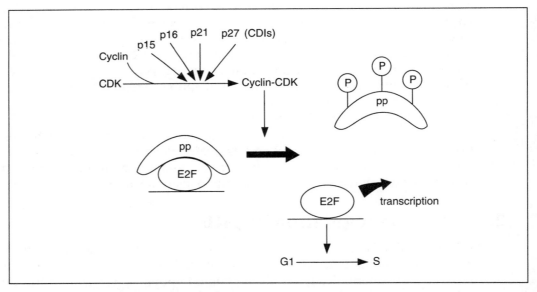

Fig. 1 Regulation of pRB during early cell cycle progression. Transcription factor E2F exists in a transcriptionally inactive state when bound to pRB or other pocket proteins (pp) such as p107 and p130. During cell cycle progression, active E2F is released due to the phosphorylation of pps by cyclin-dependent kinases (CDKs). The kinase activity of the cyclin–CDK complexes is in turn negatively regulated by an expanding group of cyclin-dependent kinase inhibitors such as p15, p16, p21, and p27. Transcriptionally active E2F increases the activity of target genes necessary for cell cycle progression

overcoming its negative growth-regulating capacity. Indeed, co-expression of cyclin D1 together with pRB can prevent pRB-dependent cell cycle arrest (18, 19), and the temporal appearance of cyclin D-dependent kinase activity during cell cycle progression (26) would be consistent with a physiological role in regulating pRB phosphorylation.

Cyclins E and A can also release a pRB-dependent cell cycle arrest (10). A preferred partner for both of these cyclins is CDK2 (11), although the exact contribution of each kinase to the phosphorylation of pRB *in vivo* remains to be established. However, given that the induction of cyclin D by mitogens is followed by an accumulation of cyclin E later in G1 (11), it is possible that the regulation of pRB is mediated by sequential phosphorylation by different cyclin–CDK complexes. For example, cyclin D–CDK4 might prime pRB for phosphorylation by other CDKs, a possibility which awaits verification.

3. Aberrant regulation in tumour cells

In tumour cells the pRB pathway is frequently deregulated. This may result from mutation directly within the *RB* gene or inactivation of the pRB protein caused, for example, by an interaction with oncoproteins (Fig. 2). It is known that mutation in *RB* can occur in a variety of tumours, such as retinoblastoma, small cell lung carcinoma, bladder carcinomas, and in many sarcomas (3). Mutational events range from point

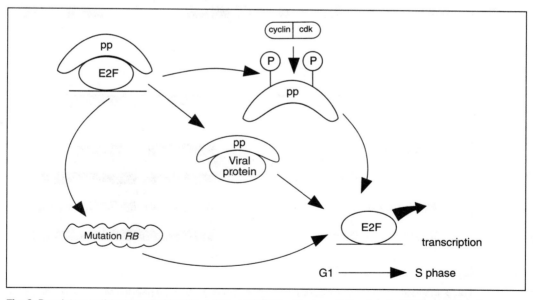

Fig. 2 Regulatory pathways controlling the activity of pRB. The kinase activity of cyclin–CDK complexes is the principal regulatory step in releasing active E2F from pp–E2F complexes. Viral oncoproteins, such as adenovirus E1A, SV40 large T antigen, and the E7 protein of 'high risk' HPVs, release E2F by physically binding pps and so preventing their association with E2F. Mutation in the *RB* gene which occurs in tumour cells (but not so far in the p107 or p130 genes) results in pRB derivatives incapable of interacting with E2F.

mutation to chromosomal deletion, and invariably affect a region referred to as the 'pocket' (Fig. 3) necessary for the biological activity of pRB (27). The pocket region was initially proposed to be an interaction domain through which pRB modulated the activity of key cellular substrates required for cell cycle progression (28), an idea borne out with the subsequent identification of target proteins (discussed later).

3.1 Regulation of pRB by the products of viral oncogenes

Interest in pRB was very much stimulated when a number of viral oncoproteins were found to sequester and inactivate the protein (29, 30). The adenovirus E1A protein, SV40 large T antigen (LT), and the E7 protein of 'high-risk' human papilloma viruses

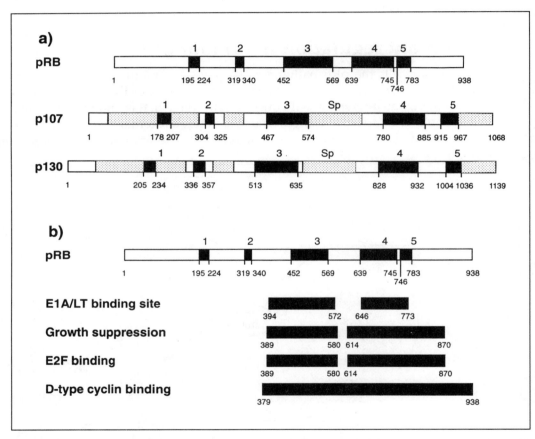

Fig. 3 Comparison of the pocket proteins pRB, p107, and p130. (a) Regions of similarity between the three proteins are indicated in black. Shaded areas indicate additional regions of similarity between p107 and p130. Numbering according to amino acid residue, and Sp indicates the location of the spacer region which in p107 and p130 stably interacts with the cyclin A or cyclin E–CDK2 kinase. (b) Functional and biochemical domains within pRB are indicated that are required for the interaction with viral oncoproteins, E2F, and D-type cyclins, and functionally required for growth suppression.

(HPV) bind pRB (Fig. 2; and see Chapter 1), an interaction dependent upon two short regions within each protein which show a remarkable degree of similarity between the different viral proteins (31–33). In the E1A protein, these regions, referred to as CR1 (conserved region 1) and CR2, are necessary for E1A to exert a range of biological effects, such as cellular immortalization and transformation in tissue culture, induction of apoptosis, promotion of DNA synthesis, and activation of transcription (34). Mutational analysis of pRB showed the pocket to be the minimal region that could bind to E1A (approximately 400 amino acid residues; Fig. 3b) and naturally occurring mutant *RB* alleles in tumour cells that disrupt the pocket region fail to bind the E1A protein (27). It is believed therefore that the ability of the viral proteins to bind pRB allows them to subvert its growth-regulating properties and promote cellular proliferation, and that mutation of the pocket region or sequestration of pRB serve a similar purpose in releasing the cell from negative growth control.

3.2 Mutation in afferent regulators of pRB

Genes encoding the afferent regulators of pRB activity may also be mutated in tumour cells. For example, amplification of the cyclin D1 gene occurs in a significant proportion of human squamous cell, oesophageal and breast carcinomas (35–37), and cyclin D1 expression is increased in some B cell lymphomas due to chromosomal translocation (38; and Chapter 1). Further, the CDK4 gene may be amplified in some tumours (39). Since it is generally believed that cyclin D–CDK complexes are key afferent regulators of pRB activity, then increased levels of cyclin D–CDK kinase potentially could accelerate growth through inactivating pRB.

The activity of the G1 cyclin-dependent kinases, such as cyclin D–CDK4, is negatively regulated by members of a group of proteins known as cyclin-dependent kinase inhibitors (CDIs; Fig. 1). The genes encoding the CDK inhibitors p15^{INK4B} and p16^{INK4A} (40–43) are mutated in certain tumour cell lines, such as those derived from oesophageal, squamous cell carcinomas, glioblastomas, lung and bladder carcinomas (42, 44–47). Mutant alleles in the p16^{INK4A} gene fail to inhibit kinase activity and arrest growth and, further, arrest by wild-type p16^{INK4A} correlates with the expression of wild-type pRB (48–50). Thus, the amplification of genes encoding cyclin D–CDK kinase, and inactivation of their inhibitory regulators p15^{INK4B} and p16^{INK4A}, are likely to affect proliferation by modulating the activity of pRB. It seems highly probable, based on current knowledge, that the *RB* pathway will be deregulated at some level in most, if not all, tumour cells.

4. Relatives of pRB

Several other cellular proteins bind to E1A via the CR1 and CR2 domains (29). The possibility was raised therefore that they share some level of structural and functional similarity with pRB. Indeed, these ideas have been confirmed through the molecular characterization of two of these proteins, called p107 and p130 (51–54), which have a significant amount of sequence, similarity with pRB (Fig. 3). The conserved domains within pRB, p107, and p130 are distributed throughout the proteins but mostly lie within the pocket region, consistent with the ability of each protein to bind to E1A. The p107 and p130 proteins are more closely related to each other than to pRB and in addition contain a 'spacer' region that divides the pocket (Fig. 3a). The p107 and p130 spacer region enables the proteins to form a stable association with either cyclin A–CDK2 or cyclin E–CDK2 kinase *in vivo* (55, 56), although a physiological role for these interactions has yet to be established.

Like pRB, the phosphorylation level of p107 and p130 is under cell cycle control, both proteins being hypophosphorylated during the early cell cycle, becoming progressively more phosphorylated as the cell cycle ensues (R. Bernards, personal communication). For p107, and probably p130, cyclin D–CDK kinases appear to be important mediators of the cell cycle-regulated phosphorylation events (57), a feature which they share with the regulation of pRB. Similarly, in certain cell types, increased levels of either p107 or p130 can cause cell cycle arrest (58, 59), although current evidence suggests that p107 contains two growth suppressing domains in contrast to the single pocket domain in pRB (60 and Fig. 3b). To date there is no evidence that mutations within the p107 or p130 genes occur in tumour cells, suggesting that within the family of pocket proteins pRB has a distinct physiological role.

5. Pocket proteins and development

Although the activity of pRB is dispensable in tumour cells, this clearly is not the case during embryonic development. Studies on the role of pRB using '*RB* knock-out' mice indicate that pRB is required during embryonic development: $RB^{-/-}$ mice fail to develop to full-term, dying *in utero* at about 12–13 days post-coitum (61–63). In these animals, the failure of cells in distinct lineages to undergo terminal differentiation, particularly within the haemopoietic and central nervous systems, together with inappropriately high levels of apoptosis, results in embryonic lethality. These observations suggest that pRB plays a crucial role in controlling cellular differentiation during development. Indeed, the frequent inactivation of *RB* in tumour cells may enable cells to avoid responding to differentiation signals and thus retain proliferative potential, a necessary prerequisite for an evolving tumour. However, it is striking that $RB^{-/-}$ mice do not suffer from retinoblastoma and further that the mouse can undergo considerable embryogenesis in the absence of pRB. We await with interest information which explains these scenarios.

In contrast to the inactivation of *RB*, mice lacking either the gene encoding p107 or p130 develop normally (personal communication). A possible explanation may be that the activity of either protein can compensate for the loss of the other and, consistent with this idea, crossing $p107^{-/-}$ with $p130^{-/-}$ mice causes a lethal phenotype (63a, 63b). Overall, the studies on 'knock-out' mice with defective pocket protein alleles suggest a physiological role for pRB which is distinct from p107 and p130 and argue that pRB plays an important role during embryonic development.

6. E2F is a principal target for pRB

A major step forward in unravelling the mechanism of action of pRB came when it was shown to form a stable physical complex with the cellular transcription factor E2F (64, 65). This observation laid the foundation for a series of exciting and provocative studies which culminated in a model to explain how pRB and its relatives mediate their physiological effects on the cell cycle.

The transcription factor E2F (also referred to as DRTF1) was initially identified as a binding activity which recognizes a functionally important DNA sequence motif in the promoters of a variety of cellular and viral genes (66, 67). However, before the connection was made between pRB and E2F, several properties of E2F implied that it performed an important physiological role, such as its regulation by the products of distinct viral oncogenes, notably adenovirus E1A, SV40 large T antigen, and the E7 protein from 'high risk' types of HPV (29). These three classes of oncoprotein release E2F from what, at the time, were believed to be inactive complexes (64, 68–70). A biological rationale for such an effect could be surmised from the identity of genes regulated by E2F since many were known to be involved in cell cycle control (29). Some E2F target genes encode enzymes which function in DNA synthesis, for example dihydrofolate reductase (DHFR), thymidylate synthase, and DNA polymerase α (29). Another group are proto-oncogenes, such as MYC and B-MYB, and others encode proteins with defined regulatory roles in cell cycle control, such as cdc2 and cyclin A (29). A particularly clear case of the functional significance of E2F sites in these promoters occurs in the DHFR gene where a region which binds E2F has been shown to be necessary for the induction of transcription towards the end of G1 (71). By releasing active E2F, the viruses overcome the cellular mechanisms which normally restrain the expression of these genes, ensuring that the levels of their products are sufficiently high so as not to become limiting.

Not surprisingly, deregulation of E2F correlates with the ability of the viral proteins to function as oncoproteins. Within the three classes of viral oncoprotein, E1A, SV40 LT, and E7, the integrity of the CR1 and CR2 homology domains, which is required for oncogenic activity, is also necessary to release transcriptionally active E2F (29). Subsequently, a series of provocative and exciting studies established that the cellular proteins known to bind E1A in a CR1- and CR2-dependent fashion interact with E2F (55, 56, 64, 65, 72–74), suggesting that E1A competes with E2F for these proteins, and thus providing an explanation for the sensitivity of complexed E2F to viral oncoproteins (Fig. 2).

The identification of E2F as a cellular target for pRB suggested that one of the levels through which pRB exerts its effects on proliferation is by regulating the transcriptional activity of E2F and indeed further experiments indicated that pRB can inactivate the transcriptional activity of E2F (75, 76). Since many cellular genes required for cell cycle progression are regulated by E2F, the interaction of pRB with E2F may limit their expression and hence lead to cell cycle arrest.

Several other observations support the importance of the pRB–E2F interaction in growth control. Of particular note is the fact that E2F binds preferentially to the hypophosphorylated form of pRB which is believed to mediate negative growth control (65). Moreover, the proteins encoded by naturally occurring mutant alleles in *RB* which fail to arrest the cell cycle cannot interact with E2F (75, 76); hence, in tumour cells carrying mutant *RB* alleles, E2F remains in a constitutively active state. Overall, current evidence implicates E2F as a key physiological target in pRB-mediated growth control.

6.1 p107 and p130 regulate E2F

The two known pRB-related proteins, p107 and p130, also bind to E2F (56, 70, 71). The interaction has similar functional consequences, namely transcriptional inactivation, and requires the integrity of the pocket region in each protein (77, 78). It is also somewhat predictable, though currently unclear, that the hypophosphorylated versions of p107 and p130 preferentially bind to E2F. However, the temporal association of each pocket protein with E2F during the cell cycle is quite different (55, 56, 78, 79). The p130–E2F complex predominates in quiescent fibroblasts and unstimulated T cells, persisting for some way into G1, after which cyclin E–CDK2 enters the complex (Fig. 4). The p107–E2F complex occurs predominantly during S phase, and pRB–E2F occurs in G1 and continues into S phase. The early form of p107–E2F (late G1) contains cyclin E–CDK2 whereas cyclin A–CDK2 is more apparent in S phase (55).

Each pocket protein therefore has its own characteristic temporal profile of interactions with E2F, although the physiological significance of multiple pocket proteins for the cell cycle has yet to be resolved. For example, it is not clear whether the pocket proteins function in parallel, overlapping, convergent, or divergent pathways, and why do tumour cells suffer mutation in *RB* rather than the genes for p107 or p130.

7. Molecular resolution of E2F

The pivotal importance of E2F in cell cycle control stimulated considerable interest in understanding its molecular composition (80). The first DNA binding component of E2F to be defined, referred to as E2F-1, was isolated by virtue of its ability to bind to the pocket region of pRB, an interaction mediated through the carboxy terminal region of E2F-1 (81–83). A potent *trans* activation domain is located within the same region, suggesting that a potential mechanism for inactivating E2F-1 may be that the binding of pRB physically prevents the *trans* activation domain from productively interacting with the transcription apparatus (84, 85).

To date, four additional cDNAs encoding proteins highly related to E2F-1 have been isolated, referred as E2F-2, -3, -4, and -5 (86) and hereafter referred to as the E2F family. Like E2F-1 the other E2F family members possess a carboxy terminal *trans* activation domain which is integrated with a pocket protein binding region, other domains such as the DNA binding domain being equally conserved between family members (Fig. 5). It is believed that E2F-1, -2, and -3 are preferentially regulated by pRB (81–83, 87, 88), and that E2F-4 and E2F-5, which at a sequence level form a subgroup of the E2F proteins, have specificity for either p107 or p130 (89–94). For E2F-

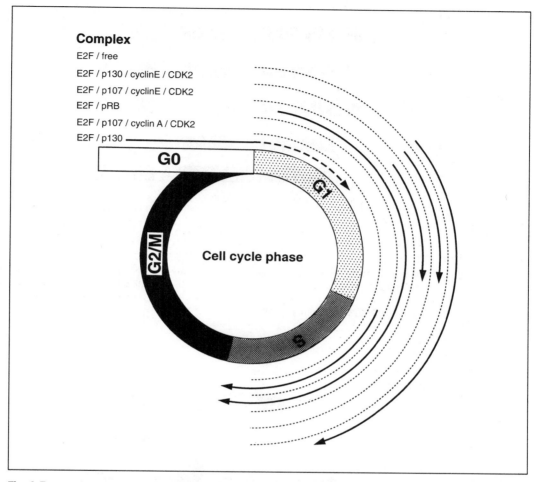

Fig. 4 Temporal appearance of the different E2F complexes during the cell cycle. The diagram, which presents a generic summary of E2F control during the cell cycle, shows free E2F (transcriptionally active) accumulating towards the end of G1 to peak during S phase. The regulation of the pRB, p107, and p130 E2F complexes are likewise indicated.

4, and possibly E2F-5, regulation by either p130 or p107 may be influenced by cell cycle progression (94). Current evidence suggests therefore that distinct pocket proteins prefer to bind to specific E2F family members, providing a potential explanation for the temporally regulated association of different pocket proteins with generic E2F during cell cycle progression (in this context generic E2F refers to the DNA binding activity in cell extracts which recognizes the E2F binding site). It is likely that these pocket protein–E2F complexes reflect the dynamically changing composition of E2F, and specifically the presence of an E2F family member which can dictate the identity of the regulatory pocket protein.

It is currently unclear, although very likely the case, that different E2F complexes

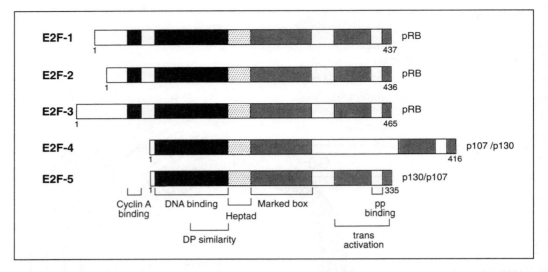

Fig. 5 E2F family members. Domains showing greatest similarity are indicated by the shading. Note that E2Fs-1, -2, and -3 preferentially bind to pRB, E2F-4 to p107 and p130, and E2F-5 to p130 and p107. The heptad and marked box are both areas of sequence similarity which as yet have no clear function. The DP similarity is a region with greatest similarity to the DP family members.

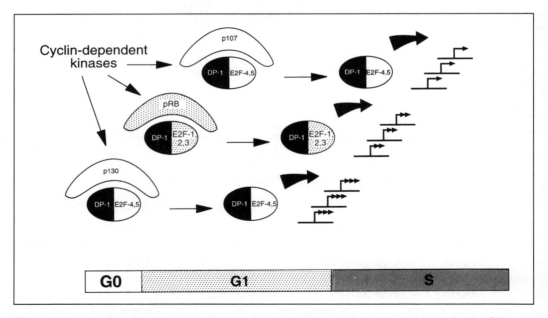

Fig. 6 Integrating cell cycle progression with transcription. In this model the kinase activities of cyclin–CDK complexes regulate the ability of pps to bind to distinct DP-1/E2F heterodimers where the E2F partner dictates the identity of the pp. It is envisaged that such a situation would allow distinct afferent signals to be transduced to pps and consequently to different DP-1/E2F heterodimers. It is unclear whether the various DP-1/E2F heterodimers have distinct, similar, or overlapping target genes.

will have functionally distinct effects on target genes, perhaps through subtle differences in E2F binding site preferences. Some evidence suggests that E2F-1 can activate through some, but not all, types of E2F site (95) and other studies indicate that E2F binding sites can have functionally diverse effects on promoters. As an example, the E2F site in the E2F-1 promoter acts in *cis* to repress promoter activity, since mutation in the E2F site constitutively increases promoter activity (96–98) whereas in other promoters, such as that of the DHFR gene, the E2F site appears to play a positive role (71). Indeed, promoter specificity would enable the activity of pocket proteins to be integrated with subsets of E2F-regulated genes, and could perhaps be responsible for temporal differences in the transcriptional activity of target genes (Fig. 6). However, such possibilities are hypothetical and await to be resolved.

8. DP-1: a widespread component of E2F

It is now clear that the generic E2F activity assayed in cell extracts is a heterodimeric DNA binding complex in which an E2F family member interacts with a DP family member (80). The first member of the DP family identified, called DP-1 (Fig. 7), can form heterodimers with each of the identified E2F family members and in many different cell types is a frequent, near universal component of generic E2F (99–101). Physiological E2F is thus a DP/E2F heterodimer. The interaction between DP-1 and E2F-1 is co-operative in both DNA binding and transcriptional activity (100–103). The DP-1/E2F-1 heterodimer can also bind pRB efficiently and is specifically recognized by the adenovirus E4 orf 6/7 (101–103), and thus possesses the hallmarks expected for a physiologically relevant and important form of E2F.

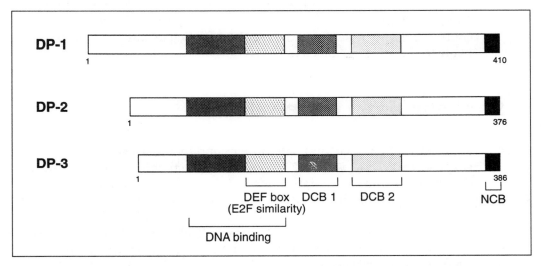

Fig. 7 DP family members. Domains showing greatest similarity are indicated by the shading. The DEF box, which resides in the carboxy region of the DNA binding domain, contains a conserved region with greatest similarity to E2F family members.

Although DP-1 is a frequent component of generic E2F, it is regulated at the level of phosphorylation during cell cycle progression; it appears in a hypophosphorylated state early during cell cycle progression and is phosphorylated at later times (101). One of the kinases implicated in the late phosphorylation control of DP-1 is the cyclin A-CDK2 complex, which locates the heterodimer and subsequently phosphorylates DP-1 by virtue of a cyclin A binding domain within the amino terminal region of E2F-1 (104). As this same domain is shared with E2F-2 and -3, the DP-1/E2F-2 and DP-1/E2F-3 heterodimers are likely to be regulated in a similar fashion, but the domain is absent from E2F-4 and -5 (Fig. 5). Phosphorylation of DP-1 reduces the DNA binding activity of the heterodimer when assayed *in vitro* and this regulation may be important therefore in down-regulating the transcription of target genes during the later stages of the cell cycle. Perhaps the cyclin A-binding members of the E2F family regulate a set of genes which, once induced, need to be down-regulated to allow progress through the cell cycle.

As might be expected, DP-1 is representative of a family of evolutionarily conserved proteins (105, 106). *Xenopus* DP-2 and murine DP-3 are well conserved across the region involved in dimerization and DNA binding (Fig. 7) and, like DP-1, can form heterodimers with all known members of the E2F family (105, 106). In addition, studies on DP-3 have indicated another level of complexity in that DP-3 RNA is alternatively spliced (106). The 5' untranslated region is spliced in a tissue-dependent fashion which together with alternative splicing within the coding sequence causes important changes in the expression and functional properties of DP-3 proteins (de la Luna and La Thangue, unpublished data). Thus, the activity of generic E2F is subject to different levels of control: its varied subunit composition made up by members of the DP and E2F families, variations in the properties of these proteins as a result of alternative splicing and subsequent regulation of the complexes by pocket proteins and phosphorylation. Given the overriding importance of the pathway in cell cycle control, it has to be said that the regulatory mechanisms influencing E2F activity are likely to show increasing complexity.

9. Evolutionary conservation

In view of the central importance of E2F in the mammalian cell cycle, the evolutionary conservation of DP and E2F proteins and their pathway of control comes as little surprise. In *Xenopus laevis*, E2F DNA binding activity is regulated during embryonic development and two members of the *X. laevis* DP family, DP-1 and DP-2, have been molecularly characterized (105, 107). In contrast, single DP and E2F genes exist in *Drosophila melanogaster* (108–110). The importance of these genes for cell cycle control has been demonstrated in flies carrying a null allele of E2F where E2F-regulated genes remain transcriptionally inactive and the consequent failure to replicate DNA causes a lethal phenotype (111).

During *Drosophila* embryogenesis the cell cycle becomes progressively more complex, developmental modifications which, interestingly, are reflected in differences in the control of E2F. For example, in endoreplicating cells where S and G phases alternate without intervening mitoses, E2F is an upstream regulator of the cyclin E gene, cyclin E being necessary for progression into S phase (112). A contrasting situation occurs in certain cells in the nervous system which employ a more sophisticated cell cycle and where cyclin E plays an upstream role in regulating E2F activity (112). These are exciting and provocative studies and it will be interesting to determine whether analogous differences exist in regulatory pathways which control mammalian E2F.

Another level of conservation is apparent from the recent studies of *Drosophila* which suggest that pocket proteins are conserved and like their mammalian counterparts are capable of interacting with and regulating E2F (110). The evolutionary conservation of molecules within the E2F pathway underscores its pivotal role in cell cycle control.

10. Integration with p53

Although interruption of the pRB–E2F pathway by tumour viruses implicates the pathway in oncogenesis, it is becoming clear that aberrant regulation of E2F can have diverse physiological outcomes. For example, an expanding body of evidence indicates that apoptosis or programmed cell death is one of the potential outcomes and that this process can be influenced by p53 (Fig. 8, and Chapter 9). Hints that this was the case came from studies on the E1A oncoprotein, where high level expression of E1A correlates with an increased frequency of apoptosis (113–115) and, further, extensive apoptosis is apparent in $RB^{-/-}$ mice (see earlier discussion). Since both treatments deregulate E2F, the results imply a role for the E2F pathway in regulating apoptosis.

Further evidence for this idea has come from studies on E2F-1 in which it was found that cells that overexpress E2F-1 apoptose in a p53-dependent fashion (116, 117). In $RB^{-/-}$ mice, lens fibre cells, which normally differentiate, continue to synthesize DNA and suffer inappropriate levels of apoptosis that is dependent upon wild-type p53; in embryos which are doubly-null for pRB and p53 apoptosis is suppressed (118).

In tumour cells, therefore, it makes very good sense that the p53 gene is frequently inactivated (see Chapter 9) and this commonly goes hand in hand with mutation in *RB*. Further, oncogenic viruses, such as adenoviruses and HPV, have evolved proteins that specifically inactivate p53 and which co-operate with either the E1A or E7 proteins in cellular transformation (30). A clear demonstration of this phenomenon occurs when the expression of the HPV E6 oncoprotein (which inactivates p53) together with E7 is targeted to lens fibre cells using the approach of transgenesis: alone the E7 protein causes increased levels of apoptosis in lens tissue whereas both proteins expressed together cause an increased frequency of lens tumours (119).

It is a currently popular view that the ability of p53 to function as a sequence-specific transcription factor is involved in p53-induced apoptosis (see Chapter 9). Recent studies do, however, suggest that other mechanisms may contribute to this

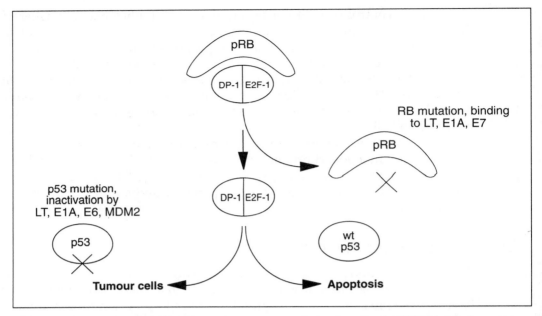

Fig. 8 Integration of E2F and p53 pathways of growth control. During the cell cycle DP/E2F heterodimers play an important physiological role in driving cells through early cell cycle transitions. In some circumstances, perhaps when cell cycle progression is not compatible with the physiological environment, cells can apoptose in a p53-dependent fashion, for example, upon the appearance of transcriptionally active DP/E2F heterodimers due to mutation in *RB* or the action of viral oncoproteins such as E1A or E7. However, if wild-type p53 activity is also absent (due to mutation in the p53 gene or amplification of the *MDM2* oncogene) then active E2F will contribute to the uncontrolled proliferation.

process since p53 molecules compromised in their ability to activate transcription can still promote apoptosis (120, 121). Although we await clarification regarding these additional mechanisms an interaction between p53 and the E2F pathway cannot be ruled out.

Overall, these results argue that the pathways regulated by p53 and pRB are physiologically integrated. Although the mechanistic details of the integration process are not yet clear, the MDM2 protein physically associates with proteins in both pathways. Human *MDM2* is an oncogene frequently amplified in certain types of tumour cells, particularly sarcomas (122). It has been shown to bind to and inactivate the transcriptional activity of p53, an interaction believed to overcome the growth suppressing properties of p53 and thus to contribute to the oncogenic properties of MDM2 (123). Recent studies have defined two further targets for MDM2, both being regulatory molecules in the pRB–E2F pathway. In the first, the MDM2 protein was found to bind to the DP-1 protein, with the functional consequence of increasing the transcriptional activity of a DP-1/E2F-1 heterodimer (124). Secondly, a stable interaction between MDM2 and pRB has been detected, and MDM2 can partly overcome the transcriptional inactivity imposed by pRB on the DP/E2F heterodimer (125). Both these interactions could theoretically enhance the activity of E2F and thus promote cell cycle progression. By combining p53 inactivation with E2F stimulation, MDM2 appears to be a sophisticated oncoprotein which in normal cells may play a role in integrating these two principal pathways of growth control.

In addition to a role in regulating apoptosis, members of both DP and E2F protein families are endowed with proto-oncogenic activity (126). When expressed at high levels, the E2F-1 protein can co-operate with an oncogenic form of *H-RAS* in the transformation of rat embryo fibroblasts, an activity that can be further enhanced by attaching the very strong VP16 transcriptional activation domain to E2F-1 (127). These results therefore suggest that the proto-oncogenic activity of E2F-1 may be exerted through its capacity to transcriptionally activate cell cycle-regulated genes whose increased levels would promote cell proliferation. However, and in contrast, the proto-oncogenic activity of the DP family of proteins is exerted through a pathway in which the regulation of E2F site-dependent transcription is not the primary target (128); the interaction of DP-1 with MDM2 (124) may be more important in the oncogenic process. It should be noted that despite these studies demonstrating the proto-oncogenic properties of E2F and DP proteins, evidence for mutation of their genes in tumour cells is lacking.

In conclusion, studies on the physiological outcomes of deregulating the E2F pathway suggest that in conditions where E2F in inappropriately activated, a pathway involving p53 (though not necessarily only p53) leads to apoptosis. In cells lacking the attention of p53, deregulating E2F, through mutation in *RB* or effects on another regulatory protein favours the production of tumour cells.

11. Other cellular targets of pRB

Although E2F is very probably the major physiological target through which pRB and related pocket proteins exert their effects on the cell cycle, pRB has nevertheless been implicated in the regulation of other transcription factors and additional proteins with important regulatory roles (Table 1).

It has been suggested that pRB plays an important role during the differentiation of muscle cells through an interaction with muscle-specific transcription factors and the subsequent activation of muscle-restricted genes (129). Thus, the activation of muscle-specific genes in SAOS-2 cells ($RB^{-/-}$) by the transcription factor MyoD is augmented by co-expression of pRB or p107 (130, 131), and MyoD and pRB can interact *in vitro* (130). However, $RB^{-/-}$ fibroblasts can undergo differentiation to myotubes although the differentiated phenotype does not appear to be stable (131). Interestingly, such cells express high levels of p107, suggesting that p107 may partially compensate for the loss of pRB. In the muscle cell lineage, the evidence suggests that pRB may be involved with commitment and differentiation but the precise role of the physical interaction between MyoD and pRB in the physiological process of muscle differentiation remains to be resolved.

Another series of provocative studies imply that the interaction of pRB with the c-ABL tyrosine kinase may be of importance in cell cycle control. A ubiquitously expressed tyrosine kinase, c-ABL is located in the cytoplasm and nucleus (132, and

Table 1 Cellular proteins interacting with pocket proteins

	Interacting protein	Function
pRB	E2F-1, -2, -3	Transcription factor, partner for DPs (82–84, 88)
	DP-1, -2, -3	Transcription factor, partner for E2Fs (99, 105, 106)
	c-MYC, N-MYC	Transcription factor (143)
	ELF-1	Transcription factor (144)
	RBP1, RBP2	Unknown (145)
	PU-1	Transcription factor (146)
	Cyclins D1, D2, and D3	Regulatory subunits for CDK (18, 19)
	RBAP48	G protein-like (147)
	PP1	Protein phosphatase (148)
	c-ABL	Tyrosine kinase (133)
	MyoD	Transcription factor (130)
	ATF2	Transcription factor (139)
	Id-2	Transcription factor (149)
	Laminin C	Nuclear structure (83)
	UBF	Transcription factor (142) (RNA polymerase I)
	BRM	Chromatin modelling (141)
	MDM2	Transcription factor (125)
p107	E2F-4, -5	Transcription factor, partner for DPs (89–94)
	DP-1, -2, -3	Transcription factor, partner for E2Fs (99, 105, 106)
	c-MYC	Transcription factor (150)
	Cyclins A, D1, D2, D3, E	Regulatory subunits of CDK (19, 55, 73)
p130	E2F-4, -5	Transcription factor, partner for DPs (91–94)
	DP-1, -2, -3	Transcription factor, partner for E2Fs (99, 105, 106)
	Cyclins A, D1, D2, D3, E	Regulatory subunits of CDK (53, 54)

see Chapter 4). The nuclear kinase activity of c-ABL is under cell cycle control, being low during the early cell cycle and increased during cell cycle progression, and c-ABL has been shown to bind to the carboxy terminal region of pRB (133, 134), a region of pRB necessary for its growth-regulating activity (135). Interestingly, c-ABL can simultaneously interact with pRB when the pocket region is occupied by E2F (134).

Although a likely explanation for the inactivation of E2F by pocket proteins can be proposed from the overlapping location of the *trans* activation and pocket protein binding domains, pRB additionally has an autonomous activity which can repress *trans* activation by some, but not all, transcription factors (136, 137). Further, in the context of certain promoters, for example *B-MYB* and *E2F-1*, the E2F site negatively regulates promoter activity (96–98, 138), suggesting that the activity of other transcription factors located on these promoters can be overridden in *cis* by the E2F binding site. Perhaps these promoters bind a particular constellation of transcription factors which are susceptible to transcriptional inactivation by pocket proteins recruited to the promoter by E2F.

Besides a capacity to inactivate transcription, pRB can increase the activity of certain transcription factors, such as ATF2 (139). This may be mediated by a direct physical interaction, as in the case of ATF2 (139), or in a more indirect fashion.

Indirect effects may be mediated through brama (BRM), a mammalian protein likely to be a homologue of the *Saccharomyces cerevisiae* (SNF2/SWI2 protein (140), and one capable of interacting with pRB (141). In yeast, the SNF2/SWI2 protein is believed to be involved in remodelling chromatin structure and perhaps altering its accessibility to transcription factors. Human BRM can co-operate with pRB in the transcriptional activation of the glucocorticoid receptor (141), suggesting a mechanism through which pRB may affect transcription by altering chromatin structure.

Finally, our discussion so far has centred around the role of pocket proteins in the regulation of RNA polymerase II-dependent transcription. Recent results do however suggest that transcription mediated by RNA polymerase I is also subject to control by pRB (142). Thus, during the differentiation of U937 myeloid progenitor cells pRB becomes localized to nucleoli (142), regions of the nucleus which are the major sites of ribosomal gene transcription by RNA polymerase I. Transcription factor UBF1, also localized to nucleoli, has a key role in activating ribosomal genes. Subsequent studies have indicated that pRB and UBF1 can bind to each other, and that the transcriptional activity of UBF1 is compromised upon this interaction (142) which could potentially be responsible for the reduced ribosomal gene expression during differentiation. Given the regulation of RNA polymerase I- and II-dependent transcription by pRB, we may anticipate similar regulatory interactions for transcription driven by RNA polymerase III.

12. Conclusion

It is an exciting era in cell cycle research. We are now uncovering the molecular details of a critical pathway which regulates early cell cycle progression by integrating signals emanating from proteins which drive the cell cycle with the transcription apparatus and the consequent control of downstream target genes. Molecules which function to positively regulate, such as cyclin–CDK complexes, and negatively regulate, such as CDIs, converge on the pathway and in turn regulate the activity of the pRB tumour suppressor gene product and related proteins. A principal role of pRB is in the regulation of the E2F transcription factor, the activity of which influences cell cycle progression. Importantly, many of the proteins in this pathway are encoded by genes which are frequently mutated in tumour cells, a feature which emphasizes a critical role in orchestrating early cell cycle control. In fact, it seems likely that the pathway is, at some point, aberrantly regulated in most, if not all, human tumour cells.

We are, however, left with an increasing number of questions which have to be answered before we can begin to visualize the complete picture. Why do humans invariably suffer retinoblastoma upon inactivation of *RB*, in contrast to, for example, the $RB^{-/-}$ mice? Is it something concerned with the susceptibility of human retinoblasts to mutation in *RB*, or is it indicating a more general difference concerned with the properties of pRB in each species? We know, from the phenotype of the $RB^{-/-}$ mice, that the activity of pRB can be dispensed with up to a mid-embryonic stage. Is this because a related protein can compensate for its loss, or is it truly telling us that pRB plays a minor role up to this developmental stage? And why do these embryos suffer such high levels of apoptosis and aberrant differentiation, and how does the phenotype relate to the physiological role of pRB?

It is principally E2F that pRB seeks out to exert its effect on the cell cycle, whilst the physiological significance of other targets awaits clarification. However, many questions remain, such as why is there such a plethora of E2F/DP heterodimers under the E2F umbrella; different genes, different targets, or different pathways of control? In human tumour cells, why is *RB* so frequently mutated, whereas the genes encoding p107 and p130 are apparently not? Does this imply that the physiological roles of p107 and p130 are of overwhelming importance that cells cannot accommodate mutations in either gene, or do they take on such minor roles that their mutation in tumour cells would be of incidental consequence.

Finally, and importantly, we should never forget that the increasing knowledge on the mechanisms of cell cycle control has profound implications for the treatment of proliferative disease. The progress and insights into the physiological pathways which regulate cell cycle progression offer a new and exciting range of realistic targets through which oncogenesis and other proliferative diseases may, in the near future, be effectively controlled. Without any doubt, the mechanistic and structural information which is rapidly accumulating offers new promise in the search for clinically viable small molecule drugs.

Acknowledgements

Thanks to Debbie Duthie for help with preparation of the manuscript, to my colleagues for stimulating discussions and the Medical Research Council, Leukaemia Research Fund, and Human Frontiers Science Programme for supporting my research.

References

1. Knudson, A. G. (1971) Mutation and cancer: statistical study of retinoblastoma. *Proc. Natl. Acad. Sci. USA*, **68**, 820.
2. Weinberg, R. A. (1991) Tumor suppressor genes. *Science*, **254**, 1138.
3. Horowitz, J. M., Park, S.-H., Bogenmann, E., Cheng, J.-C., Yandell, D. W., Kaye, F. J., *et al.* (1990) Frequent inactivation of the retinoblastoma antioncogene is restricted to a subset of human tumor cells. *Proc. Natl. Acad. Sci. USA*, **87**, 2775.
4. Friend, S. H., Bernards, R., Rogeli, S., Weinberg, R. A., Rapaport, J. M., Albert, D. M., *et al.* (1986) Identification of a human DNA segment having properties of the gene that predisposes to retinoblastoma and osteosarcoma. *Nature*, **323**, 643.
5. Friend, S. H., Horowitz, J. M., Gerber, M. R., Wang, X.-F., Bogenmann, E., Li, F. P., *et al.* (1987) Deletions of a DNA sequence in retinoblastomas and mesenchymal tumors: Organization of the sequence and its encoded protein. *Proc. Natl. Acad. Sci. USA*, **84**, 9059.
6. Bernards, R., Schackleford, G. M., Gerber, M. R., Horowitz, J. M., Friend, S. H., Schartl, M., *et al.* (1989) Structure and expression of the murine retinoblastoma gene and characterization of its encoded protein. *Proc. Natl. Acad. Sci. USA*, **86**, 6474.

7. DeCaprio, J. A., Ludlow, J. W., Lynch, D., Furukawa, Y., Griffin, J., Piwnica-Worms, H., et al. (1989) The product of the retinoblastoma gene has properties of a cell cycle regulatory element. *Cell*, **58**, 1085.

8. Chen, P.-L., Scully, P., Shew, J.-Y., Wang, J. Y. J., and Lee, W.-H. (1989) Phosphorylation of the retinoblastoma gene product is modulated during the cell cycle and cellular differentiation. *Cell*, **58**, 1193.

9. Buchkovich, K. J., Duffy, L. A., and Harlow, E. (1989) The retinoblastoma protein is phosphorylated during specific phases of the cell cycle. *Cell*, **58**, 1097.

10. Hinds, P. W., Mittnacht, S., Dulic, V., Arnold, A., Reed, S. I., and Weinberg, R. A. (1992) Regulation of retinoblastoma protein functions by ectopic expression of human cyclins. *Cell*, **70**, 993.

11. Sherr, C. J. (1993) Mammalian G1 cyclins. *Cell*, **73**, 1059.

12. Pines, J. (1995) Cyclins, CDKs and cancer. *Semin. Cancer Biol.*, **6**, 63.

13. Matsushime, H., Roussel, M. F., Ashmun, R. A., and Sherr, C. J. (1991) Colony-stimulating factor 1 regulates novel cyclins during the G1 phase of the cell cycle. *Cell*, **65**, 701.

14. Xiong, Y., Zhang, H., and Beach, D. (1992) D type cyclins associate with multiple protein kinases and the DNA replication and repair factor PCNA. *Cell*, **71**, 504.

15. Bates, S., Bonetta, L., MacAllan, D., Parry, D., Holder, A., Dickson, C., et al. (1994) CDK6 (PLSTIRE) and CDK4 (PSK-J3) are a distinct subset of the cyclin-dependent kinases that associate with cyclin D1. *Oncogene*, **9**, 71.

16. Meyerson, M. and Harlow, E. (1994) Identification of G1 kinase activity for cdk6, a novel cyclin D partner. *Mol. Cell. Biol.*, **14**, 2077.

17. Kato, J., Matsushime, H., Hiebert, S. W., Ewen, M. E., and Sherr, C. J. (1993) Direct binding of cyclin D to the retinoblastoma gene product (pRb) and pRb phosphorylation by the cyclin D-dependent kinase (CDK4). *Genes Dev.*, **7**, 331.

18. Dowdy, S. F., Hinds, P. W., Louie, K., Reed, S. I., Arnold, A., and Weinberg, R. A. (1993) Physical interaction of the retinoblastoma protein with human cyclins. *Cell*, **73**, 449.

19. Ewen, M. E., Sluss, H. K., Sherr, C. J., Matsushime, H., Kato, J. Y., and Livingston, D. M. (1993) Functional interactions of the retinoblastoma protein with mammalian D-type cyclins. *Cell*, **73**, 487.

20. Lovec, H., Sewing, A., Lucibello, F. C., Müller, R., and Moroy, T. (1994) Oncogenic activity of cyclin D1 revealed through cooperation with Ha-*ras*: link between cell cycle control and malignant transformation. *Oncogene*, **9**, 323.

21. Jiang, W., Kahn, S. M., Zhou, P., Zhang, T.-J., Cacace, A. M., Infante, A. S., et al. (1993) Overexpression of cyclin D1 in rat fibroblasts causes abnormalities in growth control, cell cycle progression and gene expression. *Oncogene*, **8**, 3447.

22. Hinds, P. W., Dowdy, S. F., Eaton, E. N., Arnold, A., and Weinberg, R. A. (1994) Function of a human cyclin gene as an oncogene. *Proc. Natl. Acad. Sci. USA*, **91**, 709.

23. Bodrug, S. E., Warner, B. J., Bath, M. L., Lindeman, G. J., Harris, A. W., and Adams, J. M. (1994) Cyclin D1 transgene impedes lymphocyte maturation and collaborates in lymphomagenesis with the *myc* gene. *EMBO J.*, **13**, 2124.

24. Wang, T. C., Cardiff, R. D., Zukerberg, L., Lees, E., Arnold, A., and Schmidt, E. V. (1994) Mammary hyperplasia and carcinoma in MMTV-cyclin D1 transgenic mice. *Nature*, **369**, 669.

25. Quelle, D. E., Ashmun, R. A., Shurtleff, S. A., Kato, J.-Y., Bar-Sagi, D., Roussel, M. F., et al. (1993) Overexpression of mouse D-type cyclin accelerates G1 phase in rodent fibroblasts. *Genes Dev.*, **7**, 1559.

26. Matsushime, H., Ewen, M. E., Strom, D. K., Kato, J. Y., Hanks, S. K., Roussel, M. F., *et al.* (1992) Identification and properties of an atypical catalytic subunit (p34^{PSK-J3}/cdk4) for mammalian D type G1 cyclins. *Cell*, **71**, 323.

27. Hu, Q. J., Dyson, N., and Harlow, E. (1990) The regions of the retinoblastoma protein needed for binding to adenovirus E1a or SV40 large T antigen are common sites for mutations. *EMBO J.*, **9**, 1147.

28. Chittenden, T., Livingston, D. M., and Kaelin, W. G. (1991) The T/E1A-binding domain of the retinoblastoma product can interact selectively with a sequence-specific DNA binding protein. *Cell*, **65**, 1073.

29. Nevins, J. R. (1992) E2F: a link between the Rb tumor suppressor protein and viral oncoproteins. *Science*, **258**, 424.

30. Vousden, K. H. (1995) Regulation of the cell cycle by viral oncoproteins. *Semin. Cancer Biol.*, **6**, 109.

31. Whyte, P., Buchkovich, K. J., Horowitz, J. M., Friend, S. H., Raybuck, M., Weinberg, R. A., *et al.* (1988) Association between an oncogene and an anti-oncogene: the adenovirus E1A proteins bind to the retinoblastoma gene product. *Nature*, **334**, 124.

32. DeCaprio, J. A., Ludlow, J. W., Figge, J., Shew, J. Y., Huang, C. M., Lee, W. H., *et al.* (1988) SV40 large tumor antigen forms specific complex with the product of the retinoblastoma susceptibility gene. *Cell*, **54**, 275.

33. Dyson, N., Howley, P. M., Munger, K., and Harlow, E. (1989) The human papilloma virus-16 E7 oncoprotein is able to bind to the retinoblastoma gene product. *Science*, **243**, 934.

34. Moran, E. (1993) DNA tumour virus transforming proteins and the cell cycle. *Curr. Opin. Genet. Dev.*, **3**, 63.

35. Bates, S. and Peters, G. (1995) Cyclin D1 as a cellular proto-oncogene. *Semin. Cancer Biol.*, **6**, 73.

36. Lammie, G., Fantl, V., Smith, R., Schuuring, E., Brookes, S., Michalides, R., *et al.* (1991) D11S287, a putative oncogene on chromosome 11q13, is amplified and expressed in squamous cell and mammary carcinomas and linked to BCL-1. *Oncogene*, **6**, 439.

37. Jiang, W., Kahan, S., Tomita, N., Zhang, Y., Lu, S., and Weinstein, B. (1992) Amplification and expression of the human cyclin D gene in esophageal cancer. *Cancer Res.*, **52**, 2980.

38. Motokura, T., Bloom, T., Kim, G., Juppner, H., Ruderman, J. V., Kronenberg, H. M., *et al.* (1991) A novel cyclin encoded by a *bcl1*-linked candidate oncogene. *Nature*, **350**, 512.

39. He, J., Allen, J. R., Collins, V. P., Allalunis-Turner, M. J., Godbout, R., Day, R. S., *et al.* (1994) CDK4 amplification is an alternative mechanism to p16 gene homozygous deletion in glioma cell lines. *Cancer Res.*, **54**, 5804.

40. Sherr, C. J. and Roberts, J. M. (1995) Inhibitors of mammalian G1 cyclin-dependent kinases. *Genes Dev.*, **9**, 1149.

41. Serrano, M., Hannon, G. J., and Beach, D. (1993) A new regulatory motif in cell-cycle control causing specific inhibition of cyclin D/CDK4. *Nature*, **366**, 704.

42. Schmidt, E. E., Ichimura, K., Reifenberger, G., and Collins, V. P. (1994) CDKN2 (p16/MTS1) gene deletion or CDK4 amplification occurs in the majority of glioblastomas. *Cancer Res.*, **54**, 6321.

43. Hannon, G. J. and Beach, D. (1994) p15^{INK4b} is a potential effector cell cycle arrest mediated by TGFβ. *Nature*, **371**, 257.

44. Kamb, A., Gruis, N. A., Weaver-Feldhaus, J., Liu, Q., Harshman, K., Tavitian, S. V., *et al.*

(1994) A cell cycle regulator potentially involved in genesis of many tumor types. *Science*, **264**, 436.

45. Nobori, T., Miura, K., Wu, D. J., Lois, A., Takbayashi, K., and Carson, D. A. (1994) Deletion of the cyclin-dependent kinase-4 inhibitor gene in multiple human cancers. *Nature*, **368**, 753.

46. Zhou, X., Tarmin, L., Yin, J., Jiang, H.-Y., Suzuki, H., Rhyu, M.-G., *et al.* (1994) The *MTS1* gene is frequently mutated in primary human esophageal tumors. *Oncogene*, **9**, 9737.

47. Jen, J., Harper, J. W., Bigner, S. H., Bigner, D. D., Papadopoulos, N., Markowitz, S., *et al.* (1994) Deletion of p15 and p16 genes in brain tumors. *Cancer Res.*, **54**, 6353.

48. Serrano, M., Gomez-Lahoz, E., DePinho, R. A., Beach, D., and Bar-Sagi, D. (1995) Inhibition of ras-induced proliferation and cellular transformation by p16^{INK4}. *Science*, **267**, 249.

49. Lukas, J., Parry, D., Aagaard, L., Mann, D. J., Bartkova, J., Strauss, M., *et al.* (1995) Retinoblastoma-protein-dependent cell-cycle inhibition by the tumour suppressor p16. *Nature*, **375**, 503.

50. Koh, J., Enders, G. H., Dynlacht, B. D., and Harlow, E. (1995) Tumour-derived p16 alleles encoding proteins defective in cell-cycle inhibition. *Nature*, **375**, 506.

51. Ewen, M. E., Xing, Y., Lawrence, J. B., and Livingston, D. M. (1991) Molecular cloning, chromosomal mapping and expression of the cDNA for p107, a retinoblastoma gene product-related protein. *Cell*, **66**, 1155.

52. Mayol, X., Grana, X., Baldi, A., Sang, N., Hu, Q., and Giordano, A. (1993) Cloning of a new member of the retinoblastoma gene family (pRb2) which binds to the E1a transforming domain. *Oncogene*, **8**, 2561.

53. Li, Y., Graham, C., Lacy, S., Duncan, A. M. V., and Whyte, P. (1993) The adenovirus E1A-associated 130-kD protein is encoded by a member of the retinoblastoma gene family and physically interacts with cyclins A and E. *Genes Dev.*, **7**, 2366.

54. Hannon, G. J., Demetrick, D., and Beach, D. (1993) Isolation of the Rb-related p130 through its interaction with CDK2 and cyclins. *Genes Dev.*, **7**, 2378.

55. Lees, E., Faha, B., Dulic, V., Reed, S. I., and Harlow, E. (1992) Cyclin E/cdk2 and cyclin A/cdk2 kinases associate with p107 and E2F in a temporally distinct matter. *Genes Dev*, **6**, 1874.

56. Cobrinik, D., Whyte, P., Peeper, D. S., Jacks, T., and Weinberg, R. A. (1993) Cell cycle-specific association of E2F with the p130 E1A-binding protein. *Genes Dev.*, **7**, 2392.

57. Beijersbergen, R. L., Carlee, L., Kerkhoven, R. M., and Bernards, R. (1995) Regulation of the retinoblastoma protein-related p107 by G1 cyclin complexes. *Genes Dev.*, **9**, 1340.

58. Zhu, L., Van den Heuvel, S., Helin, K., Fattaey, A., Ewen, M., Livingston, D., *et al.* (1993) Inhibition of cell proliferation by p107, a relative of the retinoblastoma protein. *Genes Dev.*, **7**, 1111.

59. Wolf, D. A., Hermeking, H., Albert, T., Herzinger, T., Kind, P., and Eick, D. (1995) A complex between E2F and the pRb-related protein p130 is specifically targeted by the simian virus 40 large T antigen during cell transformation. *Oncogene*, **10**, 2067.

60. Zhu, L., Enders, G., Lees, J. A., Beijersbergen, R. L., Bernards, R., and Hawlos, E. (1995) The pRB-related protein p107 contains two growth suppression domains: independent interactions with E2F and cyclin/cdk complexes. *EMBO J.*, **14**, 1904.

61. Jacks, T., Fazeli, A., Schmitt, E. M., Bronson, R. T., Goodell, M. A., and Weinberg, R. A. (1992) Effects of an Rb mutation in the mouse. *Nature*, **359**, 295.

62. Lee, E. Y-H. P., Chang, C-Y., Hu, N., Wang, Y-C. J., Lai, C-C., Herrup, K., *et al.* (1992) Mice deficient for Rb are nonviable and show defects in neurogenesis and haematopoiesis. *Nature*, **359**, 288.

63. Clarke, A. R., Maandag, E. R., Van Roon, M., Van der Luft, N. M. T., Van der Valk, M., Hooper, *et al.* (1992) Requirement for a functional *Rb-1* gene in murine development. *Nature*, **359**, 328.

63a. Lee, M. H., Williams, B. O., Mulligan, G., Mukai, S., Bronson, R. T., Dyson, N., Harlow, E. and Jacks, T. (1996) Targeted disruption of p107: functional overlap between p107 and Rb genes. *Genes Dev.*, **10**, 1621–32.

63b. Cobrinik, D., Lee, M. H., Hannon, G., Mulligan, G., Bronson, R. T., Dyson, N., Harlow, E., Beach, D., Weinberg, R. A. and Jacks, T. (1996) Shared role of the pRb-related p130 and p107 proteins in limb development. *Genes Dev.*, **10**, 1633–44.

64. Bandara, L. R. and La Thangue, N. B. (1991) Adenovirus E1a prevents the retinoblastoma gene product from complexing with a cellular transcription factor. *Nature*, **351**, 494.

65. Chellappan, S. P., Hiebert, S., Mudryj, M., Horowitz, J. M., and Nevins, J. R. (1991) The E2F transcription factor is a cellular target for the Rb protein. *Cell*, **65**, 1053.

66. Kovesdi, I., Reichel, R., and Nevins, J. R. (1986) Identification of a cellular transcription factor involved in E1A *trans*-activation. *Cell*, **45**, 219.

67. La Thangue, N. B. and Rigby, P. W. J. (1987) An adenovirus E1A-like transcription factor is regulated during the differentiation of murine embryonal carcinoma stem cells. *Cell*, **49**, 507.

68. Bagchi, S., Raychaudhuri, P., and Nevins, J. R. (1990) Adenovirus E1A proteins an dissociate heteromeric complexes involving the E2F transcription factor: A novel mechanism for E1A *trans*-activation. *Cell*, **62**, 659.

69. Morris, J. D., Crook, T., Bandara, L. R., Davies, R., La Thangue, N. B., and Vousden, K. H. (1993) Human papillomavirus type 16 E7 regulates E2F and contributes to mitogenic signalling. *Oncogene*, **8**, 893.

70. Chellappan, S., Kraus, V. B., Kroger, Bu., Munger, K., Howley, P. M., Phelps, W. C., *et al.* (1992) Adenovirus E1A, simian virus 40 tumor antigen, and human papillomavirus E7 protein share the capacity to disrupt the interaction between transcription factor E2F and the retinoblastoma gene product. *Proc. Natl. Acad. Sci. USA*, **89**, 4549.

71. Means, A. L., Slansky, J. E., McMahon, S. L., Snuth, M. W., and Farnham, P. J. (1992) The HIP1 binding site is required for growth regulation of the dihydrofolate reductase gene promoter. *Mol. Cell. Biol.*, **12**, 1054.

72. Bandara, L. R., Adamczewski, J. P., Hunt, T., and La Thangue, N. B. (1991) Cyclin A and the retinoblastoma gene product complex with a common transcription factor. *Nature*, **352**, 249.

73. Cao, L., Faha, B., Dembski, M., Tsai, L.-H., Hawlow, E., and Fattaey, A. (1992) Independent binding of the retinoblastoma protein and p107 to the transcription factor E2F. *Nature*, **355**, 176.

74. Devoto, S. H., Mudryj, M., Pines, P., Hunter, T., and Nevins, J. R. 91992) A cyclin A-specific protein kinase complex possesses sequence-specific DNA binding activity: p33^{cdk2} is a component of the E2F-cyclin A complex. *Cell*, **68**, 167.

75. Zamanian, M. and La Thangue, N. B. (1992) Adenovirus E1A prevents the retinoblastoma gene product from repressing the activity of a cellular transcription factor. *EMBO J.*, **11**, 2603.

76. Hiebert, S. W., Chellappan, S. P., Horowitz, J. M., and Nevins, J. R. (1992) The interaction of Rb with E2F coincides with an inhibition of the transcriptional activity of E2F. *Genes Dev.*, **6**, 177.

77. Zamanian, M. and La Thangue, N. B. (1993) Transcriptional repression by the Rb-related protein p107. *Mol. Biol. Cell*, **4**, 389.

78. Schwarz, J. K., Devoto, S. H., Smith, E. J., Chellappan, S. P., Jakoi, L., and Nevins, J. R. (1993) Interactions of the p107 and Rb proteins with E2F during the cell proliferation response. *EMBO J.*, **12**, 1013.

79. Shirodkar, S. M., Ewen, J. A., DeCaprio, J. A., Morgan, J., Livingston, D. M., and Chittenden, T. (1992) The transcription factor E2F interacts with the retinoblastoma product and a p107-cyclin A complex in a cell cycle-regulated manner. *Cell*, **68**, 157.

80. La Thangue, N. B. (1994) DRTF1/E2F: an expanding family of heterodimeric transcription factors implicated in cell-cycle control. *Trends Biochem. Sci.*, **19**, 108.

81. Helin, K., Lees, J. A., Vidal, M., Dyson, N., Harlow, E., and Fattaey, A. (1992) A cDNA encoding a pRb-binding protein with properties of the transcription factor E2F. *Cell*, **70**, 337.

82. Kaelin, W. G., Krek, W., Sellers, W. R., DeCaprio, J. A., Ajchenbaum, F., Fuchs, C. S., *et al.* (1992) Expression cloning of a cDNA encoding a retinoblastoma-binding protein with E2F-like properties. *Cell*, **70**, 351.

83. Shan, B., Zhu, X., Chen, P.-L., Durfee, T., Yang, Y., Sharp, D., *et al.* (1992) Molecular cloning of cellular genes encoding retinoblastoma-associated proteins: identification of a gene with properties of the transcription factor E2F. *Mol. Cell. Biol.*, **12**, 5620.

84. Helin, K., Harlow, E., and Fattaey, A. R. (1993) Inhibition of E2F-1 trans-activation by direct binding of the retinoblastoma protein. *Mol. Cell. Biol.*, **13**, 6501.

85. Flemington, E. K., Speck, S. H., and Kaelin, W. G. (1993) E2F-1-mediated transactivation is inhibited by complex formation with the retinoblastoma susceptibility gene product. *Proc. Natl. Acad. Sci. USA*, **90**, 6914.

86. Lam, E. W.-F. and La Thangue, N. B. (1994) DP and E2F proteins: coordinating transcription with cell cycle progression. *Curr. Opin. Cell. Biol.*, **6**, 859.

87. Ivey-Hoyle, M., Conroy, R., Huber, H. E., Goodhart, P. J., Oliff, A., and Heimbrook, D. C. (1993) Cloning and characterization of E2F-2, a novel protein with the biochemical properties of transcription factor E2F. *Mol. Cell. Biol.*, **13**, 7802.

88. Lees, J. A., Saito, M., Vidal, M., Valentine, M., Look, T., Harlow, E., *et al.* (1993) The retinoblastoma protein binds to a family of E2F transcription factors. *Mol. Cell. Biol.*, **13**, 7813.

89. Beijersbergen, R. L., Kerkhoven, R. M., Zhu, L., Carlee, L., Voorhoeve, P. M., and Bernards, R. (1994) E2F-4, a new member of the E2F gene family, has oncogenic activity and associates with p107 *in vivo*. *Genes Dev.*, **8**, 2680.

90. Ginsberg, D., Vairo, G., Chittenden, T., Xiao, Z.-X., Xu, G., Wydner, K. K., *et al.* (1994) E2F-4, a new E2F transcription factor family member, interacts with p107 and has transforming potential. *Genes Dev.*, **8**, 2939.

91. Buck, V., Allen, K. E., Sørensen, T., Bybee, A., Hijmans, E. M., Voorhoeve, P. M., *et al.* (1995) Molecular and functional characterisation of E2F-5, a new member of the E2F family. *Oncogene* **11**, 31.

92. Hijmans, E. M., Voorhoeve, P. M., Beijersbergen, R. L., van't Veer, L. J., and Bernards, R. (1995) E2F-5, a new E2F family member that interacts with p130 *in vivo*. *Mol. Cell. Biol.*, **15**, 3082.

93. Sardet, C., Vidal, M., Cobrinik, D., Geng, Y., Onufryk, C., Chen, A., *et al.* (1995) E2F-4 and E2F-5, two members of the E2F family, are expressed in the early phases of the cell cycle. *Proc. Natl. Acad. Sci. USA*, **92**, 2403.

94. Vairo, G., Livingston, D. M., and Ginsberg, D. (1995) Functional interaction between E2F-4 and p130: evidence for distinct mechanisms underlying growth suppression by different retinoblastoma protein family members. *Genes Dev.*, **9**, 869.

95. Slansky, J. E., Li, Y., Kaelin, W. G., and Farnham, P. J. (1993) A protein synthesis-dependent increase in E2F1 mRNA correlates with growth regulation of the dihydrofolate reductase promoter. *Mol. Cell. Biol.*, **13**, 1610.

96. Johnson, D. G., Ohtani, K., and Nevins, J. R. (1994) Autoregulatory control of *E2F1* expression in response to positive and negative regulators of cell cycle progression. *Genes Dev.*, **8**, 1514.

97. Hsiao, K.-M., McMahon, S. L., and Farnham, P. J. (1994) Multiple DNA elements are required for the growth regulation of the mouse *E2F1* promoter. *Genes Dev.*, **8**, 1526.

98. Neuman, E., Flemington, E. K., Sellers, W. R., and Kaelin, W. G. (1994) Transcription of the E2F-1 gene is rendered cell cycle dependent by E2F DNA-binding sites within its promoter. *Mol. Cell. Biol.*, **14**, 6607.

99. Girling, R., Partridge, J. F., Bandara, L. R., Burden, N., Totty, N. F., Hsuan, J. J., *et al.* (1993) A new component of the transcription factor DRTF1/E2F. *Nature*, **362**, 83.

100. Bandara, L. R., Buck, V. M., Zamanian, M., Johnston, L. H., and La Thangue, N. B. (1993) Functional synergy between DP-1 and E2F-1 in the cell cycle-regulating transcription factor DRTF1/E2F. *EMBO J.*, **13**, 4317.

101. Bandara, L. R., Lam, E. W.-F., Sørensen, T. S., Zamanian, M., Girling, R., and La Thangue, N. B. (1994) DP-1: a cell cycle-regulated and phosphorylated component of transcription factor DRTF1/E2F which is functionally important for recognition by pRb and the adenovirus E4 orf 6/7 protein. *EMBO J.*, **13**, 3104.

102. Helin, K., Wu, C.-L., Fattaey, A. R., Lees, J. A., Dynlacht, B. D., Ngwu, C., *et al.* (1993) Heterodimerization of the transcription factors E2F-1 and DP-1 leads to cooperative *trans*-activation. *Genes Dev.*, **7**, 1850.

103. Krek, W., Livingston, D. M., and Shirodkar, S. (1993) Binding to DNA and the retinoblastoma gene product promoted by complex formation of different E2F family members. *Science*, **262**, 1557.

104. Krek, W., Ewen, M. E., Shirodkar, S., Arany, Z., Kaelin, W. G., and Livingston, D. M. (1994) Negative regulation of the growth-promoting transcription factor E2F-1 by a stably bound cyclin A-dependent protein kinase. *Cell*, **78**, 161.

105. Girling, R., Bandara, L. R., Ormondroyd, E., Lam, E. W.-F., Kotecha, S., Mohun, T., *et al.* (1994) Molecular characterization of *Xenopus laevis* DP proteins. *Mol. Biol. Cell*, **5**, 1081.

106. Ormondroyd, E., de la Luna, S., and La Thangue, N. B. (1995) A new member of the DP family, DP-3, with distinct protein products suggests a regulatory role for alternative splicing in the cell cycle transcription factor DRTF1/E2F. *Oncogene*, **11**, 1437.

107. Philpot, A. and Friend, S. H. (1994) E2F and its developmental regulation in *Xenopus laevis*. *Mol. Cell. Biol.*, **14**, 5000.

108. Ohtani, K. and Nevins, J. R. (1993) Functional properties of a *Drosophila* homolog of the E2F1 gene. *Mol. Cell. Biol.*, **14**, 1603.

109. Dynlacht, B. D., Brook, A., Dembski, M., Yenush, L., and Dyson, N. (1994) DNA-binding and trans-activation properties of *Drosophila* E2F and DP proteins. *Proc. Natl. Acad. Sci. USA*, **91**, 6359.

110. Hao, X. F., Alphey, L., Bandara, L. R., Lam. E. W.-F., Glover, D., and La Thangue, N. B. (1995) Functional conservation of the cell cycle-regulating transcription factor DRTF1/E2F and its pathway of control in *Deozophila melanogaster. J. Cell. Sci.*, **108**, 2945.

111. Duronio, R. J., O'Farrell, P. H., Xie, J.-E., Brook, A., and Dyson, N. (1995) The transcription factor E2F is required for S phase during *Drosophila* embryogenesis. *Genes Dev.*, **9**, 1445.

112. Duronio, R. J. and O'Farrell, P. H. (1995) Developmental control of the G_1 to S transition in *Drosophila:* cyclin E is a limiting downstream target of E2F. *Genes Dev.*, **9**, 1456.

113. Rai, L., Debbas, M., Sabbatini, P., Hockenbery, D., Korsmeyer, S., and White, E. (1992) The adenovirus E1A proteins induce apoptosis, which is inhibited by the E1B 19-kDa and bcl-2 proteins. *Proc. Natl. Acad. Sci. USA*, **89**, 7742.

114. Lowe, S. W. and Ruley, H. E. (1993) Stabilization of the p53 tumor suppressor is induced by adenovirus 5 E1A and accompanies apoptosis. *Genes Dev.*, **7**, 535.

115. Debbas, M. and White, E. (1993) Wild-type p53 mediates apoptosis by E1A, which is inhibited by E1B. *Genes Dev.*, **7**, 546.

116. Wu, X. and Levine, A. J. (1994) p53 and E2F-1 cooperate to mediate apoptosis. *Proc. Natl. Acad. Sci. USA*, **91**, 3602.

117. Qin X.-Q., Livingston, D. M., Kaelin, W. G., and Adams, P. D. (1994) Deregulated transcription factor E2F-1 expression leads to S-phase entry and p53-mediated apoptosis. *Proc. Natl. Acad. Sci. USA*, **91**, 10918.

118. Morgenbesser, S. D., Williams, B. O., Jacks, T., and DePinho, R. A. 91994) *p53*-dependent apoptosis produced by *Rb*-deficiency in the developing mouse lens. *Nature*, **371**, 72.

119. Pan, H. and Grigs, A. E. (1994) altered cell cycle regulation in the lens of HPV-16 E6 or E7 transgenic mice: implication for tumor suppressor gene function in development. *Genes Dev.* **8**, 1285.

120. Haupt, Y., Rowan, Sh., Shaulian, E., Vousden, K. H., and Oren, M. (1995) Induction of apoptosis in Hela cells by *trans*-activation-deficient p53. *Genes Dev.*, **9**, 2170.

121. Sabbatini, P., Lin, Jiayuh, Levine, A. J., and White, E. (1995) Essential role for p53-mediated transcription in E1A-induced apoptosis. *Genes Dev.*, **9**, 2184.

122. Oliner, J. D., Kinzler, K. W., Meltzer, P. S., George, D. L., and Vogelstein, B. (1992) Amplification of a gene encoding a p53 associated protein in human sarcomas. *Nature*, **358**, 80.

123. Oliner, J. D., Pietenpol, J. A., Thiagalingam, S., Gyuris, J., Kinzler, K. W., and Vohelstein, B. (1993) Oncoprotein MDM2 conceals the activation domain of tumour suppressor p53. *Nature*, **362**, 857.

124. Martin, K., Trouche, D., Hagemeier, C., Sørensen, T. S., La Thangue, N. B., and Kouzarides, T. (1995) Stimulation of E2F1/DP1 transcriptional activity by MDM2 oncoprotein. *Nature*, **375**, 691.

125. Xiao, Z.-X., Chen, J., Levine, A. J., Modjtahedi, N., Xing, J., Sellers, W. R., *et al.* (1995) Interaction between the retinoblastoma protein and the oncoprotein MDM2. *Nature*, **375**, 694.

126. Singh, P., Wong, S. H., and Hong, W. (1994) Overexpression of E2F-1 in rat embryo fibroblasts leads to neoplastic transformation. *EMBO J.*, **14**, 3329.

127. Johnson, D. G., Cress, W. D., Jakoi, L., and Nevins, J. R. (1994) Oncogenic capacity of the E2F1 gene. *Proc. Natl. Acad. Sci. USA*, **91**, 12823.

128. Jooss, K., Lam. E. W.-F., Bybee, A., Girling, R., Müller, R., and La Thangue, N. B. (1995) Proto-oncogenic properties of the DP family of proteins. *Oncogene*, **10**, 1529.

129. Lassar, A. B., Skapek, S. X., and Novitch, B. (1994) Regulatory mechanisms that coordinate skeletal muscle differentiation and cell cycle withdrawal. *Curr. Opin. Cell. Biol.*, **6**, 788.

130. Gu, W., Schneider, J. W., Condorelli, G., Kaushal, S., Mahdavi, V., and Nadal-Ginard, B. (1993) Interaction of myogenic factors and the retinoblastoma protein mediates muscle cell commitment and differentiation. *Cell*, **72**, 309.

131. Schneider, J. W., Gu, W., Zhu, L., Mahdavi, V., and Nadal-Ginard, B. (1994) Reversal of terminal differentiation mediated by p107 in Rb$^{-/-}$ muscle cells. *Science*, **264**, 1467/

132. Wang, J. Y. L. (1994) Nuclear protein tyrosine kinases. *Trends Biochem. Sci.*, **19**, 373.

133. Welch, P. J. and Wang, J. Y. J. (1993) A C-terminal protein-binding domain in the retinoblastoma protein regulates nuclear c-Ab1 tyrosine kinase in the cell cycle. *Cell*, **75**, 779.

134. Welch, P. J. and Wang, J. Y. J. (1995) Disruption of retinoblastoma protein function by coexpression of its C pocket fragment. *Genes Dev.*, **9**, 31.

135. Qin, X. Q., Chittenden, T., Livingston, D. M., and Kaelin, W. G. (1992) Identification of a growth suppression domain within the retinoblastoma gene product. *Genes Dev.*, **6**, 953.

136. Bremner, R., Cohen, B. L., Sopta, M., Hamel, P. A., Ingles, C. J., Gallie, B. L., et al., (1995) Direct transcriptional repression by pRb and its reversal by specific cyclins. *Mol. Cell. Biol.*, **15**, 3256.

137. Weintraub, S. J., Chow, K. N. B., Luo, R. X., Zhang, S. H., He, S., and Dean, D. C. (1995) Mechanism of active transcriptional repression by the retinoblastoma protein. *Nature*, **375**, 812.

138. Lam, E. W.-F. and Watson, R. J. (1993) An E2F-binding site mediates cell-cycle regulated repression of mouse B-*myb* gene. *EMBO J.*, **12**, 2705.

139. Kim, S.-J., Wagner, S., Liu, F., O'Reilly, M. A., Robbins, P. D., and Green, M. R. (1992) Retinoblastoma gene product activates expression of the human TGF-β2 gene through transcription factor ATF-2. *Nature*, **358**, 331.

140. Peterson, C. L. and Tamkin, J. W. (1995) The SWI-SNF complex: a chromatin remodeling machine? *Trends Biochem. Sci.*, **20**, 143.

141. Singh, P., Coe, J., and Hong, W. (1995) A role for retinoblastoma protein in potentiating transcriptional activation by the glucocorticoid receptor. *Nature*, **374**, 562.

142. Cavanaugh, A. H., Hempel, W. M., Taylor, L. J., Rogalsky, V., Todorov, G., and Rothblum, L. I. (1995) Activity of RNA polymerase I transcription factor UBF blocked by Rb gene product. *Nature*, **374**, 177.

143. Rustgi, A. K., Dyson, N., and Bernards, R. (1991) Amino-terminal domains of c-myc and N-myc proteins mediate binding to the retinoblastoma gene product. *Nature*, **352**, 541.

144. Wang, C.-Y., Petryniak, B., Thompson, C. B., Kaelin, W. G., and Leiden, J. M. (1993) Regulation of the ets-related transcription factor Elf-1 by binding to the retinoblastoma protein. *Science*, **260**, 1330.

145. Defeo-Jones, D., Huang, P. S., Jones, R. E., Haskell, K. M., Vuocolo, G. A., Hanobik, M. G., et al. (1991) Cloning of cDNAs for cellular proteins that bind to the retinoblastoma gene product. *Nature*, **352**, 251.

146. Hagemeier, C., Bannister, A. J., Cook, A., and Kouzarides, T. (1993) The activation domain of transcription factor PU.1 binds the retinoblastoma (RB) protein and the transcription factor TFIID *in vitro*: RB shows sequence similarity to TFIID and TFIIB. *Proc. Natl. Acad. Sci. USA*, **90**, 1580.

147. Qian, Y.-W., Wang, Y.-C. J., Hollingsworth, R. E. Jones, D., Ling, N., and Lee, E. Y-H. (1993) A retinoblastoma-binding protein related to a negative regulator of ras in yeast. *Nature*, **364**, 648.

148. Durfee, T., Becherer, K., Chen, P.-L., Yeh, S.-H., Yang, Y., Kilburn, A. E., *et al.* (1993) The retinoblastoma protein associates with the protein phophatase type 1 catalytic subunit. *Genes Dev.*, **7**, 555.

149. Iavarone, A., Garg, P., Lasorella, A., Hsu, J., and Israel, M. A. (1994) The helix-loop-helix protein Id-2 enhances cell proliferation and binds to the retinoblastoma protein. *Genes Dev.*, **8**, 1270.

150. Gu, W., Bhatia, K., Magrath, I. T., Dang, C. V., and Dalla-Favera, R. (1994) Binding and suppression of the myc transcription activation domain by p107. *Nature*, **264**, 251.

9 | The tumour suppressor gene p53

SUMAN B. GANGOPADHYAY, JACINTH ABRAHAM, YUN PING LIN, and SAM BENCHIMOL

1. Introduction

The p53 tumour suppressor gene is frequently a target for recessive mutations in a wide range of human and rodent malignancies. The loss of wild-type p53 expression in tumour cells appears to provide these cells with a selective growth advantage *in vivo*. The existence of mice that are devoid of p53 expression indicates that p53 is not required for normal cell growth or development. However, the increased incidence of tumours in p53 null mice as well as in mutant p53 transgenic mice compared with their normal littermates demonstrates the critical role of p53 in suppressing tumour growth. Two models have been proposed to explain the role of p53 as a tumour suppressor. In one model, p53 participates in the cellular response to DNA damage by delaying cell cycle progression at a G1 checkpoint (see Chapter 7). This delay may provide time for repair of damaged DNA that might otherwise interfere with accurate DNA replication, and for repair of lesions that might be perpetuated as mutations in cells entering S phase. In a second model, p53 protein has been shown to initiate apoptosis in response to agents that cause DNA strand breakage. Failure to eliminate cells that have undergone genetic alterations following DNA damage could lead to the appearance of transformed clones. Genetic and biochemical studies indicate that two properties of p53 protein, namely site-specific binding to double-stranded DNA and transcriptional activation of genes bearing p53-responsive elements, are closely associated with its ability to act as a tumour suppressor.

2. p53 gene structure and RNA

The human p53 gene encompasses 20 kb of DNA and is located on the short arm of chromosome 17 at position 17p13.1 (1). In mouse, the gene is smaller (14 kb) and resides on chromosome 11. A p53 homologue has been found in several other species including rat, hamster, monkey, chicken, frog, and fish but has not been reported to be present in non-vertebrates. In human, mouse, and frog, the p53 gene is organized similarly into 11 exons. The first exon in each of these species is non-coding. A processed p53 pseudogene is also found in the mouse genome (2).

The p53 mRNA is ubiquitously expressed. In different species, p53 mRNA ranges in size from 2–3 kb. The human p53 mRNA is 2.8–3.0 kb in size compared with 2.0 kb for the mouse p53 mRNA. This difference is mainly due to the much longer 3' untranslated region of the human p53 transcript which contains an Alu repetitive element (2). An alternatively spliced form of p53 RNA giving rise to proteins that differ at the carboxy terminus is expressed at low levels in human and mouse cells (3, 4).

3. Protein structure

Analysis of the amino acid sequence of p53 protein from human, monkey, mouse, rat, chicken, frog, and rainbow trout, reveals five clusters of highly conserved amino acids (domains I to V, Fig. 1) (5–11). A contiguous stretch of 18 amino acids within domain IV, and a 12 amino acid stretch in domain V are conserved in all of the above species (representing amino acids 237–254 and amino acids 270–282, respectively, in human p53).

p53 protein monomers self-associate to form homo-oligomers. The predominant form *in vivo* and in solution has been found to be the tetramer (12). Oligomerization is

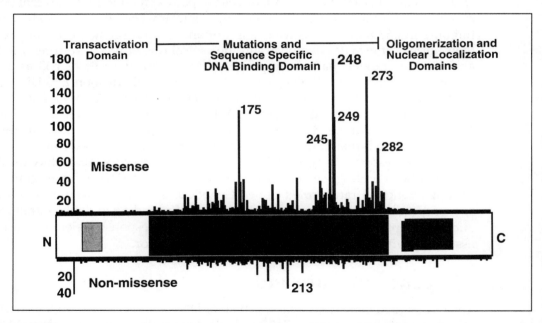

Fig. 1 Structural domains of p53. The structural regions of human p53 and distribution of mutations are shown. Functional domains include the transactivation region (amino acid 22–42, grey box), sequence-specific DNA binding region (amino acids 100–293, large black box), the nuclear localization domain (amino acids 316–325, small black box), and the oligomerization domains (amino aids 319–366, stippled box). Vertical lines represent distribution of mutations. Vertical lines above the schematic indicate missense mutations, while those below the schematic represent non-missense mutations. Seven mutational hot spot regions are indicated. This figure was generously provided by Dr C. C. Harris, and modified by Ms Dorothea Dudek, NCI, Bethesda, Maryland.

mediated by a region containing amino acids 319–366 at the carboxy terminus (13, 14). A nuclear localization sequence lies between amino acids 316–325 (15). The amino terminus of p53 contains highly charged acidic residues and is predicted to form α helical structures.

A fragment of human p53 protein corresponding to residues 94–312, which exists as a monomer in solution and binds DNA with sequence specificity, was recently crystallized in the presence of substrate DNA (16). The core domain structure consists of a sandwich of two antiparallel β sheets that acts as a scaffold for three structural elements. These structural elements include a loop–sheet–helix motif that binds to DNA within the major groove and makes contact with the bases, and two large loops that are held in part by a tetrahedrally coordinated zinc atom. One of these loops binds DNA through the minor groove. These three structural elements form the DNA binding surface of p53 and contain the majority of the p53 mutations occurring in tumours. This finding highlights the importance of DNA binding and sequence-specific transactivation for the biological activity of p53. It is interesting to note that the structural elements commonly found in other DNA binding proteins (e.g. zinc-fingers, helix–loop–helix motifs) are absent in p53.

The carboxy terminal structure of p53 has been resolved by multidimensional NMR spectroscopy (17, 18). It forms a highly symmetrical tetramer, which is composed of a dimer of dimers. Each monomeric unit contains a turn, a β strand, a second turn, and a relatively stable α helix. Each unit interacts with another unit such that the helices and β strands are antiparallel. Two such dimers interact, forming a four-helix bundle. The interactions between the helices are stabilized by several salt bridges.

Murine p53 is covalently linked to 5.8S rRNA through the phosphoserine residue at position 389 (19). The functional significance of this post-translational modification is not understood. 5.8S rRNA is a component of the ribosome where it pairs with 28S RNA in the 60S ribosomal subunit. It is also bound to the S9 and S13 proteins of the 40S ribosomal subunit suggesting that 5.8S rRNA is situated at the interface between the two subunits (20). 5.8S rRNA is believed to play an important role in ribosomal binding of tRNA (21). This finding suggests that p53 may play a role in regulating the expression, processing, or transport of 5.8S rRNA. Alternatively, p53 may be involved in translational control.

4. p53 phosphorylation

p53 protein is phosphorylated *in vivo* at multiple serine and threonine residues. The phosphorylation sites have been identified using several approaches including phosphopeptide mapping, direct sequencing of phosphopeptides, and site-directed mutagenesis. Serines 7, 9, 18, and 37 as well as two threonine residues at positions 76 and 86 are phosphorylated at the amino terminus of murine p53 (22–24); (the amino acids are numbered according to ref. 7). Peptide mapping studies have shown that serine residues 9, 15, 20, and 33 or 37 are phosphorylated at the amino terminus of monkey p53 and since the amino acid sequences of primates are highly homologous, it is likely that the same sites in human p53 are phosphorylated as in monkey (25).

Indeed, amino acids 9 and 15 of human p53 have been shown to be phosphorylated *in vivo* (26). Two serine residues at the carboxy terminus of p53 are phosphorylated, S312 and S389 in the mouse and at the corresponding amino acids S315 and S392 in primates (22, 25).

A number of kinases are implicated in p53 phosphorylation. *In vitro* studies demonstrate that the double-stranded DNA activated protein kinase (DNA-PK) can phosphorylate S15 and S37 in human and S7 and S18 in mouse p53 (23, 27). Casein kinase I (CKI) has been shown to phosphorylate mouse p53 at S7, S9, and S12 (28). The two threonine residues of mouse p53 (T76 and T86) are phosphorylated by yet another kinase—the mitogen-activated protein kinase (MAP kinase) (24). MAP kinase plays a central role in mediating the intracellular effects of a variety of mitogens and differentiating agents acting through protein tyrosine kinase receptors (see Chapter 5). Serine 315 in human p53 can be phosphorylated *in vitro* by cyclin-dependent kinases (29; see Chapter 7)). Immunodepletion of CDK1(cdc2) from cell lysates removes the kinase activity which phosphorylates S315, suggesting that CDK1 or a highly related kinase may phosphorylate this residue *in vivo*. Serine residues 389 in mouse and 392 in human p53 are targeted by casein kinase II (CKII), a serine/threonine protein kinase which targets many nuclear proteins involved in growth regulation or DNA metabolism (30, 31). Co-immunoprecipitation of p53 protein with CKII indicates that these two proteins can associate *in vivo*, and that CKII may phosphorylate p53 *in vivo*.

5. Mutations in the p53 gene

5.1 Somatic mutations

Mutations in the p53 gene are the most common genetic alterations in human cancers. Most frequently, missense mutation in one allele is accompanied by loss of the second allele, leading to a complete loss of wild-type p53 expression. This recessive mechanism for inactivation is consistent with the view of p53 as a tumour suppressor gene (32, 33). While missense mutations represent the most common type of alteration affecting the p53 gene in human cancer, nonsense mutations, deletions, gene rearrangements, and splicing mutations have also been reported albeit much less frequently (34–37).

Most point mutations are distributed between exons 5 and 9 of the p53 gene (Fig. 1). This region spans codons 126–307 and contains four of the five conserved domains of p53. Within this region, codons 175, 245, 248, 249, 273, and 282 are mutated very frequently. The frequency and distribution of p53 mutations differs from different tumour types (38).

There is now good evidence, at least in some cancers, that p53 mutations correlate with advanced pathological grade of the tumour (39). This relationship between p53 mutation and advanced tumour stage has been noted in colorectal, cervical, hepatocellular, and prostatic carcinomas, astrocytomas, melanoma, Non-Hodgkins lymphoma, multiple myeloma, and chronic myelogenous leukaemia, suggesting that for these tumours p53 mutation may be a late event contributing to tumour progression. However, alterations in the p53 gene have been detected as early events in dysplastic premalignant cell populations both in Barrett's oesophagus and in ulcerative colitis, as well as in low grade tumours of the lung, breast, head, and neck (38).

5.2 Germ-line mutations

While somatic p53 mutations are found in about 50% of human cancers, p53 mutations are also detected in the germ-line of some individuals affected with the Li–Fraumeni syndrome (LFS). LFS is a rare autosomal dominant syndrome characterized by the occurrence of diverse tumours in children and adults, including breast carcinoma, soft tissue sarcoma, brain tumour, osteosarcoma, leukaemia, and adreno-cortical carcinoma (see Chapter 10). These diverse tumours characteristically develop at an unusually early age, and multiple primary tumours are frequent (40). Affected individuals carry a constitutional heterozygous p53 mutation; when tumours develop, the wild-type p53 allele is lost (41–43).

Mice, in which both p53 alleles have been disrupted by insertional mutagenesis and homologous recombination have recently been produced (44). The viability of these mice indicates that p53 protein is not essential for normal developmental processes. The homozygous p53 null mice are developmentally normal but develop tumours spontaneously, predominantly lymphomas, and soft tissue sarcomas, by the age of three to five months. Heterozygotes develop a similar spectrum of tumours but with a longer latency period (45). The increased tumour susceptibility of p53 null mice as well as in mutant p53 transgenic mice (46) confirms the critical role of p53 as a tumour suppressor.

5.3 Dominant negative p53 mutations

Most of the p53 gene mutations found in rodent and human tumours occur in the core DNA binding domain of p53. All of these mutations disrupt the DNA binding/trans-activation activity of wild-type p53 and result in the loss of a p53 function that is required for tumour suppression. While all missense mutations found in tumours lead to the loss of the tumour suppressor function of p53, a proportion of these are dominant negative mutations (32). These dominant negative alleles encode functionally impaired p53 polypeptides that can inactivate wild-type p53 protein in *trans*. It should be noted, however, that co-expression of wild-type and mutant p53 alleles is infrequent in human tumours. In gene transfer experiments, certain missense mutant p53 alleles encode transforming p53 proteins that can co-operate with an activated *RAS* gene to transform primary rodent cells in cultures. The transforming p53 polypeptides are believed to act in a dominant negative fashion to inactivate endogenous wild-type p53 protein. The ability of the mutant protein to oligomerize with the endogenous wild-type protein has been shown to be necessary for its transforming activity.

6. Biochemical activities of p53

p53 has various biochemical activities through which it carries out its physiological functions. p53 protein exhibits double-stranded DNA binding activity that is both sequence-specific and sequence-independent (47–51). It binds to single-stranded DNA and RNA and has been shown to promote the reassociation of complementary nucleic acid molecules (52). The wild-type p53 protein is a transcription factor; it transactivates genes containing p53 responsive elements, and represses a number of genes that do not contain these elements (53–55). Whether all of these activities are required for the tumour suppressor function of p53 is not known.

6.1 Sequence-specific DNA binding

Wild-type p53 protein binds double-stranded DNA in a sequence-specific manner. The sequence-specific DNA binding domain of p53 protein has been localized to the central region of the molecule (56). Using DNase I footprinting assays, both human and murine wild-type, but not mutant, p53 proteins have been shown to bind sequences adjacent to the SV40 origin of replication (47). The region most strongly protected, while not precisely mapped, was that containing the first three of the six GC boxes (GGGCGG) on the late side of the SV40 replication origin. A human DNA sequence upstream of the transcriptional start site for the ribosomal gene cluster (RGC) was also shown to bind p53 (48). Three copies of the sequence TGCCT are found in this p53 recognition element and were shown to be necessary for binding.

El-Deiry *et al*. have identified a number of human genomic fragments that can bind to wild-type p53 protein *in vitro* by using a screening technique involving many rounds of mixing of genomic DNA fragments with p53 protein, precipitation with anti-p53 antibodies, amplification, and cloning of bound DNA (49). Analyses of binding sites within these fragments has allowed formulation of a consensus binding site with an internal symmetry. It consists of two copies of a 10 base pair (bp) motif 5′-PuPuPuC(A/T)(A/T)GPyPyPy-3′ separated by between 0 and 13 bp. One copy of the 10 bp motif is insufficient for binding, and alterations of the motif result in loss of affinity for p53. The symmetry of the four half sites within the consensus suggests that p53 interacts with DNA as a tetrameric protein which is consistent with the known structure of p53. In general, mutant p53 proteins fail to bind to this consensus sequence.

Funk *et al*., using several cycles of amplification and selection of binding targets from a large pool of random degenerate oligonucleotides mixed with nuclear extract from normal human fibroblasts as the source of p53 protein, identified a 20 bp oligonucleotide which binds to p53 (50). Their oligonucleotide sequence (GGACAT-GCCCGGGCATGTCC) perfectly matches the consensus sequence defined by El-Deiry *et al*. (49) with no intervening sequence between the two 10 bp motifs (Table 1). Interestingly the sequence identified by Funk *et al*. forms a perfect palindrome (50). When this sequence is placed upstream of a reporter gene, it confers p53-dependent activation in transient expression assays.

Several DNA sequences specifically recognized by p53 have now been identified (47–50, 57–66; see Table 1). While many of these sequences share similarity with the El-Deiry consensus sequence, others do not. For example, the p53 binding sites present in the SV40 origin of replication (47) and in the RGC sequence (48) do not fit the consensus sequence particularly well. We have carried out a search of sequences

Table 1 p53 responsive elements

Binding sequence[a]	Similarity to the p53 consensus binding site	Reference
p53 consensus binding site (the El-Deiry consensus) PuPuPuC(A/T)(T/A)GPyPyPyN{0,13}PuPuPuC(A/T)(T/A)GPyPyPy		49
SV40 origin region[b] GGGCGGAGAATGGGCGGAACTGGGCGG	–	47
Ribosomal gene cluster (RGC) CCTTGCCTGGACTTGCCTGGCCTTGCCTTTTC	19/20	48
MCK gene[c] TGGCAAGCCTATGACATGGCCGGGGCCTGCCTCTCTCTGCCTCTGACCCT	17/20	57
TGGCAAGCCTATGACATGGCCGGGGCCTGCCTCTCTCTGCCTCTGACCCT	17/20	
P53CON oligonucleotide GGACATGCCCGGGCATGTCC	20/20	50
GADD45 gene, intron 3 TGGTACAGAACATGTCTAAGCATGCTGGGGACTG	19/20	58
HTLV-I enhancer GCCCTGACGTGTCCCC	–	59
MDM2 intron1 GGTCAAGTTGGGACACGTCC	17/20	60
GAGCTAAGTCCTGACATGTCT	17/20	
GLN-LTR CCAGGACATGCCCGGGCAAGCCCATCG	20/20	61
Murine genomic DNA GACACTGGTCACACTTGGCTGCTTAGGAAT	–	62
p21/CDKN1 GAACATGTCCCAACATGTTG	18/20	63
Cyclin G AGGCCAGACCTGCCCGGGCAAGCCTTGGCA	19/20	64
BAX TCACAAGTTAGAGACAAGCCTGGGCGTGGGCTATATT	17/20	65
IGF-binding protein 3 (IGF-BP3) AAACAAGCCACCAACATGCTT	18/20	66
GGGCAAGACCTGCCAAGCCT	17/20	

[a] Underlined regions show similarity to the p53 consensus sequence and the nucleotides with asterisks represent mismatches to the consensus sequence.
[b] The region that was the most strongly protected was that containing the first three of the six GC boxes on the late side of the SV40 replication origin.
[c] This region of MCK gene contains two p53 consensus binding sites.

in Genbank which match the El-Deiry consensus perfectly, and have identified many such sequences. Nine of these sequences were examined for binding with p53 from cellular extracts, and none demonstrated any binding in electrophoretic mobility gel shift assays (Blondal and Benchimol, unpublished observations). Binding of p53 to the consensus oligonucleotide defined by Funk *et al.* was routinely observed in these experiments. These findings indicate that the parameters which govern DNA binding are not fully understood and that it will be necessary to redefine the consensus sequence more accurately.

In bacterially expressed p53 protein, the sequence-specific DNA binding activity is repressed and requires activation by cellular factors acting on the carboxy terminus of p53. Using gel mobility shift assays, Hupp *et al.* (31) have shown that recombinant wild-type human p53 has weak sequence-specific DNA binding activity which can be activated in at least four different ways:

(a) phosphorylation of S392 by CKII

(b) proteolytic removal of carboxy terminal amino acids

(c) binding to monoclonal antibody PAb421 which recognizes an epitope at the carboxy terminus of p53

(d) binding to the bacterial dnaK protein.

The carboxy terminal region of p53 likely contains a negative regulatory domain that controls the sequence-specific DNA binding property of p53.

6.2 Transcription activation

When the acidic amino terminal domain of p53 (amino acids 22–42) is fused to the DNA binding region of the yeast protein GAL4, the resulting hybrid protein activates transcription from a GAL4 operon in both yeast and mammalian cells (53, 54). This acidic region together with the central core region of wild-type p53 confer upon p53 the ability to transactivate genes that contain a p53 binding site. Co-transfection of a p53 expression vector with a plasmid containing a p53 binding site upstream of a reporter gene results in a high level of reporter gene expression in mammalian cells. Only wild-type p53 protein functions as a transcriptional activator in this type of assay (67). In contrast, a large number of cellular and viral promoters that lack a p53 binding sequence, such as the *MDR1* promoter, are repressed by wild-type p53 protein (55). It is likely that p53 functions as a tumour suppressor through its ability to be a site-specific transactivator, as well as a repressor, of transcription.

p53 forms complexes with proteins encoded by a number of DNA tumour viruses (see Chapter 1) including the SV40 large T antigen (LT), the E1B 55K protein encoded by adenovirus (Ad) type 5, and the E6 protein encoded by human papillomaviruses (HPV) (68–71; and Table 2). Binding to SV40 LT and to Ad EIB leads to p53 protein stabilization (70, 72), whereas the interaction between E6 and p53 leads to enhanced degradation of p53 by a ubiquitin-dependent pathway (73). SV40 LT binds to a region within the DNA binding domain of p53, while Ad E1B binds to the amino terminus of

Table 2 p53 associated proteins[a]

Viral proteins	Ref.	Transcription factors	Ref.	Other proteins	Ref.
SV40 large T antigen	68, 69	CCAAT box binding factor	79	MDM2	88, 89
Adenovirus type 5 E1b 55 kDa	70	Sp1	80, 81	Heat shock 70 kDa protein (hsc70)	92
Human papilloma virus E6	71	TATA binding protein	82–86	p34cdc-2 protein kinase	29
Lymphotropic papova virus large tumour antigen	75	WT1	87	Protein kinase C	93
Epstein–Barr virus nuclear antigen-5	76	p53	12	Replication protein A (RPA)	94–96
Hepatitis B virus X protein	77	TAF$_{II}$ 40 and TAF$_{II}$ 60	90	S100b	93
Human cytomegalovirus IE84 protein	78	ERCC2, ERCC3 and ERCC6	91	E. coli dnaK	97
				53 BP1 and 53 BP2	98
				Casein kinase II	30, 31
				E6-AP	99

[a] Not all of the p53 associated proteins may bind directly to p53.

p53 (47, 74). Both interactions have been shown to inhibit the transactivation function of p53. The association of HPV E6 with p53 results in a reduction in the level of functional p53 (73).

A number of genes have now been identified, whose expression appears to be positively regulated by wild-type p53 protein (Table 2 and refs 12, 29–31, 68–71, 75–99). A few of these genes are briefly described below.

6.2.1 MDM2

The first intron of the *MDM2* gene contains two p53 response elements which, when placed adjacent to a minimal promoter, can stimulate a reporter gene in a p53-dependent fashion (60). The DNA binding site contains two imperfect repeats of the El-Deiry binding consensus sequence. In transformed rat embryo fibroblasts expressing an activated *RAS* gene and a temperature sensitive (ts) mutant p53 allele (containing an A135V substitution), endogenous *MDM2* gene expression is upregulated when the temperature is shifted from 37 °C (mutant conformation) to 32 °C (wild-type conformation) (100). The *MDM2* gene is also induced in response to DNA damaging agents in a p53-dependent manner (101).

The MDM2 protein complexes with the p53 protein and this association inhibits p53-mediated transactivation (88, 89). In transient co-expression assays, MDM2 can inhibit p53-dependent transactivation of a reporter gene bearing a p53 responsive element (60). Thus, p53 activity can be regulated by MDM2. MDM2 protein binds to the amino terminus of p53 in the region of amino acids 13–41. This suggests that MDM2 may conceal the activation domain of p53 from the transcriptional machinery leading to a disruption of p53 transcriptional activity. An autoregulatory feedback loop is therefore established where the p53 protein regulates transcription of the *MDM2* gene, and the MDM2 protein regulates the activity of the p53 protein. This model implies that disruption of the loop could result in deregulation of *MDM2* gene expression and changes in cell proliferation. Indeed, the *MDM2* gene has been shown to act as an oncogene in gene transfer experiments and is amplified in certain tumours (89, 102). The model has been further strengthened by the recent generation of *MDM2* null mice (103). The loss of *MDM2* results in early embryonic lethality. However, this phenotype is rescued by deletion of p53. Mice homozygous for both the p53 and *MDM2* null alleles are viable, providing genetic evidence for an interaction of MDM2 and p53 *in vivo*.

6.2.2 GADD45

Transcription of the *GADD45* (growth arrest and DNA damage-inducible) gene is induced when cells are treated with DNA damaging agents or other treatments eliciting growth arrest. Kastan *et al*. demonstrated that the induction of *GADD45* in response to ionizing radiation is dependent on wild-type p53 expression (58). Cells lacking p53 or expressing mutant p53 protein do not show radiation-dependent induction of *GADD45*. The *GADD45* gene contains a p53 binding site within its third intron. This element matches the consensus sequence in 19 of 20 bp (Table 1) and, when placed upstream of a reporter gene construct, can promote p53-dependent expression. The discovery of *GADD45* as a p53 target gene provided a link between the transcriptional activation function of p53 and its ability to promote cell growth arrest in response to DNA damaging agents (see below).

6.2.3 p21^CIP1/WAF1 and SDI1

This gene, also designated *CDKN1*, encodes a cyclin-dependent kinase (CDK) inhibitor that was discovered in three very different systems. *SDI1* (senescent cell-derived inhibitor) was isolated by expression screening of cDNAs prepared from senescent, non-dividing human cells and identified on the basis of its DNA synthesis inhibitory activity (104). The product of the *CIP1* gene was identified in a two-hybrid genetic screen as a *c*dk-*i*nteracting *p*rotein (105). *CIP1* encodes a protein of 21 kDa (p21) that acts as a potent inhibitor of several CDKs, including cyclin D-CDK4, cyclin E–CDK2, and cyclin A–CDK2 (see Chapter 7). Cyclin D–CDK4 and cyclin E–CDK2 complexes are strongly implicated in regulation of a G1 checkpoint and in the phosphorylation of the pRB protein (see Chapter 8); cyclin A–CDK2 is required for ongoing DNA replication. *WAF1* (wild-type p53 activated fragment) was identified as a p53-inducible gene through subtraction hybridization cloning (63). This gene, hereafter referred to as *p21*^CIP1/WAF1, contains a p53 responsive element located 2.4 kb upstream of the coding region. This site differs from the consensus DNA binding site at two of 20 positions (Table 1). The *p21*^CIP1/WAF1 promoter region containing the p53 binding site was shown to stimulate expression of a promoterless luciferase reporter gene in the presence of wild-type p53 protein.

6.2.4 Cyclin G

Through a PCR-based differential display method, cyclin G mRNA was found to be overexpressed in a mouse leukaemic cell line expressing the ts p53 protein at 32 °C and in mouse embryonic fibroblasts after γ-irradiation (64). A p53 binding site, matching the consensus sequence at 19 of 20 bp (Table 1) was identified 1.5 kb upstream of the coding region of cyclin G. The role of cyclin G in regulating cell proliferation and the significance of cyclin G transactivation by p53 are not understood.

6.2.5 BAX

The human *BAX* gene was shown to be a direct target of p53 (65). Co-transfection of a wild-type p53 expression plasmid with a *CAT* reporter gene containing *BAX* promoter elements resulted in transactivation of the *CAT* gene in a p53-dependent fashion. The p53 responsive element(s) lies within a 39 bp region in the *BAX* promoter and it exhibits binding to wild-type p53 protein in an electrophoretic mobility shift assay. Mutations in this region abolish the p53 responsiveness of reporter plasmids. The responsive element differs from the consensus binding sequence at three of 20 positions (Table 1).

6.2.6 MCK

Co-transfection of the mouse wild-type p53 gene with a *CAT* reporter gene containing upstream regulatory sequences from the muscle-specific creatine kinase (*MCK*) gene resulted in p53-dependent transactivation of the *CAT* gene (106). A p53 responsive element resembling the RGC element and containing two copies of the TGCCT sequence was mapped to a region 2.8 kb upstream of the transcriptional start site (57).

6.2.7 IGF-BP3

Using a subtractive cDNA cloning approach, Buckbinder *et al.* identified the gene coding for insulin-like growth factor binding protein 3 (IGF-BP3) as being p53 regulated (66). IGF-BP3 has a high affinity for insulin-like growth factors (IGFs), interferes with IGF signalling, and is believed to be an autocrine/paracrine growth regulator (see Chapter 8). Two p53 binding sites, differing by two or three nucleotides from the p53 consensus binding sequence, reside in the first and second introns respectively (Table 1). IGF-BP3 has been implicated in p53-mediated cellular growth control.

6.2.8 GLN/RAL

Zauberman *et al.* used an immune selection procedure to identify an endogenous retrovirus-like element (GLN) in mouse genomic DNA that could bind to p53 protein (61). A p53 binding site resides within the LTR of this retrovirus-like element which shares perfect homology with the p53 consensus binding sequence (Table 1). We have used a PCR-based differential display strategy to identify a p53-regulated transcript in rat cells encoded by a member of the RAL family (107) of endogenous retroviral-like sequences (Gangopadhyay and Benchimol, in press). Since very little is known about the transcripts and proteins encoded by GLN and the RAL elements, it is not possible to assess the biological significance of these findings.

6.3 Transcription repression

In addition to the ability of wild-type p53 to act as a positive regulator of certain genes bearing p53 binding sites, it can also repress transcription from a large number of promoters that lack p53 binding sites. Transient expression studies utilizing reporter gene constructs have shown that several promoters are transcriptionally repressed by wild-type but not mutant p53 proteins (108). Some of these promoters regulate the expression of genes whose activity is associated with cell proliferation, transformation, or malignant progression including, *JUN, FOS, PCNA* (proliferating cell nuclear antigen) *MYC, BCL2*, cyclin A, and *MDR1* (multidrug resistance gene 1) (55, 108–112). Repression has also been observed in cells expressing a p53ts allele (110, 111, 113) and in cells where wild-type p53 expression is regulated by an inducible promoter (114). Interestingly, p53 missense mutants have been shown to activate a number of promoters including those present in the *PCNA* and *MDR1* genes (55, 109, 115).

It is pertinent to consider the physiological relevance of assays in which constitutively overexpressed p53 protein acts on plasmid-borne extrachromosomal copies of a promoter–reporter gene. It has been demonstrated, for example, that certain promoters that are inhibited by p53 protein in transient transfection assays are not inhibited in their native state implying that regulation of genes by p53 is subject to the natural chromatin state of the endogenous gene. Indeed, no correlation between p53 gene status and *MDR1* expression has been observed in breast, endometrial, and cervical tumours, nor in B cell chronic lymphocytic leukaemia (116, 117).

p53 responsive elements required for transcriptional repression by p53 protein have been identified in the promoters of the *RB* and *BCL2* genes (118, 119). However, binding of p53 to these elements has not been demonstrated and the mechanism by which these promoter elements confer p53 responsiveness is not understood. It should be noted that promoters which are normally repressed by p53, can be activated after insertion of a p53 responsive element (120, 121).

6.4 Mechanism of p53-mediated transcriptional regulation

p53 has been shown to bind to three subunits of the multisubunit basal transcription initiated factor TFIID. these subunits include the TATA box binding protein (TBP) and two TBP-associated factors, $TAF_{II}40$ and $TAF_{II}60$ (82–86, 90). TFIID is required to initiate transcription from promoters that contain a TATA box motif as well from promoters that utilize pyrimidine-rich initiator elements but no upstream TATA box. Transcriptional activator proteins are sequence-specific DNA binding proteins; some of these have been shown to interact with general transcription factors (TFIID or TFIIB) to initiate transcription. As suggested by Greenblatt (122), interaction of certain site-specific transcriptional activator proteins with TFIID or with TBP or with TAFs could explain the involvement of TFIID in transcriptional activation.

Two different regions of p53 protein bind independently to amino acids 220–271 of TBP. One of these regions lies at the amino terminal end of p53 and includes amino acids 20–57; the other region involves amino acids 318–393 at the carboxy terminal end (86). The first 42 amino acids of the transactivation domain of p53 at the amino terminus are also sufficient for binding to $TAF_{II}40$ and $TAF_{II}60$ (90). Both TBP and TFIID have been shown to stimulate binding of p53 protein to its responsive element (RGC DNA fragment) lacking a TATA box (86). This stimulatory activity of TBP and TFIID may be important for p53-mediated transcriptional activation and may accelerate the formation of productive promoter–transcription initiation complexes. Evidence obtained using a reconstituted *in vitro* transcription system indicated that activation of transcription by p53 is mediated at least in part by $TAF_{II}40$ and $TAF_{II}60$ (90).

Interestingly, the ability of p53 to bind TBP and TFIID has also been used to explain the transcriptional repressor activity of p53. It has been suggested that p53-mediated repression could involve interference with or disruption of TBP or TFIID binding to the TATA region (110). Both the amino terminal and carboxy terminal domains of p53 appear to be needed for its repressor activity (123). Using a 110 bp DNA fragment containing a *FOS* TATA element, Chen *et al.* showed that p53 inhibited the binding of TBP to this element but did not inhibit the binding of partially purified (TBP-containing) TFIID to the same DNA fragment (86). Thus, transcriptional repression by p53 may require additional functions other than inhibiting TBP binding.

Mack *et al.* (124) have suggested that promoter sequences that use a TATA box element to direct transcription are specifically repressed by wild-type p53 whereas promoters containing initiator elements are not affected by p53. The ability of p53 to inhibit the *MDR1* promoter which lacks a TATA box challenges this generalization (112). Specificity may be determined, however, by the specific TAFs that are involved in the formation of the initiation complexes and by the involvement of other transcription factors binding to adjacent sites on the promoter. In this regard, it is important to note that p53 protein binds a number of other transcription factors including SP1, CBF, and ERCC3, a component of TFIIH (77, 79–81). TFIIH is a complex of proteins that binds to the transcriptional initiation complex. Interaction of p53 with these factors could be involved in p53-mediated transcriptional activation/repression.

One could imagine another model for repression in which p53, acting through CIP1, inhibits the phosphorylation of pRB and the subsequent release and activation of the transcription factor E2F (Chapter 8). E2F regulates the expression of various genes required for entry into S phase (125). Hence, overexpression of p53 could reduce the amount of free E2F in a cell and lead to the transcriptional repression of E2F-dependent genes.

6.5 Non-sequence-specific RNA/DNA binding

In addition to its sequence-specific DNA binding activity, p53 can also bind non-specifically to double-stranded DNA, single-stranded DNA, and RNA.

Recombinant wild-type murine p53 as well as immunopurified mutant p53 was shown to associate with MAR (nuclear matrix attachment region DNA) elements from various sources (51). MARs play an important role in anchoring cellular DNA loops to the nuclear matrix, and are believed to coordinate DNA replication and gene expression during the cell cycle (126). Replication and transcription are believed to initiate at the base of these loops. Loops replicating early during S phase contain genes that are expressed in a cell and tissue-specific manner, while loops replicating late during S phase contain predominantly housekeeping or non-transcribed genes. By binding to MAR elements, p53 protein may contribute to the regulation and timing of replication and transcription.

The domain of p53 protein required for binding to single-stranded nucleic acids resides in the carboxy terminus of the molecule between amino acids 311–393 (52). This domain of p53 also promotes the association of complementary single-stranded nucleic acids (127, 128). The strand reassociation activity of p53 accounts for its ability to inhibit the helicase activity of SV40 large T antigen *in vivo* and *in vitro*. It has been speculated that this activity of p53 protein might also be involved in DNA repair and replication.

7. Biological functions of p53

The role of p53 as a negative growth regulator was first demonstrated by gene transfer experiments in which a functional wild-type p53 gene was reintroduced into transformed cells which had lost endogenous p53 gene expression by recessive mutation. The most common outcome of these studies was growth arrest of the recipient cells in the G0/G1 phase of the cell cycle (109, 129–133). In other studies, wild-type p53 protein expression resulted in apoptosis (134–137) which was preceded by a transient delay in G1 in some, but not all cell types. A third outcome of p53 expression in p53-negative tumour cells was the induction of differentiation (137, 138). It is pertinent to note that terminal differentiation is associated with loss of proliferative capacity and that it is often accompanied by growth arrest in G1. Moreover, in many cell types terminal differentiation culminates in apoptosis. Hence, the three seemingly disparate activities that have been associated with wild-type p53 protein in reconstituted cells (i.e. G1 growth arrest, differentiation, and apoptosis) may be linked and may be dependent on the lineage and maturation potential of the recipient cells.

7.1 p53-dependent G1 checkpoint arrest

Cells exposed to various DNA damaging agents invariably respond by delaying cell cycle progression. For example, after exposure to ionizing radiation, the transient delays observed in both G1 and in G2 are believed to provide time for repair of damage before the cell re-initiates replicative DNA synthesis and/or begins mitosis. Failure to repair DNA damage prior to DNA replication or mitosis could result in propagation of mutagenic lesions, and contribute to the progressive accumulation of genetic changes involved in neoplastic transformation. Numerous studies indicate that p53 protein plays a key role in regulating a G1 checkpoint in response to DNA damage in mammalian cells.

Early studies by Maltzman and Czyzyk in 1984 demonstrated that treatment of mouse cells with either ultraviolet (UV) light or with a UV-mimetic carcinogen induced accumulation of p53 protein through a post-translational mechanism (139). A wide variety of DNA damaging agents have now been shown to induce p53 protein expression in cells. Kastan *et al.* (140) showed that in normal human haematopoietic progenitor cells or in wild-type p53 expressing ML-1 cells (myeloblastic leukaemia cells), γ-irradiation resulted in an increase in the level of p53 protein and a transient inhibition of replicative DNA synthesis. Haematopoetic cells possessing wild-type p53 exhibited irradiation induced G1 and G2 arrest, whereas, cells with no p53 genes or those overexpressing mutant p53 genes exhibited only the G2 arrest. Insertion of wild-type p53 genes into HL60 cells (myeloid leukaemic cells lacking functional p53) led to partial restoration of γ-irradiation induced G1 arrest, whereas overexpression of mutant p53 in RKO cells (colorectal carcinoma cells expressing wild-type p53) abrogated the G1 arrest (141). These studies provided compelling evidence for a role of p53 in mediating a G1 checkpoint in response to γ-irradiation.

The involvement of p53 in regulating a G1 checkpoint was also demonstrated in studies of cells exposed to metabolic inhibitors (142, 143). Normal fibroblasts expressing wild-type p53 arrested in G1 when exposed to the uridine biosynthesis inhibitor PALA (*N*-phosphonacetyl-L-aspartate) and failed to demonstrate PALA-selected *CAD* (trifunctional enzyme carbamoyl-P synthetase, aspartate transcarbamylase, dihydroorotase) gene amplification. Amplification of the *CAD* gene represents the sole recognized mechanism by which PALA-resistant clones arise. The increase in gene copy number that arises through gene amplification represents one type of genomic instability. Consequently, the frequency with which PALA-resistant cells arise provides an accurate measurement of *CAD* gene amplification and provides a reflection of genomic integrity. Cells lacking wild-type p53 expression or expressing mutant p53 protein failed to arrest when placed in drug and inappropriately entered S phase. These cells displayed *CAD* gene amplification at high frequency. Hence, increased genetic instability appears to be one consequence of loss of p53-mediated G1 checkpoint function.

The observation that wild-type p53 protein has site-specific double-stranded DNA biding activity and that it possesses transcription regulatory activities suggested that the p53-mediated G1 checkpoint might involve downstream effector genes (49, 50, 144, 145; see Fig. 2). The p53-regulated *GADD45* gene contains a well conserved p53 binding motif in its third intron (58) and induction of *GADD45* by ionizing radiation is strictly dependent on normal p53 function. In gene transfer experiments, *GADD45* gene expression resulted in growth inhibition as measured by [^{3}H] thymidine incorporation (146). A second gene whose expression is regulated by p53 is *p21*[CIP1/WAF1] (63). As discussed earlier, the product of this gene, p21, inhibits the activity of cyclin-dependent kinases necessary for the G1–S transition (104, 105, 147, and Chapter 7), and is considered to be a critical downstream effector in the p53-specific pathway of growth control (63, 148, 149).

The p53-mediated G1 checkpoint can be disrupted in a number of different ways including mutation of the p53 gene, by expression of certain cellular or viral proteins that interact with p53 protein and interfere with its transactivation function, as well as by other mechanisms that affect upstream or downstream components of the p53 growth control pathway. For example, overexpression of MDM2 protein in RKO cells results in p53–MDM2 interaction and loss of p53-mediated transactivation and G1 checkpoint function in response to irradiation (101). Cells from individuals with ataxia-telangiectasia (AT) show an abnormal response to irradiation; higher doses of irradiation are required for p53 induction in these cells compared with normal cells (150). It has been suggested that the ATM gene product is required for the induction of p53 protein. Expression of exogenously transfected HPV E6 and E7 sequences abrogates the p53-dependent G1 checkpoint in a number of human cells treated with PALA, γ-irradiation, and actinomycin D (149, 151–153) although this is less evident in HPV-positive cervical tumour cells in which E6 and E7 expression is driven from the homologous viral promoter (154). In these models it has been suggested that E6 promotes the degradation of p53 while E7 protein binds and inactivates pRB. Interestingly, we have found that rat embryo fibroblast clones expressing wild-type p53, HPV16 E6, and activated *RAS* maintain the p53-dependent G1 checkpoint in response to γ-irradiation (155). We are not certain why E7 can disrupt the p53-mediated G1 checkpoint in human cells but not in rat cells.

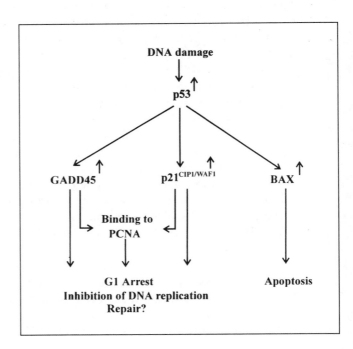

Fig. 2 p53-dependent responses following DNA damage.

7.2 p53-dependent apoptosis

Gene transfer experiments showed that ectopic wild-type p53 expression in p53-negative recipient cell lines was not compatible with continued cell growth (131, 156, 157). Conditional expression of p53, using a ts p53 allele or inducible promoters, demonstrated that p53 promoted cell death through an apoptosis pathway (134–137, 158–161).

Subsequent experiments showed that endogenous wild-type p53 protein also has this activity. Normal murine thymocytes exposed to ionizing radiation in culture undergo apoptosis whereas thymocytes obtained from p53 null mice remain viable after irradiation on the basis of short-term membrane permeability assays. In contrast, dexamethasone induction of apoptosis was observed in thymocytes obtained from both normal and p53 null mice indicating a lack of involvement by p53 (162, 163). This indicates that at least two mechanisms can lead to apoptosis in thymocytes. In addition, expression of oncogenes such as *MYC*, *E1A*, and *H-RAS* can result in apoptosis, particularly in cells that have been deprived of serum, and this form of apoptosis has also been shown to be p53-dependent (164, 165). It is possible that failure to eliminate cells that have sustained irreparable DNA damage and failure to eliminate cells undergoing inappropriate cell growth may contribute to tumorigenesis. Recent *in vivo* studies on p53-deficient mice confirmed that loss of p53 leads to increased susceptibility to chemically-induced and radiation-induced tumorigenesis (45). Since ionizing radiation and many chemotherapeutic agents induce DNA damage, the status of p53 in tumour cells is likely to play an important role in determining sensitivity to cytotoxic anti-cancer agents. Recent experiments using clonogenic assays to measure cell survival following ionizing radiation indicate that loss of wild-type p53 expression is associated with increased radioresistance (166, 167). Whether loss of the p53-mediated apoptosis pathway provides the sole explanation for increased radioresistance of cells expressing mutant p53 remains to be proven.

The molecular mechanism through which p53-mediated apoptosis occurs is starting to be unravelled. The product of the *BCL2* gene is known to play a role in promoting cell survival and inhibiting apoptosis induced by numerous stimuli (168, 169). *BCL2* has been shown to block p53-dependent apoptosis (170, 171). The *BAX* gene encodes a dominant inhibitor of the BCL2 protein. BAX can homodimerize and can also form heterodimers with BCL2. It has been suggested that the ratio of BCL2 to BAX protein determines survival or death following an apoptotic stimulus (172). Recently, an intriguing association was reported for p53, BAX, and BCL2 (111, 173). Cells expressing high levels of wild-type p53 had increased levels of BAX and decreased levels of BCL2 suggesting that the *BAX* and *BCL2* genes are transcriptionally regulated by p53.

There is no satisfactory explanation for the observation that certain cells (such as fibroblasts) respond to DNA damage by arresting in G1 (174) while other cells (such as thymocytes) respond by undergoing apoptosis. It is not known if the ability of p53 to mediate G1 arrest or to promote apoptosis represents two separate functions of p53 or one single function. The connection between these two p53-related responses is uncertain. One possibility is that the response depends on the cell type and/or physiological state of the cells. Another possibility is that apoptosis occurs only after repair fails, although it has not yet been demonstrated that DNA repair occurs during the p53-mediated delay in G1. A third possibility is that prolonged residency in G1 leads to apoptosis. Yet a fourth possibility, is that p53-dependent apoptosis occurs when cells inappropriately exit from G1 under conditions that normally suppress growth.

Recent reports indicate that p53-induced apoptosis is distinct from p53-induced G1 arrest. We have shown that apoptosis and G1 arrest can be uncoupled by addition of a cytokine in culture medium in murine erythroleukaemia cells transfected with a temperature sensitive p53 allele (175). At the permissive temperature, in response to p53, these cells undergo G1 arrest, apoptosis, and differentiation. However, addition of a cytokine (erythropoietin, KIT-ligand, or interleukin-3; see Chapter 2) to the culture medium blocks p53-mediated apoptosis and differentiation but not the p53-mediated G1 arrest.

It is not clear whether apoptosis mediated by p53 is dependent on its transactivation function. Reports indicate that p53-dependent apoptosis occurs in the presence of the transcription inhibitor actinomycin D and the protein synthesis inhibitor cycloheximide (176, 177). Shen *et al.* have also shown that BCL2 and E1B 19 kDa protein, both of which can suppress p53-induced apoptosis, do not interfere with the transcriptional activation function of p53 (178). These proteins, however, do inhibit p53-mediated repression of promoters that lack a p53 consensus site. This study raises the possibility that p53 promotes apoptosis by repressing transcription of specific genes; *BCL2* may represent a critical target in this process.

7.3 p53 and differentiation

Any discussion concerning a putative role for p53 in cellular differentiation must be prefaced with the statement that p53 is clearly not required during embryogenesis. This was convincingly demonstrated by the generation of p53 null mice that are completely devoid of p53 gene expression (44). The possibility that alternative pathways compensate for the lack of p53 protein in these mice has neither been confirmed nor rejected.

Overexpression of wild-type p53 protein in the p53-negative and Abelson virus-transformed pre-B cell line L12, resulted in increased cell surface expression of the B220 antigen and expression of cytoplasmic immunoglobulin μ heavy chain, two markers for B cell differentiation (138). In pre-B cells expressing endogenous wild-type p53, treatment with agents that induce differentiation resulted in kappa immunoglobulin expression that was preceded by increased expression of native p53 (179). Wild-type p53 protein has been shown to transactivate the promoter element of the kappa light chain gene. Pre-B cells induced to undergo differentiation following expression of p53 were shown to have decreased tumorigenic potential.

Friend virus-transformed erythroleukaemia cells expressing a p53ts allele were also shown to express globin RNA and protein, a marker for erythroid differentiation, when the cells were incubated at 32 °C (the temperature at which the p53ts protein behaves as wild-type) but not at 37 °C (137).

In transgenic mice carrying a p53 promoter fused to a reporter gene, expression of the reporter gene is highest in the testes and is confined to the primary spermatocytes. On the basis of this finding, Rotter and her colleagues have suggested that p53 may play a role in the meiotic process of spermatogenesis (180).

7.4 p53 in DNA replication and repair

p53 protein inhibits the initiation of SV40 origin-dependent DNA replication *in vitro* and *in vivo*. The interaction between p53 protein and the SV40 LT is critical for this activity of p53. p53 protein, through its ability to bind to single-stranded DNA and promote strand reassociation, interferes with the helicase activity of LT, which is required to unwind the SV40 origin of replication. The last 27 amino acids of p53 are important for this activity. In addition, p53 was shown to compete with DNA polymerase α, an essential component of the DNA replication machinery, for binding to SV40 LT (181–184). In this way, p53 interferes with the ability of LT to recruit DNA polymerase α to the replication origin.

p53 protein binds to replication protein A (RPA), the single-stranded DNA binding protein complex that is required for DNA unwinding during replication. Binding of p53 to RPA inhibits the ability of RPA to bind single-stranded DNA. The extent to which this interaction contributes to the ability of p53 to inhibit the onset of DNA replication in S phase is difficult to assess since both mutant and wild-type p53 proteins can bind RPA (94–96).

The product of the p53 inducible gene *p21*$^{CIP1/WAF1}$ was recently shown to interact directly with PCNA (185). PCNA is a component of the DNA replication machinery which is required by DNA polymerase delta for its processive polymerase activity. SV40 origin-dependent DNA replication reconstituted with purified replication proteins is inhibited by addition of p21. Hence, p21 inhibits CDK activity as well as PCNA-dependent DNA replication. Both of these separate functions of p21 may facilitate p53-mediated suppression of cell proliferation in G1.

PCNA also interacts with the product of another p53-inducible gene, *GADD45* (146). Overexpression of GADD45 leads to growth arrest, preventing the progression of cells into the S phase. The interaction of GADD45 with PCNA could mediate its role in negatively regulating DNA synthesis. It should be noted that both *GADD45* and *p21*$^{CIP1/WAF1}$ can be induced in p53-dependent and p53-independent pathways. Hence, the activities of these two genes need not always reflect p53 function.

Recently, important evidence for the role of p53 gene in DNA repair has emerged. Disruption of p53 in human colon carcinoma RKO cells results in an enhanced sensitivity to UV-induced damage (186). Furthermore, extracts from cell lines with disrupted p53 function show a loss of induced repair following cellular UV irradiation. Similarly, loss of normal functional p53 in human fibroblasts renders the cells more sensitive to the chemotherapeutic agent taxol (187). Enhanced sensitivity towards cisplatin (a DNA damaging drug) was also observed when p53 function was disrupted in the breast cancer cell line MCF-7. The DNA lesions induced by cisplatin are repaired exclusively by nucleotide excision and p53 is known to associate with nucleotide excision repair factors ERCC2, ERCC3, and ERCC6 (91). Only wild-type p53 and not the mutant form can inhibit ERCC2 and ERCC3 DNA helicase activities. These observations strengthen the role for p53 in DNA repair.

8. p53 and the future

In recent years, research in the p53 field has generated considerable interest, mainly due to its role in tumour suppression. A number of biological and biochemical properties of p53 have been elucidated. However, in order to fully understand the role of p53 in cancer, and to develop therapeutic strategies that target p53, a number of questions remain to be answered. While it is clear that p53 acts as a transcriptional factor, it is not certain that this property of p53 alone is sufficient for G1 arrest and apoptosis. Does p53 play a more direct role in blocking DNA replication and in the repair of DNA damage? While *p21*$^{CIP1/WAF1}$ and *GADD45* have been shown to play important roles in p53-induced G1 arrest, it is important to determine if additional target genes exist that are regulated by p53. The p53-dependent and p53-independent pathways of apoptosis are poorly defined; how do seemingly divergent pathways lead to a common signal that initiates the cell death program? How is p53 gene expression regulated particularly in response to certain DNA damaging agents which have been shown to increase the intracellular amount of p53 protein? Is the functional state of p53 protein regulated during the cell cycle? The answers to these questions will improve our understanding of oncogenesis and provide insight into the growth advantage incurred by tumour cells that have lost wild-type p53 gene expression.

Acknowledgements

We would like to thank Dr C. C. Harris and Ms Dorothea Dudek, NCI, Bethesda, for Fig. 1. This work was supported by grants from the Medical Research Council of Canada and the National Cancer Institute of Canada. S. G. was supported by a fellowship from the Cancer Research Society and Y. P. L. was supported by an Ontario Graduate Scholarship.

References

1. Benchimol, S., Lamb, P., Crawford, L. V., Sheer, D., Shows, T. B., Bruns, G. A. P., *et al.* (1985) Transformation associated p53 protein is encoded by a gene on human chromosome 17. *Somatic Cell Mol. Genet.*, **11**, 505.
2. Soussi, T., Caron de Fromentel, C., and May, P. (1990) Structural aspects of the p53 protein in relation to gene evolution. *Oncogene*, **5**, 945.
3. Matlashewski, G., Pim, D., Banks, L., and Crawford, L. (1987) Alternative splicing of human p53 transcripts. *Oncogene Res.*, **1**, 77.

4. Arai, N., Nomura, P., Yokota, K., Wolf, D., Brill, E., Shohat, O., *et al.* (1986) Immunologically distinct p53 are generated by alternative splicing. *Mol. Cell. Biol.*, **6**, 3232.

5. Matlashewski, G., Lamb, P., Pim, D., Peacock, J., Crawford, L., and Benchimol, S. (1984) Isolation and characterization of the human p53 cDNA clone: expression of the human gene. *EMBO J.*, **3**, 3257.

6. Rigaudy, P. and Eckhart, W. (1989) Nucleotide sequence of a cDNA encoding the monkey cellular phosphoprotein p53. *Nucleic Acids Res.*, **17**, 8375.

7. Jenkins, J. R., Rudge, K. I., Redmond, S., and Wade-Evans, A. (1984) Cloning and expression analysis of full length mouse cDNA sequence encoding the transformation associated protein p53. *Nucleic Acids Res.*, **12**, 5609.

8. Soussi, T., Caron de Fromentel, C., Brengnot, C., and May, P. (1988) Nucleotide sequence of a cDNA encoding the rat p53 nuclear oncoprotein. *Nucleic Acid Res.*, **16**, 11384.

9. Soussi, T., Begue, A., Stachelin, D., and May, P. (1988) Nucleotide sequence of a cDNA encoding the chicken p53 nuclear oncoprotein. *Nucleic Acids Res.*, **16**, 11383.

10. Soussi, T., Caron de Fromentel, C., Méchali, M., May, P., and Kress, M. (1987) Cloning and characterization of a cDNA from *Xenopus laevis* coding for a protein homologous to human and murine p53. *Oncogene*, **1**, 71.

11. Caron de Fromentel, C., Pakdel, F., Chapus, A., Baney C., May, P., and Soussi, T. (1992) Rainbow trout p53: cDNA cloning and biochemical characterisation. *Gene*, **112**, 241.

12. Kraiss, S., Quaiser, A., Oren, M., and Montenarh, M. (1988) Oligomerization of oncoprotein p53. *J. Virol.*, **62**, 4737.

13. Sturzbecher, H. W., Brain, R., Addison, C. C., Rudge, K., Remm, M., Grimaldi, M., *et al.* (1992) A C-terminal α-helix plus basic region motif is the major structural determinant of p53 tetramerization. *Oncogene*, **7**, 1513.

14. Slingerland, J. M., Jenkins, J. R., and Benchimol, S. (1993) The transforming and suppressor functions of p53 alleles: effects of mutations that disrupt phosphorylation, oligomerization and nuclear translocation. *EMBO J.*, **12**, 1029.

15. Shaulsky, G., Goldfinger, N., Ben Ze'ev, A., and Rotter, V. (1990) Nuclear accumulation of p53 protein is mediated by several nuclear localization signals and plays a role in tumorigenesis. *Mol. Cell. Biol.*, **10**, 6565.

16. Cho, Y., Gorina, S., Jeffrey, P. C., and Pavletich, N. P. (1994) Crystal structure of p53 tumour suppressor–DNA complex: understanding tumorigenic mutations. *Science*, **265**, 346.

17. Clore, G. M., Omichinski, J. G., Sakaguchi, K., Zaubarno, N., Sakamoto, H., Appella, E., *et al.* (1994) High-resolution structure of the oligomerization domain by multidimensional NMR. *Science*, **265**, 386.

18. Lee, W., Harvey, T. S., Yin, Y., Yau, P., Litchfield, D., and Arrowsmith, C. H. (1994) Solution structure of the tetrameric minimum transforming domain of p53. *Nature Genet.*, **1**, 877.

19. Fontoura, B. M. A., Sorokina, E. A., David, E., and Carroll, R. B. (1992) p53 is covalently linked to 5.8S rRNA. *Mol. Cell. Biol.*, **12**, 5145.

20. Ullrich, N., Lin, A., and Wool, I. G. (1979). Identification by affinity chromatography of the eukaryotic ribosomal proteins that bind to 5.8S ribosomal ribonucleic acid. *J. Biol. Chem.*, **254**, 8641.

21. Walker, K., Elela, S. A., and Nazaar, R. N. (1990) Inhibition of protein synthesis by anti 5.8S rRNA oligodeoxyribonucleotides. *J. Biol. Chem.*, **265**, 2428.

22. Meek, D. and Eckhart, W. (1988) Phosphorylation of p53 in normal and Simian virus 40-transformed NIH 3T3 cells. *Mol. Cell. Biol.*, **8**, 461.

23. Wang, Y. and Eckhart, W. (1992) Phosphorylation sites in the amino-terminal region of mouse p53. *Proc. Natl. Acad. Sci. USA*, **89**, 4231.

24. Milne, D. M., Campbell, D. G., Caudwell, F. B., and Meek, D. W. (1994) Phosphorylation of the tumour suppressor protein p53 by mitogen-activated protein kinases. *J. Biol. Chem.*, **269**, 9253.

25. Tack, L. C. and Wright, J. H. (1992) Altered phosphorylation of free and bound forms of monkey p53 and simian virus 40 large T antigen during lytic infection. *J. Virol.*, **66**, 1312.

26. Ullrich, S. J., Sakaguchi, K., Lees-Miller, S. P., Fiscella, M., Mercer, W. E., Anderson, C. W., *et al.* (1993) Phosphorylation at ser-15 and ser-392 in mutant p53 molecules from human tumours is altered compared to wild-type p53. *Proc. Natl. Acad. Sci. USA*, **90**, 5954.

27. Lees-Miller, S. P., Sakaguchi, K., Ullrich, S. J., Appella, E., and Anderson, C. W. (1992) Human DNA-activated protein kinase phosphorylates serines 15 and 37 in the amino-terminal transactivation domain of human p53. *Mol. Cell. Biol.*, **12**, 5041.

28. Milne, D. M., Palmer, R. H., Campbell, D. G., and Meek, D. W. (1992) Phosphorylation of the p53 tumour suppressor protein at three N-terminal residues by a novel casein kinase I-like enzyme. *Oncogene*, **7**, 1361.

29. Bischoff, J. R., Friedman, P. N., Marshak, D. R., Prives, C., and Beach, D. (1990) Human p53 is phosphorylated by p60-cdc2 and cyclin B-cdc2. *Proc. Natl. Acad. Sci. USA*, **87**, 4766.

30. Meek, D. W., Simon, S., Kikkawaa, U., and Eckhart, W. (1990) The p53 tumour suppressor protein is phosphorylated at serine 389 by casein kinase II. *EMBO J.*, **9**, 3253.

31. Hupp, T. R., Meek, D. W., Midgley, C. A., and Lane, D. P. (1992). Regulation of the specific DNA binding function of p53. *Cell.* **71**, 875.

32. Lane, D. P. and Benchimol, S. (1990) p53: oncogene or anti-oncogene? *Genes Dev.*, **4**, 1.

33. Hollstein, M., Sidransky, D., Vogelstein, B., and Harris, C. C. (1991) p53 mutation in human cancer. *Science*, **253**, 49.

34. Masuda, H., Miller, C., Koeffler, H. P., Battifora, H., and Cline, M. J. (1987) Rearrangements of the p53 gene in human osteogenic sarcomas. *Proc. Natl. Acad. Sci. USA*, **84**, 7716.

35. Miller, C. W., Aslo, A., Tsay, C., Slamon, D., Ishizaki, K., Toguchida, Y., *et al.* (1990) Frequency and structure of p53 rearrangements in human osteosarcomas. *Cancer Res.*, **50**, 7950.

36. Ahuja, H., Bar-Eli, M., Advani, S. M., Benchimol, S., and Cline, M. J. (1989) Alterations in the p53 gene and the clonal evolution of the blast crisis of chronic myelocytic leukaemia. *Proc. Natl. Acad. Sci. USA*, **86**, 6783.

37. Ahuja, H., Bar-Eli, M., Arliln, Z., Advani, S., Allan, S. L., Goldman, J., *et al.* (1991) The spectrum of molecular alterations in the evolution of chronic myelocytic leukaemia. *J. Clin. Invest.*, **87**, 2042.

38. Greenblatt, M. S., Bennett, W. P., Hollstein, M., and Harris, C. C. (1994) Mutations in the p53 tumor suppressor gene: clues to cancer etiology and molecular pathogenesis. *Cancer Res.*, **54**, 4855.

39. Blondal, J. A. and Benchimol, S. (1994) The role of p53 in tumour progression. *Semin. Cancer Biol.*, **5**, 177.

40. Li, F. P., Fraumeni, J. F., Mulvihill, J., Blattner, W. A., Dreyfus, M. G., Tuacker, M. A., *et al.* (1988) A cancer family syndrome in twenty four kindreds. *Cancer Res.*, **48**, 5358.

41. Malkin, D., Li, F. P., Strong, L. C., Fraumeni, J. F., Nelson, C. E., Kim, D. H., *et al.* (1990) Germ-line p53 mutation in a familial syndrome of breast cancer, sarcomas and other neoplasms. *Science*, **250**, 1233.

42. Srivastava, S., Zon, Z., Pirollo, K., Blattner, W., and Chang, E. H. (1990) Germ-line transmission of a mutated p53 gene in a cancer-prone family with Li-Fraumeni syndrome. *Nature*, **348**, 747.

43. Malkin, D., Jolly, K. W., Barbier, N., Look, A. T., Friend, S. H., Gebhardt, M. C., *et al.* (1992) Germline mutations of the p53 tumour suppressor gene in children and young adults with second malignant neoplasms. *N. Engl. J. Med.*, **326**, 1309.

44. Donehower, L. A., Harvey, M., Slagle, B. L., MacArthur, M. J., Montgomery, C. A., Butel, J. S., *et al.* (1992) Mice deficient for p53 are developmentally normal but susceptible to spontaneous tumours. *Nature*, **356**, 215.

45. Kemp, C. J., Donehower, L., Bradley, A., and Balmain, A. (1993) Reduction of p53 dosage does not increase initiation or promotion but enhances malignant progression of chemically induced skin tumours. *Cell*, **74**, 813.

46. Lavigueur, A., Maltby, V., Mock, D., Rossant, J., Pawson, T., and Bernstein, A. (1989) High incidence of lung, bone, and lymphoid tumours in transgenic mice overexpressing mutant alleles of the p53 oncogene. *Mol. Cell. Biol.*, **9**, 3982.

47. Bargonetti, J., Friedman, P. N., Kern, S. E., Vogelstein, B., and Prives, C. (1991) Wild-type but not mutant p53 immunopurified proteins bind to sequences adjacent to the SV40 origin of replication. *Cell*, **65**, 1083.

48. Kern, S. E., Kinzler, K. W., Bruskin, A., Jarosz, D., Friedman, P., Prives, C., *et al.* (1992) Identification of p53 as a sequence-specific DNA binding protein. *Science*, **252**, 1708.

49. El-Deiry, W. S., Kern, S. E., Pietenpol, J. A., Kinzler, K. W., and Vogelstein, B. (1992) Definition of a consensus binding site for p53. *Nature Genet.*, **1**, 45.

50. Funk, W. D., Pak, D. T., Karas, R. H., Wright, W. E., and Shay, J. W. (1992) A transcriptionally active DNA binding site for human p53 protein complexes. *Mol. Cell. Biol.*, **12**, 2866.

51. Weissker, S. N., Muller, B. F., Homfeld, A., and Deppert, W. (1992) Specific and complex interactions of murine p53 with DNA. *Oncogene*, **7**, 1921.

52. Oberosler, P., Hloch, P., Ramsperger, W., and Stahl, H. (1993) p53-catalyzed annealing of complementary single-stranded nucleic acids. *EMBO J.*, **12**, 2389.

53. Fields, S. and Jang, S. K. (1990) Presence of a potent transcription activating sequence in the p53 protein. *Science*, **249**, 1046.

54. Raycroft, L., Wu, H., and Lozano, G. (1990) Transcriptional activation by wild-type but not transforming mutants of the p53 anti-oncogene. *Science*, **249**, 1049.

55. Chin, K-V., Ueda, K., Pastan, I., and Gottesman, M. M. (1992) Modulation of activity of the promoter of the human mdr 1 gene by ras and p53. *Science*, **255**, 459.

56. Wang, Y., Reed, M., Wang, P., Stenger, J. E., Mayr, G., Anderson, M. E., *et al.* (1993) p53 domains: identification and characterization of two autonomous DNA-binding regions. *Genes Dev.*, **7**, 2575.

57. Zambetti, G. P., Bargonetti, J., Walker, K., Prives, C., and Levine, A. J. (1992) Wild-type p53 mediates positive regulation of gene expression through a specific DNA sequence element. *Genes Dev.*, **6**, 11443.

58. Kastan, M. B., Zhan, Q., El-Deiry, W. S., Carrier, F., Jacks, T., Walsh, W. V., *et al.* (1992)

A mammalian cell cycle checkpoint pathway utilizing p53 and GADD45 is defective in Ataxia-telangiectasia. *Cell*, **71**, 587.

59. Aoyama, N., Nagase, T., Sawazaki, T., Mizuguchi, G., Nakagoshi, H., Fujkisawa, J., *et al.* (1992) Overlap of the p53 responsive element and cAMP responsive element in the enhancer of human T cell leukemia virus type I. *Proc. Natl. Acad. Sci. USA*, **89**, 5403.

60. Wu, X., Bayle, J. H., Olson, D., and Levine, A. J. (1993) The p53-mdm-2 autoregulatory feedback loop. *Genes Dev.*, **7**, 1126.

61. Zauberman, A., Barak, Y., Ragimov, N., Levy, N., and Oren, M. (1993) Sequence-specific DNA binding by p53: identification of target sites and lack of binding to p53-mdm-2 complexes. *EMBO J.*, **12**, 2799.

62. Foord, O., Navot, N., and Rotter, V. (1993) Isolation and characterisation of DNA sequences that are specifically bound by wild-type p53 protein. *Mol. Cell. Biol.*, **13**, 1378.

63. El-Deiry, W. S., Tokino, T., Velculescu, V. E., Levy, D. B., Parsons, R., Trent, J. M., *et al.* (1993) WAF1, a potential mediator of p53 tumour suppression. *Cell*, **75**, 817.

64. Okamoto, K. and Beach, D. (1994) Cyclin G is a potential target of the p53 tumour suppressor protein. *EMBO J.*, **13**, 4816.

65. Miyashita, T. and Reed, J. C. (1995) Tumour suppressor p53 is a direct transcriptional activator of the human Bax gene. *Cell*. **80**, 293.

66. Buckbinder, L., Talbott, R., Velasco-Miguel, S., Takenaka, I., Faha, B., Seizinger, B. R., *et al.* (1995) Induction of the growth inhibitor IGF-binding protein 3 by p53. *Nature*, **377**, 646.

67. Farmer, G., Bargonetti, J., Zhu, H., Friedman, P., Prywes, R., and Prives, C. (1992) Wild-type p53 activates transcription *in vitro*. *Nature*, **358**, 83.

68. Lane, D. P. and Crawford, L. V. (1979) T antigen is bound to a host protein in SV40-transformed cells. *Nature*, **278**, 261.

69. Linzer, D. I. H. and Levine, A. J. (1979) Characterization of a 54 K dalton cellular SV40 tumour antigen present in SV40-transformed cells and uninfected embryonal carcinoma cells. *Cell*, **17**, 43.

70. Sarnow, P., Ho, X. S., Williams, J., and Levine, A. J. (1982) Adenovirus E1B-58 kd tumour antigen and SV40 large tumour antigen are physically associated with same 54 kd cellular protein in transformed cells. *Cell*, **28**, 387.

71. Crook, T., Wrede, D., Tidy, J., Scholefield, J., Crawford, L., and Vousden, K. H. (1991) Status of c-myc, p53 and retinoblastoma genes in human papillomavirus positive and negative squamous cell carcinomas of the anus. *Oncogene*, **6**, 1251.

72. Reihaus, E., Kahler, M., Kraiss, S., Oren, M., and Montenarh, M. (1990) Regulation of the level of the oncoprotein p53 in non-transformed and transformed cells. *Oncogene*, **5**, 137.

73. Scheffner, M., Werness, B. A., Huibregste, J. M., Levine, A. J., and Howley, P. M. (1990) The E6 oncoprotein encoded by human papillomavirus types 16 and 18 promotes degradation of p53. *Cell*, **63**, 1129.

74. Yew, P. R., and Berk, A. J. (1992) Inhibition of p53 transactivation required for transformation by adenovirus early 1B protein. *Nature*, **357**, 82.

75. Symonds, H., Chen, J., and Van Dyke, T. (1991) Complex formation between the lymphotropic papovavirus large tumour antigen and the tumour suppressor protein p53. *J. Virol.*, **65**, 5417.

76. Szekely, L., Selivanova, G., Magnusson, K. P., Klein, G., and Wiman, K. G. (1993) EBNA-5, an Epstein–Barr virus-encoed nuclear antigen, binds to the retinoblastoma and p53 proteins. *Proc. Natl. Acad. Sci. USA*, **90**, 5455.

77. Wang, X. W., Forrester, K., Yeh, H., Feitelson, M. A., Gu, J-R., and Harris, C. C. (1994) Hepatitis B virus X protein inhibits p53 sequence-specific DNA binding, transcriptional activity, and association with transcription factor ERCC3. *Proc. Natl. Acad. Sci. USA*, **91**, 2230.

78. Speir, E., Modali, R., Huang, E-S., Leon, M. B., Shwl, F., Finkel, T., *et al.* (1994) Potential role of human cytomegalovirus and p53 interaction in coronary restenosis. *Science*, **265**, 391.

79. Agoff, S. N., Hou, J., Linzer, D. I. H., and Wu, B. (1993) Regulation of the human hsp 70 promoter by p53. *Science*, **259**, 84.

80. Macleod, M. C. (1993) Identification of a DNA structural motif that includes the binding sites for Sp1, p53 and GA-binding protein. *Nucleic Acids Res.*, **21**, 1439.

81. Borellini, F. and Glazer, R. I. (1993) Induction of sp1-p53 DNA-binding hetercomplexes during graunulocyte/macrophage colony-stimulating factor-dependent proliferation in human erythroleukemia cell line TF-1. *J. Biol. Chem.*, **268**, 7923.

82. Seto, E., Usheva, A., Zambetti, G. P., Momand, J., Horikoshi, N., Weinman, R., *et al.* (1992) Wild-type p53 binds to the TATA-binding protein and represses transcription. *Proc. Natl. Acad. Sci. USA*, **89**, 12028.

83. Truant, R., Xiao, H., Ingles, C. J., and Greenblatt, J. (1993) Direct interaction between the transcriptional activation domain of human p53 and the TATA box-binding protein. *J. Biol. Chem.*, **268**, 2284.

84. Liu, X., Miller, P. H., Koeffler, P. H., and Berk, A. J. (1993) p53 activtion domain binds to the TATA-box binding polypeptide and a neighbouring p53 domain inhibits transcription. *Mol. Cell. Biol.*, **13**, 3291.

85. Martin, D. W., Munoz, R. M., Subler, M. A., and Deb, S. (1993) p53 binds to the TATA-binding protein – TATA complex. *J. Biol. Chem.*, **268**, 13062.

86. Chen, X., Farmer, G., Prywes, R., and Prives, C. (1993) Cooperative DNA binding of p53 with TFIID (TBP): a possible mechanism for transcriptional activation. *Genes Dev.*, **7**, 1837.

87. Maheswaran, S., Park, S., Bernard, A., Morris, J. F., Rauscher, F. J., Hill, D. E., *et al.* (1993) Physical and functional interaction between WT1 and p53 proteins. *Proc. Natl. Acad. Sci. USA*, **90**, 5100.

88. Momand, J., Zambetti, G. P., Olson, D. C., George, D., and Levine, A. J. (1992) The mdm-2 oncogene product forms a complex with the p53 protein and inhibits p53-mediated transactivation. *Cell*, **69**, 1237.

89. Oliner, J. D., Kinzler, K. W., Meltzer, P. S., George, D., and Vogelstein, B. (1992) Amplification of a gene encoding a p53-associated protein in human sarcomas. *Nature*, **358**, 80.

90. Thut, C. J., Chen, J-L., Klemm, R., and Tjian, R. (1995) p53 transcriptional activation mediated by coactivators $TAF_{II}40$ and $TAF_{II}60$. *Science*, **267**, 100.

91. Wang, X. W., Yeh, H., Schaeffer, L., Roy, R., Moncollin, V., Egly, J-M., *et al.* (1995) p53 modulation of TFIIH-associated nucleotide excision repair activity. *Nature Genet.*, **10**, 188.

92. Pinhasi-Kimhi, O., Michalovitz, D., Ben-Zeev, A., and Oren, M. (1986) Specific interaction between the p53 cellular tumour antigen and major heat shock proteins. *Nature*, **320**, 182.

93. Baudier, J., Delphin, C., Grunwald, D., Khochbin, S., and Lawrence, J. J. (1992) Characterization of the tumour suppressor protein p53 as a protein kinase C substrate and a S100b-binding protein. *Proc. Natl. Acad. Sci. USA*, **89**, 11627.

94. Dutta, A., Ruppert, J. M., Aster, J. C., and Winchester, E. (1993) Inhibition of DNA replication factor RPA by p53. *Nature*, **365**, 79.

95. He, Z., Brinton, B. T., Greenblatt, J., Hassell, J. A., and Ingles, C. J. (1993) The transactivator proteins VP16 and GAL4 bind replication factor A. *Cell*, **73**, 1223.

96. Li, R. and Botchan, M. R. (1993) The acidic transcriptional activation domains of VP16 and p53 bind the cellular replication protein A and stimulate *in vitro* BPV-1 DNA replication. *Cell*, **73**, 1207.

97. Clarke, C. F., Heng, K., Frey, A. B., Stein, R., Hinds, P. W., and Levine, A. J. (1988) Purification of complexes of nuclear oncogene p53 with rat and *Escherichia coli* heat shock proteins: *in vitro* dissociation of hsc70 and dnaK from murine p53 by ATP. *Mol. Cell. Biol.*, **8**, 1206.

98. Takimoto, M., Sermsuvitayawong, K., and Matsubara, K. (1994) Identification of cellular proteins that bind the central conserved region of p53. *Biochem. Biophys. Res. Commun.*, **202**, 490.

99. Huibregtse, J. M., Scheffner, M., and Howley, P. M. (1993) Localization of the E6-AP regions that direct human papillomavirus E6 binding, association with p53, and ubiquitination of associated proteins. *Mol. Cell. Biol.*, **13**, 4918.

100. Barak, Y., Juven, T., Haffner, R., and Oren, M. (1993) mdm-2 expression is induced by wild-type p53 activity. *EMBO J.*, **12**, 461.

101. Chen, C-Y., Oliner, J. D., Zhan, Q., Fornace, A. J., Vogelstein, B., and Kastan, M. B. (1994) Interactions between p53 and mdm-2 in a mammalian cell cycle checkpoint pathway. *Proc. Natl. Acad. Sci. USA*, **91**, 2684.

102. Fakharzadeh, S. S., Trusko, S. P., and George, D. L. (1991) Tumorigenic potential associated with enhanced expression of a gene that is amplified in a mouse tumour cell line. *EMBO J.*, **10**, 1565.

103. Montes de Oca Luna, R., Wagner, D. S., and Lozano, G. (1995) Rescue of early embryonic lethality in mdm2-deficient mice by deletion of p53. *Nature*, **378**, 203.

104. Noda, A., Ning, Y., Venable, S. F., Pereira-Smiith, O. M., and Smith, J. R. (1994) Cloning of senescent cell-derived inhibitors of DNA synthesis using an expression screen. *Exp. Cell Res.*, **211**, 90.

105. Harper, J. W., Adami, G. R., Wei, N., Keyomarsi, K., and Elledge, S. J. (1993) The p21 cdk-interacting protein Cip1 is a potent inhibitor of G1 cyclin-kinases. *Cell*, **75**, 805.

106. Weintraub, H., Hauschka, S., and Tapscott, S. J. (1991) The mck enhancer contains a p53 responsive element. *Proc. Natl. Acad. Sci. USA*, **88**, 4570.

107. Nakamuta, M., Furuich, M., Takahashi, K., Suzuki, N., Endo, H., and Yamamoto, K. (1989) Isolation and characterization of a family of rat endogenous retroviral sequences. *Virus Genes*, **3**, 69.

108. Ginsberg, D., Mechta, F., Yaniv, M., and Oren, M. (1991) Wild-type p53 can down-modulate the activity of various promoters. *Proc. Natl. Acad. Sci. USA*, **88**, 9979.

109. Mercer, W. E., Shields, M. T., Lin, D., Appella, E., and Ullrich, S. J. (1991) Growth suppression induced by wild-type p53 protein is accompanied by selective down-regulation of proliferating-cell nuclear antigen expression. *Proc. Natl. Acad. Sci. USA*, **88**, 1958.

110. Ragimov, N., Krauskopf, A., Navot, N., Rotter, V., Oren, M., and Aloni, Y. (1993) Wild-type but not mutant p53 can repress transcription initiation *in vitro* by interfering with the binding of the basal transcription factors to TATA motif. *Oncogene*, **8**, 1183.

111. Miyashita, T., Krajewski, S., Krajewska, M., Wang, H. G., Lin, H. K., Leibermann, D. A.,

et al. (1994) Tumour suppressor p53 is a regulator of bcl-2 and bax gene expression *in vitro* and *in vivo*. *Oncogene*, **9**, 1799.

112. Yamamoto, M., Yoshida, M., Ono, K., Fujita, T., Ohtani-Fujita, N., Sakai, T., *et al.* (1994) Effect of tumour suppressors on cell cycle-regulatory genes: RB suppresses p34^{cdc2} expression and normal p53 suppresses cyclin A expression. *Exp. Cell Res.*, **210**, 94.

113. Ginsberg, D., Michael-Michalovitz, D., Ginsberg, D., and Oren, M. (1991) Induction of growth arrest by a temperature-sensitive p53 mutant is correlated with increased nuclear-localization and decreased stability of the protein. *Mol. Cell. Biol.*, **11**, 582.

114. Mercer, W. E., Shields, M. T., Amin, M., Sauve, G. J., Appella, E., Romano, J. W., *et al.* (1990) Negative growth regulation in a glioblastoma tumour cell line that conditionally expresses human wild-type p53. *Proc. Natl. Acad. Sci. USA*, **87**, 6166.

115. Zastawny, R. L., Salvino, R., Chen, J., Benchimol, S., and Ling, V. (1993) The core promoter region of the P-glycoprotein gene is sufficient to confer differential responsiveness to wild-type and mutant p53. *Oncogene*, **8**, 1529.

116. Andreeff, M., Zhao, S., Drach, D., Hegewisch-Becker, S., Rees, J. H. K., Lin, Y., *et al.* (1993) Expression of multidrug resistance (mdr-1) and p53 genes in hematologic cell systems: implications for biology and gene therapy. *Cancer Bull.*, **45**, 131.

117. El Rouby, S., Thomas, A., Costin, D., Rosenbeg, C. R., Potmesil, S., Silber, R., *et al.* (1993) p53 gene mutation in B-cell chronic lymphocytic leukemia is associated with drug resistance and is independent of mdr1/mdr3 gene expression. *Blood*, **82**, 3452.

118. Shiio, Y., Yamamoto, T., and Yamaguchi, M. (1992) Negative regulation of Rb expression by the p53 gene product. *Proc. Natl. Acad. Sci. USA*, **89**, 5206.

119. Miyashita, T., Harigai, M., Hanada, M., and Reed, J. C. (1994) Identification of a p53-dependent negative response element in the bcl-2 gene. *Cancer Res.*, **54**, 3131.

120. Yuan, J.-N., Liu, B.-H., Lee, H., Shaw, Y.-T., Chiou, S.-T., Chang, W.-T., *et al.* (1993) Release of the p53-induced repression on thymidine kinase promoter by single p53-binding sequence. *Biochem. Biophys. Res.*, **191**, 662.

121. Zhan, Q., Carrier, F., and Fornace Jr., A. J. (1993) Induction of cellular p53 activity by DNA-damaging agents and growth arrest. *Mol. Cell. Biol.*, **13**, 4242.

122. Greenblatt, J. (1991) Role of TFIID in transcriptional initiation by RNA polymerase II. *Cell*, **66**, 1067.

123. Horikoshi, N., Usheva, A., Chen, J., Levine, A. J., Weinmann, R., and Shenk, T. (1995) Two domains of p53 interact with the TATA-binding protein, and the adenovirus 13S E1A protein disrupts the association, relieving p53-mediated transcriptional repression. *Mol. Cell. Biol.*, **15**, 227.

124. Mack, D. H., Vartikar, J., Pipas, J. M., and Laimins, L. A. (1993) Specific repression of TATA-mediated but not initiator-mediated transcription by wild-type p53. *Nature*, **363**, 281.

125. Oswald, F., Lovec, H., Moroy, T., and Lipp, M. (1994) E2F-dependent regulation of human myc: transactivation by cyclins D1 and A overrides tumour suppressor protein functions. *Oncogene*, **9**, 2029.

126. Gasser, S. M. and Laemmli, U. K. (1987) A glimpse at chromosomal order. *Trends Genet.*, **3**, 16.

127. Bakalkin, G., Yakovleva, T., Selivanova, G., Magnusson, K. P., Szekely, L., Kiseleva, E., *et al.* (1994) p53 binds single-stranded DNA ends and catalyzes DNA renaturation and strand transfer. *Proc. Natl. Acad. Sci. USA*, **91**, 413.

128. Brain, R. and Jenkins, J. R. (1994) Human p53 directs DNA strand reassociation and is photolabelled by 8-Azido ATP. *Oncogene*, **9**, 1775.
129. Diller, L., Kassel, J., Camille, E. N., Gryka, M. A., Litwak, G., Gebhardt, M., *et al.* (1990) p53 functions as a cell cycle control protein in osteosarcomas. *Mol. Cell. Biol.*, **10**, 5772.
130. Martinez, J., Georgoff, I., Martinez, J., and Levine, A. J. (1991) Cellular localisation and cell cycle regulation by a temperature-sensitive p53 protein. *Genes Dev.*, **5**, 151.
131. Johnson, P., Gray, D., Mowat, M., and Benchimol, S. (1991) Expression of wild-type p53 is not compatible with continued growth of p53-negative tumor cells. *Mol. Cell. Biol.*, **11**, 1.
132. Chen, P-L., Chen, Y., Bookstein, R., and Lee, W.-H. (1990) Genetic mechanisms of tumour suppression by the human p53 gene. *Science*, **250**, 1576.
133. Michalovitz, D., Halevy, O., and Oren, M. (1990) Conditional inhibition of transformation and of cell proliferation by a temperature-sensitive mutant of p53. *Cell*, **62**, 671.
134. Yonish-Rouach, E., Resnitzky, D., Lotem. J., Sachs, L., Kimchi, A., and Oren M. (1991) Wild-type p53 induces apoptosis of myeloid leukemic cells that is inhibited by interleukin 6. *Nature*, **352**, 345.
135. Shaw, P., Bovey, R., Tardy, S., Sahli, R., Sordat, B., and Costa, J. (1992) Innduction of apoptosis by wild-type p53 in a human colon tumor-derived cell line. *Proc. Natl. Acad. Sci. USA*, **89**, 4495.
136. Ryan, J. J., Danish, R., Gottlieb, C. A., and Clarke, M. F. (1993) Cell cycle analysis of p53-induced cell death in murine erythroleukemia cells. *Mol. Cell. Biol.*, **13**, 711.
137. Johnson, P., Chung, S., and Benchimol, S. (1993) Growth suppression of Friend virus-transformed erythroleukemia cells by p53 protein is accompanied by hemoglobin production and is sensitive to erythropoietin. *Mol. Cell. Biol.*, **13**, 1456.
138. Shaulsky, G., Goldfinger, N., Peled, A., and Rotter, V. (1991) Involvement of wild-type p53 in pre-B-cell differentiation *in vitro*. *Proc. Natl. Acad. Sci. USA*, **88**, 8982.
139. Maltzman, W. and Czyzyk, L. (1984) UV irradiation stimulates levels of p53 cellular tumour antigen in non-transformed mouse cells. *Mol. Cell. Biol.*, **4**, 1689.
140. Kastan, M. B., Onyekwere, O., Sidransky, D., Vogelstein, B., and Craig, R. W. (1991) Participation of p53 protein in the cellular response to DNA damage,. *Cancer Res.*, **51**, 6304.
141. Kuerbitz, S. J., Plunkett, B. S., Walsh, W. V., and Kastan, M. B. (1992) Wild-type p53 is a cell-cycle checkpoint determinant following irradiation. *Proc. Natl. Acad. Sci. USA*, **89**, 7491.
142. Livingstone, L. R., White, A., Sprouse, J., Livanos, E., Jacks, T., and Tlsty, T. D. (1992) Altered cell cycle arrest and gene amplification potential accompany loss of wild-type p53. *Cell*, **70**, 923.
143. Yin, Y., Tainsky, M. A., Bischoff, F. Q., Strong, L. C., and Wahl, G. M. (1992) Wild-type p53 restores cell cycle control and inhibits gene amplification in cells with mutant p53 alleles. *Cell*, **70**, 937.
144. Crook, T., Marston, N. J., Sara, E. A., and Vousden, K. H. (1994) Transcriptional activation by p53 correlates with suppression of growth but not transformation. *Cell*, **79**, 817.
145. Pietenpol, J. A., Tokino, T., Thiagalingam, S., El-Deiry, W. S., Kinzler, K. W., and Vogelstein, B. (1994) Sequence specific transcriptional activation is essential for growth suppression by p53. *Proc. Natl. Acad. Sci. USA*, **91**, 1998.
146. Smith, M. L., Chen, I-T., Zhan, Q., Bae, I., Chen, C-Y., Gilmer, T. M., *et al.* (1994) Interaction of the p53-regulated protein GADD45 with the proliferating cell nuclear antigen. *Nature*, **266**, 1376.

147. Xiong, Y., Hannon, G. J., Zhang, H., Casso, D., Kobayashi, R., and Beach, D. (1993) p21 is a universal inhibitor of cyclin kinases. *Nature*, **306**, 701.

148. Dulic, V., Kaufmann, W. K., Wilson, S. J., Tlsty, T. D., Lees, E., Harper, J. W., *et al.* (1994) p53-dependent inhibition of cyclin-dependent kinase activity in human fibroblasts during radiation-induced G1 arrest. *Cell*, **76**, 1013.

149. Slebos, R. J. C., Lee, M. H., Plunkett, B. S., Kessis, T. D., Williams, B. D., Tacks, T., *et al.* (1994) p53-dependent G1 arrest involves pRB-related protein and is disrupted by the human papillomavirus 16 E7 oncoprotein. *Proc. Natl. Acad. Sci. USA*, **91**, 5320.

150. Canman, C. E., Wolff, A. C., Chen, C-Y., Fornace, A. J. Jr, and Kastan, M. B. (1994) The p53-dependent G1 cell cycle checkpoint pathway and ataxia-telangiectasia. *Cancer Res.*, **54**, 5054.

151. White, A. E., Livanos, E. M., and Tlsty, T. (1994) Differential disruption of genomic integrity and cell cycle regulation in normal human fibroblasts by the HPV oncoprotein. *Genes Dev.*, **8**, 666.

152. Demers, G. W., Foster, S. A., Halbert, C. L., and Galloway, D. A. (1994) Growth arrest by induction of p53 in DNA damaged keratinocytes is bypassed by human papillomavirus 16 E7. *Proc. Natl. Acad. Sci. USA*, **91**, 4382.

153. Hickman, E. S., Picksley, S. M., and Vousden, K. H. (1994) Cells expressing HPV16 E7 continue cell cycle progression following DNA damage induced p53 activation. *Oncogene*, **9**, 2177.

154. Butz, K., Shahabeddin, L., Geisen, C., Spitkovsky, D., Ullmann, A., and Hoppe-Seyler, F. (1995) Functional p53 protein in human papillomavirus-positive cancer cells. *Oncogene*, **10**, 927.

155. Peacock, J. W., Chung, S., Bristow, R. G., Hill, R. P., and Benchimol, S. (1995) The p53-mediated G1 checkpoint is retained in tumorigenic REF clones transformed by HPV16 E7 and EJ-ras. *Mol. Cell. Biol.*, **15**, 1446.

156. Finlay, C. A., Hinds, P. W., and Levine, A. J. (1989) The p53 proto-oncogene can act as a suppressor of transformation. *Cell*, **57**, 1083.

157. Eliyahu, D., Michalovitz, D., Eliyahu, S., Pinhasi-Kimhi, O., and Oren, M. (1989) Wild-type p53 can inhibit oncogene-mediated focus formation. *Proc. Natl. Acad. Sci. USA*, **86**, 8763.

158. Mercer, W. E., Shields, M. T., Amin, M., Sauve, G. J., Apella, E., Romano, J. W., *et al.* (1990) Negative growth regulation in a glioblastoma cell line that conditionally expresses human wild-type p53. *Proc. Natl. Acad. Sci. USA*, **87**, 6166.

159. Yonish-Rouach, E., Grunwald, D., Wilder, S., Kimchi, A., May, E., Lawrence, J. J., *et al.* (1993) p53-mediated cell death: relationship to cell cycle control. *Mol. Cell. Biol.*, **13**, 1454.

160. Ramqvist, T., Magnusson, K. P., Wang, Y., Szekely,L., Klein, G., and Wiman, K. (1993) Wild-type p53 induces apoptosis in a Burkitt lymphoma (BL) line that carries mutant p53. *Oncogene*, **8**, 1495.

161. Wang, Y., Ramqvist, T., Szekely, L., Axelson, H., Klein, G., and Wiman, K. (1993) Reconstitution of wild-type p53 expression triggers apoptosis in a p53-negative v-myc retrovirus-induced T-cell lymphoma line. *Cell Growth Diff.*, **4**, 467.

162. Lowe, S. W., Schmitt, E. M., Smith, S. W., Osborne, B. A., and Jacks, T. (1993) p53 is required for radiation-induced apoptosis in mouse thymocytes. *Nature*, **362**, 847.

163. Clarke, A. R., Purdie, C. A., Harrison, D. J., Morris, R. G., Bird, C. C., Hooper, M. L., *et al.* (1993) Thymocyte apoptosis induced by p53-dependent and independent pathways. *Nature*, **362**, 849.

164. Debbas, M. and White, E. (1993) Wild-type p53 mediates apoptosis by E1A, which is inhibited by E1B. *Genes Dev.*, **7**, 546.
165. Lowe, S. W., Jacks, T., Housman, D. E., and Ruley, H. E. (1994) Abrogation of onco-gene-associated apoptosis allows transformation of p53-deficient cells. *Proc. Natl. Acad. Sci. USA*, **91**, 2026.
166. Lee, J. M. and Bernstein, A. (1993) p53 mutations increase resistance to ionizing radia-tion. *Proc. Natl. Acad. Sci. USA*, **90**, 5742.
167. Bristow, R. G., Jang, A., Peacock, P., Chung, S., Benchimol, S., and Hill, R. P. (1994) Mutant p53 increases radioresistance in rat embryo fibroblasts simultaneously trans-fected with HPV16-E7 and/or activated H-ras. *Oncogene*, **9**, 1527.
168. Korsmeyer, S. J. (1992) Bcl-2: an antidote to programmed cell death. *Cancer Surv.*, **15**, 105.
169. Hockenbery, D. M., Oltvai, Z. N., Yin, X. M., Milliman, C. L., and Korsmeyer, S. J. (1993) Bcl-2 functions in an antioxidant pathway to prevent apoptosis. *Cell*, **75**, 241.
170. Wang, Y., Szekely, L., Okan, I., Klein, G., and Wiman, K. G. (1993) Wild-type p53-trig-gered apoptosis is inhibited by bcl-2 in a v-myc-induced T-cell lymphoma line. *Onco-gene*, **8**, 3427.
171. Chiou, S. K., Rao, L., and White, E. (1994) Bcl-2 blocks p53-dependent apoptosis. *Mol. Cell. Biol.*, **14**, 2556.
172. Oltvai, Z. N., Milliman, C. L., and Korsmeyer, S. J. (1993) Bcl-2 heterodimerizes *in vivo* with a conserved homolog, Bax that accelerates programed cell death. *Cell*, **74**, 609.
173. Selvakumaran, M., Lin, H. K., Miyashita, T., Wang, H. G., Krajewski, S., Reed, J. C., *et al.* (1994) Immediate early up-regulation of bax expression by p53 but not TGFβ1: a paradigm for distinct apoptotic pathways. *Oncogene*, **9**, 1791.
174. Di Leonardo, A., Linke, S. P., Clarkin, K., and Wahl, G. M. (1994) DNA damage triggers a prolonged p53-dependent G1 arrest and long-term induction of Cip1 in normal human gibroblasts. *Genes Dev.*, **8**, 2540.
175. Lin, Y. and Benchimol, S. (1995) Cytokines inhibit p53-mediated apoptosis but not p53-mediated G1-arrest. *Mol. Cell. Biol.*, **15**, 6045.
176. Caelles, C., Helmberg, A., and Karin, M. (1994) p53-dependent apoptosis in the absence of transcriptional activation of p53-target genes. *Nature*, **370**, 220.
177. Wagner, A. J., Kokontis, J. M., and Hay, N. (1994) Myc-mediated apoptosis requires wild-type p53 in a manner independent of cell cycle arrest and the ability of p53 to induce p21$^{waf1/cip1}$. *Genes Dev.*, **8**, 2817.
178. Shen, Y. Q. and Shenk, T. (1994) Relief of p53-mediated transcriptional repression by the adenovirus E1B 19-kDa protein or the cellular Bcl-2 protein. *Proc. Natl. Acad. Sci. USA*, **91**, 8940.
179. Aloni-Grinstein, R., Zan-Bar, I., Alboum, I., Goldfinger, N., and Rotter, V. (1993) Wild-type p53 functions as a control protein in the differentiation pathway of the B-cell lineage. *Oncogene*, **8**, 3297.
180. Almon, E., Goldfinger, N., Kapon, A., Schwartz, D., Levine, A. J., and Rotter, V. (1993) The p53 suppressor is expressed in spermatogenesis. *Dev. Biol.*, **156**, 107.
181. Gannon, J. V. and Lane, D. P. (1987) p53 and DNA polymerase alpha compete for bind-ing to SV40 T antigen. *Nature*, **329**, 456.
182. Braithwaite, A. W., Sturzbecher, H.-W., Addison, C., Palmer, C., Rudge, K., and Jenkins, J. R. (1987) Mouse p53 inhibits SV40 origin-dependent DNA replication. *Nature*, **329**, 458.

183. Wang, E. H., Friedman, P. N., and Prives, C. (1989) The murine p53 protein blocks replication of SV40 DNA in vitro by inhibiting the initiation functions of SV40 large T antigen. *Cell*, **57**, 379.
184. Tack, L. C., Wright, J. H., Deb, S. P., and Tegtmeyer, P. (1989) The p53 complex from monkey cells modulates the biochemical activities of simian virus 40 large T antigen. *J. Virol.*, **63**, 1310.
185. Waga, S., Hannon, G. J., Beach, D., and Stillman, B. (1994) The p21 inhibitor of cyclin-dependent kinase controls DNA replication by interaction with PCNA. *Nature*, **369**, 574.
186. Smith, M. L., Chen, I-T., Zhan, Q., O'Conner, P. M., and Fornace, A. J. Jr. (1995) Involvement of the p53 tumour suppressor in repair of UV-type DNA damage. *Oncogene*, **10**, 1053.
187. Wahl, A. F., Donaldson, K. L., Fairchild, C., Lee, F. Y. F., Foster, S. A., Demers, G. W., *et al.* (1995) Loss of normal p53 function confers sensitization to taxol by increasing G2/M arrest and apoptosis. *Nature Med.*, **2**, 72.

10 | Tumour suppressor genes and inheritance of cancer

DONALD M. BLACK

1. Introduction

Several genes have been identified which confer an inherited predisposition to cancer. Although the susceptibility is usually inherited as a dominant trait, at the cellular level the susceptibility mutations are almost always recessive. Therefore, for the cancer to develop, the dominant wild-type copy of the gene must be mutated or deleted. Such genes are called tumour suppressors. They encode proteins of diverse function which need to be inactivated for the initiation and progression of malignancy. The existence of families with susceptibility to cancer are important in two ways. First, they give us additional insights into the molecular events which underlie the transformation from normal to tumour cells; and secondly, they allow the possibility of genetic testing for cancer risk.

2. Tumour suppressor genes

Most cancers occur in both familial and sporadic forms (1). Families affected with an inherited genetic predisposition to one or multiple forms of cancer are rare, but together may account for about 10% of the common cancers. The prototypical inherited cancer syndrome is familial retinoblastoma, and the epidemiological study of this tumour and mathematical modelling of the age of onset in the familial versus sporadic cases led Knudson to propose the now classical 'two-hit' hypothesis for inherited cancers (2). Two rate limiting mutational events were proposed; the first mutation is either germ-line (inheritable retinoblastoma) or somatic (in non-familial cases), and the second event is always somatic (Fig. 1). We now know that in almost all heritable cancers, the first mutation inactivates a single allele of a tumour suppressor gene and that the rate limiting second mutation is the loss of the remaining normal allele. The predisposing inherited lesions are proposed to be recessive, since the loss of function of one copy of the gene remains latent until the normal allele is inactivated. Therefore, even though the susceptibility to cancer is inherited as an autosomal dominant trait, the susceptibility allele is actually recessive at the cellular level.

The two-hit hypothesis also fits the epidemiological data for familial cancers other than retinoblastoma, including neuroblastoma, pheochromocytoma, and Wilms'

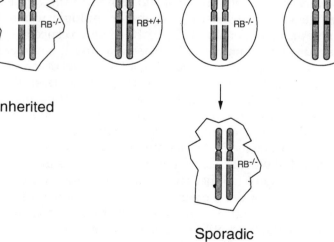

Fig. 1 The 'two-hit' model of cancer-specific mutations. The figure shows cells containing a generic pair of chromosomes in which a marker gene (*RB*) is either wild-type (black boxes) or mutant (white boxes). The homozygous wild-type and heterozygous cells have the same normal phenotype, demonstrating the recessive nature of the mutant allele. Tumorigenesis will only ensue if both copies of the gene are mutated or deleted. In an individual who inherits a mutant copy from one parent, only a single somatic mutation is needed to lead to tumorigenesis. In individuals carrying two wild-type alleles, both copies must sustain independent somatic mutations.

tumour (3, 4). A broader version of this model can be applied to cancers which require the accumulation of more than two mutations before expression of the fully malignant phenotype. Colorectal carcinoma occurs in both familial and sporadic forms but the epidemiological data suggests the accumulation of approximately six independent mutational events (5). Comparison of the age of diagnosis for sporadic colorectal carcinoma with that for the familial disease implied that one or two fewer mutations were necessary in patients carrying an inherited mutation (6). The epidemiological analysis of colorectal carcinoma, retinoblastoma, and other tumours suggests that inactivation of a single allele of a tumour suppressor locus followed by somatic inactivation of the remaining allele, with or without the requirement for alterations in other dominant or recessive oncogenes, is a common mechanism in the development of human malignancy. This model suggests that some familial cancers result from recessive mutations which increase the risk of tumorigenesis above that of the normal population by producing target cells requiring one less mutation to initiate malignancy.

An additional manifestation of the two-hit hypothesis which has influenced the search for tumour suppressor genes in both familial and sporadic cancers is 'loss of heterozygocity' or LOH. This reflects the fact that one of the simplest ways to sustain the second somatic mutation is either to lose the entire chromosome carrying the normal allele or a large section of it, or to eliminate the normal allele by recombination events that duplicate the mutant allele. In situations in which these events can be traced at the DNA level, for example by monitoring restriction fragment length or CA repeat-type of polymorphism, the outcome is that the tumour appears to be homozygous (or hemizygous) for markers in or close to the relevant tumour suppressor gene.

To date, at least 19 genes which can predispose to cancer when mutated in the germ-line have been identified and additional candidates that have been mapped to specific chromosomal regions are currently the subjects of extensive cloning efforts (Table 1).

3. Identified familial cancer genes

Genes responsible for familial cancers (see Table 1) have been isolated by three different strategies. The majority of the familial cancer genes cloned to date (*APC, ATM, BRCA1, BRCA2, NF1, NF2, RB1, TSC2, VHL,* and *WT1*) were identified by a positional cloning approach based on knowledge of the gene's location, often in conjunction with overlapping deletions and/or translocations. An approach based on the joint knowledge of chromosomal position and candidate genes in that region led to the

Table 1 Genes involved in hereditary predisposition to cancer

Gene	Cancer type[a]	Chromosomal location	Protein function	Type of mutation
APC	Colon	5q21	Cell adhesion	Loss of function
ATM	Multiple	11q21	DNA repair checkpoint	Loss of function
BRCA1	Breast and ovary	17q21	Granin	Loss of function
BRCA2	Breast and ovary	13q13	Unknown	Loss of function
CDK4	Melanoma	12q13	Cyclin D kinase	Missense
CDKN2	Melanoma	9p21	CDK inhibitor	Loss of function
IGF2	Multiple	11p15	Growth factor	Loss of imprinting
hMLH1	HNPCC	3p21	DNA mismatch repair	Loss of function
hMSH2	HNPCC1	2p16	DNA mismatch repair	Loss of function
hPMS1	HNPCC	2q31	qDNA mismatch repair	Loss of function
hPMS2	HNPCC	7p22	DNA mismatch repair	Loss of function
MEN1	Thyroid	11q13	Unknown	Unknown
NF1	Neural crest	17q11	GTPase	Loss of function
NF2	Schwannoma	22q12	Cell adhesion	Loss of function
RB1	Retinoblastona	13q14	Cell cycle checkpoint	Loss of function
RET	MEN2A and 2B	10q11	Growth factor receptor	Missense
TSC1	Multiple	9q34	Unknown	Unknown
TSC2	Multiple	16p13	GTPase	Loss of function
TP53	Multiple	17p13	DNA repair checkpoint	Loss of function
VHL	Renal	3p25	Transcription factor	Loss of function
WT1	Renal	11p13	Transcription factor	Loss of function

[a] HNPCC, hereditary non-polyposis colon cancer. MEN, multiple endocrine neoplasia.

implication of *p53* in Li–Fraumeni syndrome (see Chapter 9), *RET* in multiple endocrine neoplasia type 2A (MEN2A; see Chapter 3), *CDKN2A* in familial melanoma (see Chapter 7), and *hMSH2* in hereditary non-polyposis colon cancer (HNPCC), as well as a suggestion that *IGFII* is involved in Beckwith–Wiedemann syndrome (BWS; see Chapter 2). A knowledge of the likely function of the gene product led to the identification of a germ-line *CDK4* mutation in familial melanoma and to additional genes (*hMLH1*, *hPMS1*, and *hPMS2*) encoding DNA mismatch repair proteins in families that do not show linkage to chromosome 2p16 colon cancer.

Functionally, these loci encode components of cellular pathways that transduce regulatory signals (as discussed in other chapters). Biochemically, the encoded proteins include growth factors and receptors, membrane-bound and cytosolic signalling molecules, proteins involved in cell to cell contacts, transcription factors, cell cycle regulators, and components of the DNA synthesis and repair apparatus.

3.1 Genes encoding nuclear proteins

3.1.1 The retinoblastoma susceptibility locus

Retinoblastoma results from the mutation of a single gene (formally designated *RB1*) on chromosome 13q14. Inheritance of a mutant *RB* allele predisposes to retinoblastoma (7) and a limited repertoire of second tumours (8). However, there are only about 15 cases of familial retinoblastoma in the UK per annum, the vast majority of cases being sporadic.

As discussed extensively in Chapters 7 and 8, pRB acts predominantly as a negative regulator of the E2F and DP-1 families of transcription factors and is itself regulated by phosphorylation by cyclin-dependent kinases (9–12). Its ubiquitous distribution implies that the pRB product has an important role in the development and maintenance of a broad range of tissues. Indeed, *RB* mutations occur at high frequency in a variety of tumour types as part of their malignant progression (12). It therefore remains enigmatic that the inheritance of a mutant allele predisposes specifically to retinoblastoma, to a lesser extent osteosarcoma, and even more rarely to other tumour types (7, 8). One possibility is that a limited number of cell types, including retinoblasts and osteoblasts, may be particularly dependent on pRB-mediated regulation of the G1 to S checkpoint in the cell cycle. In other cell types, with redundant regulatory pathways, loss of pRB may only be effective in conjunction with mutational disruption of other pathways, such as that regulated by p53, so that mutation of *RB* is observed only at later stages of malignant progression.

3.1.2   p53 mutations and Li–Fraumeni syndrome

While somatic mutations in the *p53* gene (formally designated *TP53*) are implicated in the progression of more than 30 types of human malignancy (13, 14), germ-line mutations in *p53* confer an autosomal dominant predisposition to cancer of the breast, brain, bone, soft tissues, haematopoietic system, and adrenal cortex, termed the Li–Fraumeni syndrome (15, 16).

Like pRB, p53 is a ubiquitously expressed transcription factor which appears to be involved in cell cycle progression and apoptosis (see Chapter 9). The fact that DNA tumour viruses have developed mechanisms to circumvent the regulatory functions of both of these proteins implies that while they regulate the cell cycle at the same checkpoint they most likely affect different pathways (Chapters 8 and 9). p53 appears to accomplish its regulatory role either by interacting with other proteins, including heat shock proteins, the oncoprotein MDM2 (17), and the product of the *WT1* locus (18, and see below), or by transcriptional activation of a variety of target genes including *MDM2*, *GADD45*, cyclin G, and *CIP1* (see Chapter 9). Overexpression of MDM2 in tumours occurs in the absence of p53 mutations, suggesting that the two are alternative mechanisms which serve the purpose of inactivating p53 (19). A more specific role for p53 may be as part of the cell's response to DNA damaging agents, restricting cell cycle progression until DNA repair is complete (20). One of the mechanisms by which this is likely to be achieved is through the induction of the $p21^{CIP1/WAF1}$ gene which encodes the p21 inhibitor of G1-specific CDKs (21). $p21^{CIP1/WAF1}$ is itself an attractive candidate for a familial cancer gene and although there is no evidence as yet, it will be interesting to see if any families which are phenotypically Li–Fraumeni, but do not have p53 mutations have alterations in either $p21^{CIP1/WAF1}$ or *MDM2*.

The presence of a single mutant *p53* allele can result in a dominant negative phenotype (22) by the formation of inactive p53 oligomers between mutant and wild-type proteins (23). Point mutations leading to inactivation of the oligomeric complex may have a more severe phenotype than deletion of the entire allele or point mutations that only affect the function of the p53 molecule carrying the mutation (as in some cases of Li–Fraumeni syndrome). In support of this is the relatively mild phenotype observed in mice that are heterozygous for a null *p53* allele (24).

3.1.3 Wilms' tumour and 11p13

Wilms' tumour or nephroblastoma, is the commonest solid paediatric tumour, affecting 1 in 10 000 children, usually during the first five years of life. Most cases are sporadic and unilateral, but about 7% are bilateral, and a further 1% show familial clustering (25). Wilms' tumour occurs both in a simple familial form and as one phenotypic manifestation of three distinct growth abnormality syndromes: WAGR, Denys–Drash syndrome (DDS), and Beckwith–Wiedemann syndrome (BWS). The WAGR syndrome is characterized by Wilms' tumour, aniridia (malformation of the irises), genito-urinary abnormalities, and mental retardation (26, 27), whereas in DDS, Wilms' tumour occurs in association with pseudohermaphroditism and progressive renal failure (28, 29). Although no candidate gene (nor even chromosomal position) has yet been proposed for simple familial Wilms' tumour, the gene on chromosome 11p13 implicated in both WAGR and DDS has been identified and designated *WT1* (30–32). Whereas WAGR is associated with constitutional deletion of the 11p13 region that includes *WT1* (29), DDS is associated with point mutations of *WT1* (32).

The *WT1* gene encodes a nuclear transcription factor which is related to the EGR and KROX family of transcription factors (33, 34; and Chapter 6). WT1 binds to the same DNA sequence as EGR1 (34) causing transcriptional repression (35). There is also some evidence that WT1 can act as a transcriptional activator upon binding to p53 (18). These data suggest that WT1, like p53 and pRB, is involved in cell cycle control. However, the narrow expression profile of WT1 in the developing fetal kidney and gonads (36, 37) suggests that WT1 most likely exerts its effect in a very limited repertoire of cell types and is involved in the differentiation process of these tissues, whereas p53 and pRB are thought to function in all cell types.

While the loss of normal WT1 function can contribute to tumorigenesis, WT1 does not always function as a classic tumour suppressor. Like p53, a dysfunctional WT1 protein can produce more severe abnormalities than expected for simple reduction in the level of the protein, presumably by sequestering other cellular proteins into inactive complexes or by altering the profile of target genes recognized.

3.1.4 *CDKN2A* and familial melanoma

Each year there are approximately 30 000 new cases of cutaneous malignant melanoma diagnosed in the USA, and about 5000 in the UK. It is estimated that 10% of these cases are the result of a familial susceptibility (38). To date, two susceptibility genes have been identified: the *CDKN2A* gene, on 9p21, which encodes the p16[INK4A] inhibitor of CDK4 and CDK6 (21, 39, 40), and more rarely the *CDK4* gene itself on chromosome 12q13 (41). There is also linkage to a susceptibility locus on chromosome 1 in some melanoma families. The susceptibility to melanoma is conferred by loss of function mutations in *CDKN2A*, which result in either the absence of a gene product or the production of a mutant form which is unable to bind to and inhibit CDK4 and CDK6. Only one susceptibility mutation has so far been identified in the *CDK4* gene, a missense mutation that results in a form of CDK4 that is no longer susceptible to inhibition by p16 (41). The role of CDKs and CDK inhibitors in controlling progress through the cell cycle is covered in detail elsewhere in this book (Chapter 7).

3.1.5 HNPCC and DNA repair

The majority of hereditary non-polyposis colon cancer (HNPCC) families show linkage to a locus on chromosome 2p16 (*COCA1*; ref. 42). Pre-cancerous lesions and colorectal tumours from these patients consistently show instability of microsatellite and monotonic DNA sequences throughout the genome, indicating that the predisposing allele is associated with a greatly decreased genetic stability (43–45). In these families inheritance of a mutant *COCA1* allele results in the acquisition of a DNA replication or repair defect. The *COCA1* gene was identified by a combination of positional cloning and candidate gene strategies (46, 47) and since it was found to be the human homologue of the bacterial *mutS* and yeast *MSH2* genes, it is now called *hMSH2*. The bacterial *mutS* gene product binds to DNA mismatches as part of the repair mechanism. In yeast, mismatch repair additionally requires the *HML1* and *PMS1* gene products and since many HNPCC families do not show genetic linkage to *hMSH2* (48), the human homologues of these and other mismatch repair enzymes were obvious candidates for the aberrant genes in these families. The respective human genes were identified by searching the cDNA databases for sequences related to the known yeast and *E. coli* mismatch repair enzymes (49–51). The *hMLH1*, *hPMS1*, and *hPMS2*, which map to chromosomes 3p21, 2q31, and 7p22 respectively, were each shown to sustain germ-line mutations in HNPCC families (49–51).

3.1.6 Von Hippel–Lindau disease

It has been known for many years that oncogenes can encode transcription factors that act by regulating the expression of target genes at the level of transcription initiation. However, it has only recently become apparent that a tumour suppressor gene product, namely the gene responsible for Von Hippel–Lindau disease (*VHL*), can also operate at this level by interacting with the proteins that regulate transcription.

Von Hippel–Lindau disease is a dominantly inherited syndrome that affects a minimum of 1 in 35 000 people and predisposes individuals to a variety of tumours. The most frequent tumours are haemangiomas of the central nervous system and retina, renal cell carcinoma, and phaeochromocytoma (52). The *VHL* gene was identified by a positional cloning strategy (53) and shown to be the target of mutations both in VHL-associated tumours and in sporadic renal cell carcinomas. A putative role in signal transduction or cell adhesion was implied by a region of homology with a surface membrane protein of *Trypanosoma brucei* (53). However, when the VHL protein was first identified, it was shown to be associated with two small proteins: elongin B and elongin C, which are components of the cellular transcription factor, elongin (SIII) (54).

Elongin (SIII) was originally identified as an enzyme activity that increases the rate of the RNA polymerase complex movement along the DNA template (55). It was subsequently shown to be a heterotrimeric complex, consisting of subunits A, B, and C. The binding of VHL to elongin B and C suggests two putative mechanisms to explain how VHL operates as a tumour suppressor. One possibility is that the wild-type VHL protein competes with the elongin A protein for binding to elongin B and C. Thus, in the absence of wild-type VHL, elongin B and C are free to associate with elongin A, resulting in an active transcription factor and presumably increased transcription of as yet unknown target genes. The second possibility is that the VHL–elongin B–elongin C heterotrimer also operates as a transcription factor, and VHL mutants alter the specificity or activity of this complex. This suggestion is supported by the finding that in sparsely growing cells, VHL is located in the nucleus, but once a culture becomes confluent, the protein is relocalized to the cytoplasm. VHL may therefore regulate gene expression in response to other cellular conditions, such as contact inhibition.

3.1.7 Ataxia telangiectasia

Ataxia telangiectasia (AT) is a rare progressive disorder in which there is variable immune dysfunction, an excess sensitivity to ionizing radiation, and two distinct patterns of susceptibility to malignancy (56). AT is familial and shows an autosomal recessive pattern of inheritance, with a mutant gene frequency of between 1 in 100 and 1 in 200. There is evidence of genetic heterogeneity and the disease has been divided into four complementation groups which are based on the resistance of fibroblasts from patients with AT to exhibit inhibition of DNA synthesis immediately following exposure to ionizing radiation. Fusion of fibroblasts from different groups will correct this radiation sensitivity. However, linkage studies show that most AT families are due to a locus on human chromosome 11q22-q23 (56). The *ATM* (for AT-mutated) gene was identified by a positional cloning strategy (57, 58) and was surprisingly found to be mutated in all four AT complementation groups, indicating that although phenotypically heterogeneous, AT is likely to be a single gene defect.

In the homozygous state, *ATM* mutations predispose individuals to a 70-fold increased risk of leukaemia and a 250-fold increased risk of lymphoma. Additionally, carriers of one mutant copy of the gene (heterozygotes) have a significantly increased susceptibility to many solid tumours including bladder, ovarian, pancreatic, prostate, and stomach cancer. Most notably, female *ATM* heterozygotes have been found to have an approximately fivefold increased risk to breast cancer. Based on the estimations of the *ATM* mutation frequency (1 in 200) and incidence of breast cancer (1 in 11), it has been calculated that as many as 9% of women in the UK and USA with breast cancer may be *ATM* heterozygotes (57).

The *ATM* gene specifies a 12 kb transcript, encoding a 3056 amino acid polypeptide (57, 58) that shows similarities to a number of proteins in yeast and *Drosophila* that have been implicated in cell cycle regulation, particularly the checkpoints that sense DNA damage. A common feature of these proteins is the presence of a domain that shows striking homology to the kinase domain of phosphatidylinositol-3' kinase (59; see Chapters 4 and 5).

3.2 Cytoplasmic and membrane-associated proteins

A number of the cloned tumour suppressor loci identified in Table 1 encode proteins that are localized outside the nucleus. Proposed functions for these proteins include the physical linkage of integral membrane proteins to the cytoskeleton (NF2), cytoskeletal organization and adhesion (APC), cell–cell or cell–matrix interactions (DCC), and cytoplasmic signalling (NF1). In general, these classes of protein would be expected to be involved in regulation of cell shape, motility, and anchorage, the reorganization of the cytoplasm, and organelles during cell division, and extra- and intracellular communication.

3.2.1 The *APC* gene in colorectal carcinoma

Three chromosomal regions frequently undergo loss of heterozygocity in colorectal carcinoma, 5q, 17q, and 18q (60). Of these, 5q is now recognized as the site of the predisposing genetic lesions associated with familial adenomatous polyposis (FAP) and Gardiner syndrome (GS) although 5q allele loss is also observed in sporadic colorectal carcinoma, consistent with the inactivation of a tumour suppressor locus. The target gene on 5q has been identified and takes its name, *APC* from the familial condition (adenomatous polyposis coli) in which patients develop pre-cancerous hyperproliferative lesions (polyps) in their colons (61–63). About 70 FAP patients in the UK develop colorectal carcinoma each year. Mutations in *APC* occur in early, benign, adenomas (64, 65) indicating that inactivation of *APC* is a key step in early stages of tumorigenesis. Further progression to the carcinoma stage correlates with LOH affecting 18q and 17p (66). In addition, activation of the dominantly acting onco-gene *RAS* (Chapter 5) appears to be associated with the transition from early to late stage adenomas (67, 68).

APC encodes a 300 kDa cytoplasmic protein (69) which has homology to myosins and keratins in regions that are predicted to form coiled-coil structures. The APC protein can form homo-oligomers via interactions of these amino terminal sequences (70). The potential to form inactive oligomers suggests that a mutant APC molecule could function in a dominant negative fashion, reminiscent of p53 and WT1.

The APC protein binds β-catenin (71), a protein which is part of adherens junctions. These structures are known to mediate adhesion between cells, to communicate signals between neighbouring cells, and to anchor the actin cytoskeleton. In serving these roles, adherens junctions regulate normal cell growth and differentiation. It is possible that the APC–catenin complex regulates transmission of the contact inhibition signal into the cell. This is consistent with the observation that *APC* mutations are associated with the development of hyperplastic lesions (polyps), an early event in tumorigenesis. Inactivation of *APC* may disrupt normal interactions between cells, or between cells and the extracellular matrix, thereby providing a growth advantage.

The two other tumour suppressor loci have been implicated in colorectal carcinoma, *p53* (13, 14) and *DCC* (72), which stands for 'deleted in colorectal carcinoma'. *DCC* encodes a membrane-bound protein related to cellular adhesion molecules (73). However, no colon cancer families have been identified which show linkage to *DCC* and no germ-line *DCC* mutations have been identified. Interestingly, although p53 mutations are common in colorectal carcinoma, very few cases of colorectal carcinoma are seen in Li–Fraumeni families, suggesting that p53 mutations are only advantageous in later stages in the progression of this tumour.

3.2.2 Neurofibromatosis type 2

Neurofibromatosis type 2 (NF2) is characterized by the development of bilateral vestibular schwannomas (74). It occurs at an incidence of 1 in 30 000, and the NF2 susceptibility gene was mapped to chromosome 22 and identified by a positional cloning strategy (75, 76).

The suppressor gene predisposing to Neurofibromatosis type 2 (*NF2* or *SCH*) encodes a protein (merlin/schwannomin) with homology to the erthyrocyte band 4.1 family, suggesting that, like APC and DCC, it may function as a link between membrane proteins (perhaps integrins) and the cytoskeleton (75, 76). Other members of this family are phosphorylated in response to growth factors and may be involved in mediating signal transduction via modulation of cell–cell or cell–matrix interactions.

3.2.3 Neurofibromatosis type 1

Neurofibromatosis type 1 (NF1) is one of the commonest autosomal dominant predispositions to cancer seen in man, affecting about 1 in 2000 people and characterized by multiple benign abnormalities as well as tumours (77). The underlying tumour suppressor gene, *NF1*, has been identified and mapped to band q11.2 on human chromosome 17 (77). LOH of the proximal region of 17q is observed in *NF1*-associated tumours and inactivating mutations are present in the germ-line and in the tumours of familial patients (78–80). Benign neurofibromas and schwannomas remain heterozygous for the *NF1* region suggesting that reduced levels of the encoded protein may result in a growth advantage and complete loss may be involved in the progression of the benign lesion.

The *NF1* gene encodes a protein (neurofibromin) with homology to the yeast IRA proteins (inhibitory regulators of the RAS–cAMP pathway) and mammalian p120^{GAP} (RAS–GTPase–activating protein) (81, 82) suggesting a role in the RAS signalling pathway (see Chapter 5). The neurofibromin catalytic domain is able to compensate for *IRA1* and *IRA2* mutants of *Saccharomyces cerevisiae* and stimulates RAS–GTPase activity (83, 84). Growth stimulatory signals induce RAS to exchange GDP for GTP, switching it from an inactive to an active state. The GAP proteins may serve two functions in the RAS signalling cycle. They may release their own downstream signal as well as enhancing RAS GTPase activity, thus both transducing the signal from and regulating the levels of the effector complex. Loss of neurofibromin would therefore increase the levels of activated RAS and inactivate one of the pathways through which RAS.GTP communicates. Since there are multiple RAS signalling pathways in most cells (85), loss of one signalling pathway could result in over-stimulation of the remaining pathway(s) by the increased levels of RAS.GTP. Loss of function mutations in *NF1* and activating mutations in *RAS* appear to be mutually exclusive (86) suggesting that, as with p53 and MDM2, or p16^{INK4A} and pRB, they may represent alternative ways of achieving the same effects.

3.2.4 Tuberous sclerosis

Tuberous sclerosis is an autosomal dominant predisposition to cancer which has been mapped to two loci: *TSC1* at 9q34.3 and *TSC2* at 16p13.3. Tuberous sclerosis is characterized by the development of multiple growths, described as hamartomata, in many tissues, resulting in a wide variety of symptoms. This variability has probably led to underestimation of its prevalence, which may be as high as 1 in 5800 (87). The *TSC2* gene was recently identified by a positional cloning strategy. The gene is widely expressed and its protein product, tuberin, has a region of homology to the GTPase activating protein GAP3 (88). Like neurofibromin, tuberin is likely to have a role in RAS-dependent signalling pathways.

3.3 Growth factors and receptors

3.3.1 The *RET* gene in MEN2A

Multiple endocrine neoplasia type 2A (MEN2A) is a dominantly inherited cancer syndrome affecting neural ectoderm-derived tissues. Between 20 and 30 cases of meduallary thyroid cancer occur annually in the UK in MEN2A families (89). Like HNPCC, linkage of MEN2A to a chromosomal region (10q11.2) has not been supported by LOH for probes in the same region, suggesting that inactivation of a suppressor allele was not the mechanism predisposing to this cancer syndrome. Indeed, MEN2A is the result of germ-line mutations in the proto-oncogene *RET* (90) which encodes a cell surface receptor for an as yet unknown ligand (see Chapter 3). A high percentage (95%) of mutations in *RET* affect conserved cysteine residues in the extracellular domain of the receptor. Such alterations could modify the conformation of the protein and affect ligand specificity or affinity or change the downstream signal from RET. RET is distantly related to the cadherins, a family of transmembrane molecules that mediate homophilic calcium-dependent cell–cell adhesion (91). Thus, the ligand for RET could be a surface molecule on an adjacent cell, contact with which could result in a growth inhibitory signal. Loss of this signal in cells expressing half mutant/half wild-type RET could lead to enhanced growth. Alternatively, constitutive activation of RET tyrosine kinase activity could lead to growth stimulation of the cell in the absence of ligand.

RET is structurally rearranged in 25% of papillary thyroid carcinomas resulting in the replacement of 5′ *RET* sequences with other expressed sequences (92; and Chapters 1 and 3). These rearrangements tend to produce dominant phenotypes in transfection assays.

MEN2B, a second form of multiple endocrine neoplasia, is also linked to 10q11.2. The genetic lesion responsible for this familial cancer syndrome appears to be an exon 16-specific germ-line alteration in the *RET* gene (93). This is a T to C transition at codon 918, resulting in a methionine to threonine change in the tyrosine kinase domain of the RET protein, presumably altering substrate recognition (89).

3.3.2 *IGFII* in Beckwith Wiedemann syndrome

Beckwith Wiedemann syndrome (BWS) is associated with rearrangements of the chromosome 11p15 region, including trisomy and paternal uniparental disomy, and manifests as multiorgan developmental abnormalities, including an increased risk of Wilms' tumour (94, 95). Familial BWS is a rare autosomal dominant trait showing incomplete penetrance and genetic linkage to 11p15 (96, 97). The tumour-specific LOH that affects 11p15 in Wilms' tumours is unusual in that it is almost always the maternally-derived allele which is lose. This observation is suggestive of an imprinting effect in which the maternally-and paternally-derived alleles of a gene or genes in the region are not functionally equivalent. Thus, in BWS, allele loss does not appear to point to the presence of a tumour suppressor gene, but rather to an imprinting effect.

The gene encoding insulin-like growth factor 2 (*IGFII*) maps to the 11p15 region and the mouse homologue has been shown to be differentially imprinted, with higher levels of expression from the paternal allele (98). Thus, the loss of maternal sequences coupled with duplication of the paternal counterpart results in higher levels of IGFII in Wilms' tumours. The connection between IGFII and BWS is further supported by the observation that imprinting of the *IGFII* gene is constitutively altered in BWS patients (99). Moreover, *IGFII* imprinting is relaxed in Wilms' tumours that do not show LOH at 11p15. In these cases, expression occurs from both maternal and paternal alleles (100, 101), suggesting that overexpression of IGFII plays a role in the aetiology of Wilms' tumour, perhaps via autocrine stimulation of cell growth (see Chapter 2).

3.4 Secreted proteins

It has been suggested that at least one tumour suppressor locus (*BRCA1*) encodes a protein that is related to the granin family and is secreted. It is currently unknown whether these proteins function in an autocrine or paracrine fashion.

3.4.1 *BRCA1* and *BRCA2* in breast and ovarian cancer

Breast cancer susceptibility mutations can be divided into two types: high penetrance and low penetrance. High penetrance susceptibility mutations are extremely rare, but they are important as they are responsible for large 'breast cancer families'. Such mutations increase a woman's lifetime risk of breast cancer from about 10% to greater than 80%. Germ-line mutations in high penetrance susceptibility genes are responsible for approximately a third of breast cancers diagnosed before the age of 30. This proportion falls to about 1% of cases diagnosed after the age of 80. Overall, about 6% of breast cancer cases are due to germ-line mutations in high penetrance suscepti-bility genes (102). Three high penetrance genes have been identified in breast cancer:

p53, *BRCA1*, and *BRCA2*. However, it is probable that a greater proportion of breast cancers are attributable to genes carrying low penetrance susceptibility mutations, as they are likely to be present in the population at a higher frequency (192). The *ATM* gene (see Section 3.1.7) would be an obvious example of such a gene.

In the USA and Western Europe approximately 1 in 12 women develop breast cancer and it has been estimated that about 5% of these cases are the result of inherited mutations in either *BRCA1* or *BRCA2* (103). The *BRCA1* gene on chromosome 17q21 is responsible for an autosomal dominant susceptibility to breast and ovarian cancer and was identified by a positional cloning strategy (104, 105). *BRCA1* encodes a 1863 amino acid protein which has two regions of significant similarity to known proteins: a RING-finger motif near its amino terminus (amino acids 24–64) and a granin consensus at amino acids 1214–1223 (196). Female carriers of *BRCA1* mutations have about a 85% lifetime risk of breast cancer (103). It has been shown that in families in which the *BRCA1* mutations are in the 3' third of the gene, after the granin motif, a lower proportion of ovarian cancers is observed among the carriers (107, 108). These findings indicate that mutant BRCA1 proteins which retain the granin sequence also retain partial function in ovarian epithelial cells. *BRCA1* mRNA has been found to be expressed at five- to tenfold higher levels in normal breast tissue than in invasive breast cancer and expression is markedly decreased during the transition from carcinoma *in situ* to invasive carcinoma (109).

The *BRCA2* gene on chromosome 13q12-q13 is responsible for an autosomal dominant susceptibility to both female and male breast cancer (110). The risk of female breast cancer is similar to that conferred by *BRCA1*, but the risk of ovarian cancer is substantially lower, and the risk of male breast cancer considerably higher. The *BRCA2* gene has recently been identified, and shown to encode a 3418 amino acid protein (111, 112). The BRCA2 protein also has a granin motif, at amino acids 3334–3344 (106). Many germ-line mutations have been identified in breast cancer families, in male breast cancer cases, and in female breast and ovarian cancer cases. As these are putative loss of function mutations, it would appear that like *BRCA1*, *BRCA2* is a tumour suppressor gene. This is additionally supported by the loss of the *BRCA2* region in sporadic breast cancer and homozygous deletion of the *BRCA2* gene in a sporadic pancreatic tumour (113).

4. Conclusions

The spectrum of genes involved in familial susceptibility to cancer is broad, with functions as diverse as growth factors, receptors, cytoplasmic organizers, signal transducers, nuclear factors, and secreted growth inhibitors. The tumour suppressor genes appear to encode products that regulate unrestricted growth by transducing inhibitory growth signals or limiting the efficacy of stimulatory signals. Investigation of the mechanisms through which the tumour suppressor genes act has resulted in functional links with the dominant oncogenes. For example, both pRB and p53 are targets of oncoproteins encoded by DNA tumour viruses and may in turn regulate the expression of or bind directly to the products of cellular proto-oncogenes, such as *MDM2* (see Chapters 8 and 9). *WT1* may inhibit the expression of early response genes through binding to the same DNA sequence as the EGR1 transcription factor (Chapter 6). Neurofibromin potentiates RAS by stimulating GTPase activity and, possibly, by acting as a downstream effector molecule (see Chapter 5). In MEN2A, the target of predisposing germ-line mutations is a dominant oncogene of the tyrosine kinase receptor family, and in HNPCC a dominant alteration is expected in a DNA repair or replication gene.

The division between dominant and recessive mutations becomes blurred in some cases. For example, the oligomerization of p53 can lead to the formation of non-functional complexes between mutant and wild-type proteins. Other tumour suppressor products with the potential for protein–protein interactions, such as APC and WT1, may also act in this dominant negative fashion. The introduction of a normal allele of a tumour suppressor locus into cells lacking any normal product from that locus has unequivocally demonstrated the dominant effects of wild-type pRB and p53.

A number of additional loci that are responsible for a high penetrance predisposition to cancer are likely to be identified within the next few years. Pedigree studies indicate the presence of additional genes for breast and ovarian cancer (*BRCA3*) and for non-polyposis colon cancer. The search is already underway for a gene or genes for pancreatic cancer and for prostate cancer (*PRCA1*), the chromosome 1 melanoma susceptibility locus, a testicular cancer susceptibility locus, and the genes for MEN type 1 and Gorlin syndrome. It is possible that there are also high penetrance susceptibility genes for lung cancer and head and neck cancer, as these diseases show familial clustering. Additionally, more genes which give a low penetrance susceptibility to cancer will be mapped, probably as a result of animal studies. Although the cancer risk associated with mutant alleles at these loci will not be great, the high frequency of the mutant alleles could mean that these genes are responsible for a greater proportion of cancers than the rare high penetrance susceptibility genes.

The isolation of these genes will enable the identification of individuals who carry high risk alleles. Such individuals could then be put forward for either intensive screening (both conventional medical and molecular) and for the option of prophylactic removal of any non-essential target tissue for the disease. Additionally, new opportunities for diagnosis and possibly treatment of sporadic, as well as familial cancers will become possible. Molecular diagnosis may become available for specific cancers, by detecting the mutant genes or their products in circulating blood, smears, or microscopic quantities of biopsied material, and in the case of colorectal cancer, in cells shed into the faeces. Understanding the cellular pathways in which the products of susceptibility genes participate will clearly be important in our understanding of the molecular changes involved in carcinogenesis. Interacting proteins and downstream targets of susceptibility gene products could also provide useful markers in the early diagnosis of cancer. In the longer-term, gene therapy approaches could be used either to treat somatic disease, or to replace mutant cancer susceptibility alleles with the wild-type copy of the gene.

References

1. Knudson, A. G. (1986) Genetics of human cancer. *Annu. Rev. Genet.*, **20**, 231.
2. Knudson, A. G. (1971) Mutation and cancer: Statistical study of retinoblastoma. *Proc. Natl. Acad. Sci. USA*, **68**, 820.
3. Knudson, A. G. and Strong, L. C. (1972) Mutation and cancer: A model for Wilms' tumor of the kidney. *J. Natl. Cancer Inst.*, **48**, 313.
4. Knudson, A. G. and Strong, L. C. (1972) Mutation and cancer: Neuroblastoma and pheochromocytoma. *Am. J. Hum. Genet.*, **24**, 514.
5. Armitage, P. and Doll, R. (1954) The age distribution of cancer and a multi-stage theory of carcinogenesis. *Br. J. Cancer*, **8**, 1.
6. Ashley, D. J. B. (1969) The two 'hit' theory of carcinogenesis. *Br. J. Cancer*, **23**, 313.
7. Friend, S. H., Bernards, R., Rogeli, S., Weinberg, R. A., Rapaport, J. M., Alberts, D. M., *et al.* (1986) A human DNA segment with properties of the gene that predisposes to retinoblastoma. *Nature*, **323**, 643.
8. Friend, S. H., Horowitz, J. M., Gerber, M. R., Wang, X.-F., Bogenmann, E., Li, F. P., *et al.* (1987) Deletions of a DNA sequence in retinoblastomas and mesenchymal tumors: Organization of the sequence and its encoded protein. *Proc. Natl. Acad. Sci. USA*, **84**, 9059.
9. Weinberg, R. A. (1995) The retinoblastoma protein and cell cycle control. *Cell*, **81**, 323.
10. Wang, J. Y. J., Knudsen, E. S., and Welch, P. J. (1994) The retinoblastoma tumor suppressor protein. *Adv. Cancer Res.*, **64**, 25.
11. Sherr, C. J. (1993) Mammalian G1 cyclins. *Cell*, **73**, 1059.
12. Goddard, A. D. and Solomon, E. (1993) Genetic aspects of cancer. In *Advances in human genetics* (ed. H. H. A. K. Hirschhorn), pp. 321–76. Plenum Press: New York.
13. Hollstein, M., Sidransky, D., Vogelstein, B., and Harris, C. C. (1991) p53 mutation in human cancer. *Science*, **253**, 49.
14. de Fromentel, C. C. and Soussi, T. (1992) *TP53* tumor suppressor gene: A model for investigating human mutagenesis. *Genes Chrom. Cancer*, **4**, 1.
15. Malkin, D., Li, F. P., Strong, L. C., Fraumeni, J. F., Nelson, C. E., Kim, D. H. *et al.* Germline p53 mutations in a familial syndrome of breast cancer, sarcomas, and other neoplasms. *Science*, **250**, 1233.
16. Srivastava, S., Zou, Z., Pirollo, K., Blattner, W., and Chang, E. H. (1990) Germ-line transmission of a mutated p53 gene in a cancer-prone family with Li-Fraumeni syndrome. *Nature*, **348**, 747.
17. Oliner, J. D., Pietenpol, J. A., Thiagalingam, S., Gyuris, J., Kinzler, K. W., and Vogelstein, B. (1993) Oncoprotein MDM2 conceals the activation domain of tumour suppressor p53. *Nature*, **362**, 857.
18. Maheswaran, S., Park, S., Barnard, A., Morris, J. F., Rauscher, F. J. III, Hill, D. E., *et al.* (1993) Physical and functional interaction between WT1 and p53 proteins. *Proc. Natl. Acad. Sci. USA*, **90**, 5100.
19. Reifenberger, G., Liu, L., Ichimura, K., Schmidt, E. E., and Collins, V. P. (1993) Amplification and overexpression of the *MDM2* gene in a subset of human malignant gliomas without p53 mutations. *Cancer Res.*, **53**, 2736.
20. Lane, D. P. (1992) p53, guardian of the genome. *Nature*, **358**, 15.
21. Sherr, C. J. and Roberts, J. M. (1995) Inhibitors of mammalian G1 cyclin-dependent kinases. *Genes Dev.*, **9**, 1149.

22. Herskowitz, I. (1987) Functional inactivation of genes by dominant negative mutations. *Nature*, **329**, 219.
23. Green, M. R. (1989) When the products of oncogenes and anti-oncogenes meet. *Cell*, **56**, 1.
24. Donehower, L. A., Harvey, M., Slagle, B. L., McArthur, M. K., Montgomery, C. A. J., Butel, J. S., *et al.* (1992) Mice deficient for p53 are developmentally normal but susceptible to spontaneous tumours. *Nature*, **356**, 215.
25. Breslow, N., Beckwith, J. B., Ciol, M., and Shaples, K. (1988) Age distribution of Wilms' Tumor: Report from the National Wilms' Tumor Study. *Cancer Res.*, **48**, 1653.
26. Miller, R. W., Fraumeni, J. F. J., and Manning, M. D. (1964) Association of Wilms' tumor with aniridia, hemihypertrophy and other congenital malformations. *N. Engl. J. Med.*, **270**, 922.
27. Riccardi, V. M., Sujansky, E., Smith, A. C., and Franke, U. (1978) Chromosomal imbalance in the aniridia-Wilms' tumor association: 11p interstitial deletion. *Pediatrics*, **61**, 604.
28. Denys, P., Malvaux, P., van den Berghe, H., Tanghe, W., and Proesmans, W. (1967) Association d'un syndrome anatomo-pathologique de pseudohermaphrodisme masculin, d'une tumeur de Wilms, d'une nephropathie parenchymateuse et d'un mosaicisme XX/XY. *Arch. Fran. Ped.*, **24**, 729.
29. Drash, A., Sherman, F., Hartmann, W. H., and Blizzard, R. M. (1970) A syndrome of pseudohermaphroditism, Wilms' tumor, hypertension and degenerative renal disease. *J. Ped.*, **76**, 585.
30. Bonetta, L., Kuehn, S. E., Huang, A., Law, D. J., Kalikin, L. M., Koi, M., *et al.* (1990) Wilms tumor locus on 11p13 defined by multiple CpG island-associated transcripts. *Science*, **250**, 994.
31. Call, K. M., Glaser, T., Ito, C. Y., Buckler, A. J., Pelletier, J., Haber, D. A., *et al.* (1990) Isolation and characterization of a zinc finger polypeptide gene at the human chromosome 11 Wilms' tumor locus. *Cell*, **60**, 509.
32. Gessler, M., Poustka, A., Cavenee, W., Neve, R. L., Orkin, S. H., and Bruns, G. A. P. (1990) Homozygous deletion in Wilms' tumours of a zinc-finger gene identified by chromosome jumping. *Nature*, **343**, 774.
33. Pelletier, J., Bruening, W., Kashtan, C. E., Mauer, S. M., Manivel, J. C., Striegel, J. E., *et al.* (1991) Germline mutations in the Wilms' tumor suppressor gene are associated with abnormal urogenital development in Denys-Drash syndrome. *Cell*, **67**, 437.
34. Rauscher, F. J. III, Morris, J. F., Tournay, O. E., Cook, D. M., and Curran, T. (1990) Binding of the Wilms' tumor locus zinc finger protein to the EGR-1 consensus sequence. *Science*, **250**, 1259.
35. Madden, S. L., Cook, D. M., Morris, J. F., Gashler, A., Sukhatme, V. P., and Rauscher, F. J. III (1991) Transcriptional repression mediated by the WT1 Wilms-tumor gene-product. *Science*, **253**, 1550.
36. Pritchard-Jones, K., Fleming, S., Davidson, D., Bickmore, W., Porteous, D., Gosden, C., *et al.* (1990) The candidate Wilms' tumour gene is involved in genitourinary development. *Nature*, **346**, 194.
37. van Heyningen, V., Bickmore, W. A., Seawright, A., Fletcher, J. M., Maule, J., Fekete, G., *et al.* (1990) Role for the Wilms tumor gene in genital development? *Proc. Natl. Acad. Sci. USA*, **87**, 5383.
38. Skolnick, M. H., Cannon-Albright, L. A., and Kamb, A. (1994) Genetic predisposition to melanoma. *Eur. J. Cancer*, **30A**, 1991.

39. Hussussain, C. J., Struewing, J. P., Goldstein, A. M., Higgins, P. A. T., Ally, D. S., Shaehan, M. D., *et al.* (1994) Germline p16 mutations in familial melanoma. *Nat. Genet.*, **8**, 15.

40. Kamb, A., Shattuck-Eidens, D., Eeles, R., Liu, Q., Gruis, N. A., Ding, W., *et al.* (1994) Analysis of the p16 gene (*CDKN2*) as a candidate for the chromosome 9p melanoma susceptibility locus. *Nat. Genet.*, **8**, 22.

41. Zuo, L., Weger, J., Tang, Q., Goldstein, A. M., Tucker, M. A., Walker, G. J., *et al.* (1996) Germline mutations in the p16^{INK4a} binding domain of CDK4 in familial melanoma. *Nat. Genet.*, **12**, 97.

42. Peltomäki, P., Aaltonen, L. A., Sistonen, P., Pylkkanen, L., Mecklin, J. P., Jarvinen, H., *et al.* (1993) Genetic mapping of a locus predisposing to human colorectal cancer. *Science*, **260**, 810.

43. Aaltonen, L. A., Peltomäki, P., Leach, F. S., Sistonen, P., Pylkkanen, L., Mecklin, J. P., *et al.* (1993) Clues to the pathogenesis of familial colorectal cancer. *Science*, **260**, 812.

44. Ionov, Y., Peinado, M. A., Malkhosyan, S., Shibata, D., and Perucho, M. (1993) Ubiquitous somatic mutations in simple repeated sequences reveal a new mechanism for colonic carcinogenesis. *Nature*, **363**, 558.

45, Thibodeau, S. N., Bren, G., and Schaid, D. (1993) Microsatellite instability in cancer of the proximal colon. *Science*, **260**, 816.

46. Fishel, R., Lescoe, M. K., Rao, M. R. S., Copeland, N. G., Jenkins, N. A., Garber, J., *et al.* (1993) The human mutator gene homolog MSH2 and its association with hereditary nonpolyposis colon cancer. *Cell*, **75**, 1027.

47. Leach, F. S., Nicolaides, N. C., Papadopoulos, N., Lui, B., Jen, J., Parsons, R., *et al.* (1993) Mutations of the mutS homolog in hereditary nonpolyposis colon cancer. *Cell*, **75**, 1215.

48. Bishop, D. T. and Hall, N. R. (1994) The genetics of colorectal cancer. *Eur. J. Cancer*, **30A**, 1946.

49. Bronner, C. E., Baker, S. M., Morrison, P. T., Warren, G., Smith, L. G., Lescoe, M. K., *et al.* (1994) Mutation in the DNA mismatch repair gene homologue *hMLH1* is associated with hereditary non-polyposis colon cancer. *Nature*, **368**, 258.

50. Papadopoulos, N., Nicolaides, N. C., Wei, T-F., Ruben, S. M., Carter, K. C., Rosen, C. A., *et al.* (1994) Mutation of a *mutL* homolog in hereditary colon cancer. *Science*, **263**, 1625.

51. Nicolaides, N. C., Papadopoulos, N., Lui, B., Wei, Y-F., Carter, K. C., Ruben, S. M., *et al.* (1994) Mutations of two *PMS* homologues in hereditary nonpolyposis colon cancer. *Nature*, **371**, 75.

52. Maher, E. R. (1994) Von Hippel-Lindau Disease. *Eur. J. Cancer*, **30A**, 1987.

53. Latif, F., Tory, K., Gnarra, J., Yao, M., Duh, F. M., Orcutt, M. L., *et al.* (1993) Identification of the von Hippel-Lindau disease tumor suppressor gene. *Science*, **260**, 1317.

54. Duan, R. X., Pause, A., Burgess, W. H., Aso, J., Chen, D. T., Garrett, K. P., *et al.* (1995) Inhibition of transcription elongation by the VHL tumor suppressor protein. *Science*, **269**, 1402.

55. Krumm, A. and Groudine, M. (1995) Tumor suppression and transcription termination: the dire consequences of changing partners. *Science*, **269**, 1400.

56. Harnden, D. G. (1994) The nature of ataxia-telangiectasia: problems and perspectives. *Int. J. Radiat. Biol.*, **66**, S13.

57. Savinsky, K., Bar-Shira, A., Gilard, S., Rotman, G., Ziv, Y., Vanagaite, L., *et al.* (1995) A single ataxia-telangiectasia gene with a product similar to PI-3 kinase. *Science*, **268**, 1749.

58. Savinsky, K., Sfez, S., Tagle, D. A., Ziv, Y., Sartiel, A., Collins, F. S., *et al.* (1995) The complete sequence of the coding region of the ATM gene reveals similarity to cell cycle regulators in different species. *Hum. Mol. Genet.*, **4**, 2025.

59. Zakian, V. A. (1995) *ATM*-related genes: what do they tell us about functions of the human gene? *Cell*, **82**, 685.

60. Vogelstein, B., Fearon, E. R., Kern, S. E., Hamilton, S. R., Preisinger, A. C., Nakamura, Y., *et al.* (1989) Allelotypes of colorectal carcinomas. *Science*, **244**, 207.

61. Groden, J., Thliveris, A., Samowitz, W., Carlson, M., Gelbert, L., Albertsen, H., *et al.* (1991) Identification and characterization of the familial adenomatous polyposis coli gene. *Cell*, **66**, 589.

62. Miyoshi, Y., Ando, H., Nagese, H., Nishisho, I., Horii, A., Miki, Y., *et al.* (1992) Germline mutations of the APC gene in 53 familial adenomatous polyposis patients. *Proc. Natl. Acad. Sci. USA*, **89**, 4452.

63. Nishisho, I., Nakamura, Y., Miyoshi, Y., Miki, Y., Ando, H., Horii, A. (1991) Mutations of chromosome 5q21 genes in FAP and colorectal cancer patients. *Science*, **253**, 665.

64. Powell, S. M., Zilz, N., Beazer-Barclay, Y., Bryan, T. M., Hamilton, S. R., Thibodeau, S. N., *et al.* (1992) *APC* mutations occur early during colorectal tumorigenesis. *Nature*, **359**, 235.

65. Rees, M., Leigh, S. E. A., Delhanty, J. D. A., and Jass, J. R. (1989) Chromosome 5 allele loss in familial and sporadic colorectal adenomas. *Br. J. Cancer*, **59**, 361.

66. Vogelstein, B., Fearon, E. R., Kern, S. E., Hamilton, S. R., Preisinger, A. C., Leppert, M., *et al.* (1988) Genetic alterations during colorectal-tumor development. *N. Engl. J. Med.*, **319**, 525.

67. Bos, J. L., Fearon, E. R., Hamilton, S. R., Verlaan-de Vries, M., van Boom, J. H., van der Eb, A. J., *et al.* (1987) Prevalence of ras gene mutations in human colorectal cancers. *Nature*, **327**, 293.

68. Forrester, K., Almoguera, C., Han, K., Grizzle, W. E., and Perucho, M. (1987) Detection of high incidence of K-ras oncogene mutations during human colon tumorigenesis. *Nature*, **327**, 298.

69. Smith, K. J., Johnson, K. A., Bryan, T. M., Hill, D. E., Markowitz, S., Wilson, J. K., *et al.* (1993) The *APC* gene product in normal and tumor cells. *Proc. Natl. Acad. Sci. USA*, **90**, 2846.

70. Su, L.-K., Johnson, K. A., Smith, K. J., Hill, D. E., Vogelstein, B., and Kinzler, K. W. (1993) Association between wild type and mutant *APC* gene products. *Cancer Res.*, **53**, 2728.

71. Su, L.-K., Vogelstein, B., and Kinzler, K. W. (1993) Association of the APC tumor suppressor protein with catenins. *Science*, **262**, 1734.

72. Fearon, E. R., Cho, K. R., Nigro, J. M., Kern, S. E., Simons, J. W., Ruppert, J. M., *et al.* (1990) Identification of a chromosome 18q gene that is altered in colorectal cancers. *Science*, **247**, 49.

73. Hedrick, L., Cho, K. R., Fearon, E. R., Wu, T-C., Kinzler, K. W., and Vogelstein, B. (1994) The DCC gene product in cellular differentiation and colorectal tumorigenesis. *Genes Dev.*, **8**, 1174.

74. Thomas, G., Merel, P., Sanson, K., Hoang-Xuan, K., Zucman, J., Desmaze, C., *et al.* (1994) Neurofibromatosis type 2. *Eur. J. Cancer*, **30A**, 1981.

75. Rouleau, G. A., Merel, P., Lutchman, M., Sanson, M., Zucman, J., Marineau, C., *et al.* (1993) Alteration in a new gene encoding a putative membrane-organizing protein causes neuro-fibromatosis type 2. *Nature*, **363**, 515.

76. Trofatter, J. A., MacCollin, M. M., Rutter, J. L., Murrell, J. R., Duyao, M. P., Parry, D. M., *et al.* (1993) A novel moesin- ezrin-, radixin-like gene is a candidate for the neurofibromatosis 2 tumor suppressor. *Cell*, **72**, 791.

77. Coleman, S. D. and Wallace, M. R. (1994) Neurofibromatosis type 1. *Eur. J. Cancer*, **30A**, 1974.

78. Cawthon, R. M., Weiss, R., Xu, G. F., Viskochil, D., Culver, M., Stevens, J., *et al.* (1990) A major segment of the neurofibromatosis type 1 gene: cDNA sequence, genomic structure, and point mutations. *Cell*, **62**, 193.

79. Viskochil, D., Buchberg, A. M., Xu, G., Cawthon, R. M., Stevens, J., Wolff, R. K., *et al.* (1990) Deletions and a translocation interrupt a cloned gene at the neurofibromatosis type 1 locus. *Cell*, **62**, 187.

80. Wallace, M. R., Marchuk, D. A., Andersen, L. B., Letcher, R., Odeh, H. M., Saulino, A. M., *et al.* (1990) Type 1 neurofibromatosis gene: identification of a large transcript disrupted in three NF1 patients. *Science*, **249**, 181.

81. Buchberg, A. M., Cleveland, L. S., Jenkins, N. A., and Copeland, N. G. (1990) Sequence homology shared by neurofibromatosis type-1 gene and IRA-1 and IRA-2 negative regulators of the RAS cyclic pathway. *Nature*, **347**, 291.

82. Xu, G. F., O'Connell, P., Viskochil, D., Cawthon, R., Robertson, M., Culver, M., *et al.* (1990) The neurofibromatosis type 1 gene encodes a protein related to GAP. *Cell*, **62**, 599.

83. Wu, G. F., Lin, B., Tanaka, K., Dunn, D., Wood, D., Gesteland, R., *et al.* (1990) The catalytic domain of the neurofibromatosis type 1 gene product stimulates ras GRPase and complements ira mutants of *S. cerevisiae*. *Cell*, **63**, 835.

84. Ballester, R., Marchuk, D., Boguski, M., Saulino, A., Letcher, R., Wigler, M., *et al.* (1990) The NF1 locus encodes a protein functionally related to mammalian GAP and yeast IRA proteins. *Cell*, **63**, 851.

85. Bollag, G. and McCormick, F. (1992) NF is enough of GAP. *Nature*, **356**, 663.

86. DeClue, J. E., Papageorge, A. G., Fletcher, J. A., Diehl, S. R., Ratner, N., Vass, W. C., *et al.* (1992) Abnormal regulation of mammalian p21ras contributes to malignant tumor growth in von Recklinghausen (type 1) neurofibromatosis. *Cell*, **69**, 265.

87. Osborne, J. P., Fryer, A., and Webb, D. (1991) Epidemiology of tuberous sclerosis. *Annl. N. Y. Acad. Sci.*, **615**, 125.

88. The European chromosome 16 tuberous sclerosis consortium (1993) Identification and characterization of the tuberous sclerosis gene on chromosome 16. *Cell*, **75**, 1305.

89. Forster-Gibson, C. J. and Mulligan, L. M. (1994) Multiple endocrine neoplasia type 2. *Eur. J. Cancer*, **30A**, 1969.

90. Mulligan, L. M., Kwok, J. B. J., Healey, C. S., Elsdon, M. J., Eng, C., Gardner, E., *et al.* (1993) Germ-line mutations of the RET proto-oncogene in multiple endocrine neoplasia type 2A. *Nature*, **363**, 458.

91. Schneider, R. (1992) The human protooncogene *ret*: a communicative cadherin? *Trends Biochem. Sci.*, **17**, 468.

92. Fusco, A., Grieco, M., Santoro, M., Berlingieri, M. T., Pilotti, S., Pierotti, M. A., *et al.* (1987) A new oncogene in human thyroid papillary carcinomas and their lymph-nodal metastases. *Nature*, **328**, 170.

93. Hofstra, R. M., Landsvater, R. M., and Ceccherini, I. (1995) A mutation in the *RET* proto-oncogene associated with multiple endocrine neoplasia type 2B and sporadic medullary thyroid carcinoma. *Nature*, **367**, 375.

94. Sotelo-Avila, C. and Gooch, W. M. (1976) Neoplasms associated with the Beckwith-Wiedemann syndrome. *Perspect. Pediatr. Pathol.*, **3**, 255.

95. Henry, I., Bonaiti-Pellié, C., Chehensse, V., Beldjord, C., Schwartz, C., Utermann, G., *et al.* (1991) Uniparental paternal disomy in a genetic cancer-predisposing syndrome. *Nature*, **351**, 665.

96. Koufos, A., Grundy, P., Morgan, K., Aleck, K. A., Hadro, T., Lampkin, B. C., *et al.* (1989) Familial Wiedemann-Beckwith syndrome and a second Wilms tumor locus both map to 11p15.5. *Am. J. Hum. Genet.*, **44**, 711.

97. Ping, A. J., Reeve, A. E., Law, D. J., Young, M. R., Boehnke, M., and Feinberg, A. P. (1989) Genetic linkage of Beckwith-Wiedemann syndrome to 11p15. *Am. J. Hum. Genet.*, **44**, 720.

98. DeChiara, T. M., Robertson, E. J., and Efstratiadis, A. (1991) Paternal imprinting of the mouse insulin-like growth factor II gene. *Cell*, **64**, 849.

99. Weksberg, R., Shen, D. R., Fei, Y. L., Song, Q. L., and Squire, J. (1993) Disruption of insulin-like growth factor 2 imprinting in Beckwith-Wiedemann syndrome. *Nat. Genet.*, **5**, 143.

100. Ogawa, O., Eccles, M. R., Szeto, J., McNoe, L. A., Yun, K., Maw, M. A., *et al.* (1993) Relaxation of insulin-like growth factor II gene imprinting implicated in Wilms' tumour. *Nature*, **362**, 749.

101. Rainier, S., Johnson, L. A., Dobry, C. J., Ping, A. J., Grundy, P. E., and Feinberg, A. P. (1993) Relaxation of imprinted genes in human cancer. *Nature*, **362**, 747.

102. Black, D. M. (1994) The genetics of breast cancer. *Eur. J. Cancer*, **30A**, 1957.

103. Szabo, C. I. and King, M-C. (1995) Inherited breast and ovarian cancer. *Hum. Mol. Genet.*, **4**, 1811.

104. Hall, J. M., Lee, M. K., Newman, B., Morrow, J. E., Anderson, L. A., Huey, B., *et al.* (1990) Linkage of early-onset familial breast cancer to chromosome 17q21. *Science*, **250**, 1684.

105. Miki, Y., Swensen, J., Shattuck-Eidens, D., Futreal, P. A., Harshman, K., Tavtigian, S., *et al.* (1994) A strong candidate for the breast and ovarian cancer gene *BRCA1*. *Science*, **266**, 66.

106. Jensen, R. A., Thompson, M. E., Jettson, T. L., Szabo, C., van der Meer, R., Helou, B., *et al.* (1996) *BRCA1* is secreted and exhibits properties of a granin. *Nat. Genet.*, **12**, 303.

107. Gayther, S. A., Warren, W., Mazoyer, S., Russell, P. A., Harrington, P. A., Chiano, M., *et al.* (1995) Germline mutations of the *BRCA1* gene in breast and ovarian cancer families provide evidence for a genotype-phenotype correlation. *Nat. Genet.*, **11**, 428.

108. Holt, J. T., Thompson, M. E., Szabo, C., Robinson-Benion, C., Artega, C. L., King, M-C., *et al.* (1996) Growth retardation and tumour inhibition by *BRCA1*. *Nat. Genet.*, **12**, 298.

109. Thompson, M. E., Jensen, R. A., Obermiller, P. S., Page, D. L., and Holt, J. T. (1995) Decreased expression of *BRCA1* accelerates growth and is often present during sporadic breast cancer progression. *Nat. Genet.*, **9**, 444.

110. Wooster, R., Neuhausen, S., Mangion, J., Quirk, Y., Ford, D., Collins, N., *et al.* (1994) Localisation of a breast cancer susceptibility gene, *BRCA2*, to chromosome 13q12–13. *Science*, **265**, 2088.

111. Wooster, R., Bignel, G., Lancaster, J., Swift, S., Seal, S., Mangion, J., (1995) Identification of the breast cancer susceptibility gene *BRCA2*. *Nature*, **378**, 789.

112. Tavtigian, S., Simard, J., Rommens, J., Couch, F., Shattuck-Eidens, D., Neuhaussen, S., *et al.* (1996) The complete *BRCA2* gene sequence and mutations in chromosome 13q-linked kindreds. *Nat. Genet.*, **12**, 333.

113. Schutte, M., Rozenblum, E., Moskaluk, C. A., Juan, X., Hoque, A. T. M. S., Hahn, S. A., *et al.* (1995) An integrated high resolution physical map of the DPC/BRCA2 region at chromosome 13q12. *Cancer Res.*, **55**, 4570.

11 | Clinical relevance of oncogenes

KAROL SIKORA and HARDEV PANDHA

1. Introduction

In most developed countries, one person in three will develop cancer during their lifetime. This will increase to one in two by the year 2010, reflecting shifts in the age characteristics of the population. The disease represents a considerable public health problem. The term 'cancer' comprises over 200 disorders which differ in their genetic basis, aetiology, clinical characteristics, patterns of progression, and final outcome to sufficient degrees to be classified as separate entities. Genetic alterations are at the very centre of tumorigenesis so that, at a cellular level, cancer can be designated a genetic disorder. As we have seen from the preceding chapters, the last decade has witnessed remarkable progress in our understanding of the molecular pathogenesis of cancer. This knowledge, however, has yet to have a significant positive impact on the treatment and survival of affected individuals. It is clear that we are poised to exploit our new knowledge across the whole field of oncology—from prevention through screening and diagnosis to the development of logically based molecular therapies. Here we will consider current clinical problems and discuss how a greater understanding of the molecular biology of specific cancer types could help in their management in the clinic. We then consider colorectal cancer in some detail as an example of how molecular technology is beginning to impinge on clinical practice.

2. Current clinical problems

The last two decades have brought little gain in terms of survival benefit to patients with most types of cancer. We urgently need new approaches to solve many dilemmas in cancer patient care and to reduce the incidence of the disease in the population.

2.1 Prevention

The prevention of cancer requires a detailed understanding of the potentially reversible lifestyle factors involved in the aetiology of specific tumours. Whilst epidemiological investigations can be informative, it may be possible to explore certain questions in greater depth using molecular techniques. This in turn could lead to more precise targeting of educational and public health intervention. The discovery, for example, that certain *RAS* mutations are more frequently associated with radon-induced lung cancer may refine the relationship between exposure to environmental radon and cancer, leading to new guidelines (1). Similarly, an understanding of the progressive genetic changes in colorectal cancer could help in monitoring interventional dietary manipulation studies in high risk patient groups (2). There is good evidence for the existence of cancer preventing agents in plants (3). Their mode of action is unclear but they are almost certainly responsible for beneficial effects of a high fruit and vegetable-containing diet on cancer incidence in a population. A detailed analysis of the genetic mechanisms involved in their action could lead to new approaches to promote genetic stability, so reducing cancer incidence.

2.2 Screening

Whereas local tumours can be destroyed effectively by surgery or radiotherapy, metastatic disease requires systemic therapy. As this is relatively ineffective in patients with common solid tumours, it is logical to try to identify patients with early stage disease, so improving the chances of local control and thus cure. Unfortunately many of the current screening programmes are not very efficient. Mammographic screening for breast cancer is a good example (4). Taking multiple X-rays of the breast is a time-consuming and costly method to try to reduce the stage of presentation of breast cancer in a population. Regular screening is relatively non-specific, identifying many benign lesions requiring further investigation and biopsy. Large studies have shown that mammographic screening has only a small effect on overall breast cancer mortality and only in the 50–64 age group. Another example of relatively ineffective screening is the use of the biochemical tumour marker, prostate-specific antigen (PSA), to identify men with asymptomatic prostate cancer (5). A large percentage of men over 50 years old actually have prostate cancer, but it remains confined to the prostate gland and is of no significance to their health. Identifying and removing these localized tumours may not have any beneficial effect on overall survival as death is mainly caused by the effects of metastatic disease. Molecular techniques could resolve some of these dilemmas in several ways. First, genetic screening could identify high risk patient groups who might benefit from more intensive screening as well as inclusion in trials of preventive agents. Secondly, true indicators of the likely metastatic potential of a cancer may become available and provide a rationale for more aggressive therapy. Again an understanding of the progressive accumulation of genetic damage seen in breast, pancreatic, thyroid, and colorectal cancer could lead to novel pre-cancer detection systems. An example would be the identification by PCR of mutant *RAS* sequences in faecal material (6).

2.3 Diagnosis

The diagnosis of cancer is usually based on the recognition of aberrant cellular patterns in a biopsy sample by a histopathologist. Increasingly, the cytological examination of fine needle aspirates is being used not only to make the diagnosis but also to evaluate the sites of spread, a process called staging. Fine needles can be inserted, often under radiological guidance, into any part of the body. The problem of course is that the aspirated material may contain only very few cells and these may be structurally damaged by the aspiration process. Although immunocytochemistry may be of help, it often produces confusing results because of the altered nature of the removed material. DNA or protein-based assays may be more effective under these circumstances. The use of PCR to detect mutant *RAS* genes in a fine needle aspirate from a pancreatic mass is one example of attempts to use our knowledge of oncogenes for clinical purposes (7).

2.4 Guiding treatment decisions

Individualizing the treatment plan is based on a combination of diagnostic information, clinical experience, and a retrospective review of similar patient groups. Information on the abnormal expression of oncogenes and tumour suppressor genes may provide additional guidance. The biggest problem is the choice of whether to give adjuvant systemic therapy after apparently successful tumour resection. In breast cancer, for example, a variety of criteria are used including the patient's menopausal status, the differentiation of the tumour, and the presence of micrometastases in axillary lymph nodes (8). There are many possible adjuvant therapies which vary considerably in their toxicity, ranging from oral tamoxifen, through combination chemotherapy, to bone marrow ablation with peripheral blood stem cell rescue. Although clinical trials are now well established, their power would be enhanced if further subgrouping of patients could be made using molecular prognostic factors derived from the growth control apparatus of the cell. Examples could include the amplification of *MYC*, *ERBB2*, or cyclin D1 and the status of the pRB, p53, and p16 tumour suppressors, as discussed in other chapters.

Similarly, in colorectal cancer, adjuvant therapy with 5-fluorouracil has been shown to increase survival when the primary tumour extends through the bowel wall (9). Refining subgroups here could lead to better guidance. It is also possible that new molecular markers could provide better prognostic indicators generally—information that the patient might find valuable in planning for their future.

2.5 New systemic treatments

Ultimately the dissection of the oncogene pathway, as discussed in previous chapters, should lead to novel targets for logical drug design. Many groups are active in this area and potential targets for development include:

- synthetic growth factor receptor inhibitory ligands
- receptor dimerization inhibitors
- cell adhesion stabilizers
- tyrosine kinase inhibitors
- RAS inhibitors
- MAP kinase blockers
- transcription factor blockers
- small molecule mimicry of tumour suppressor products
- apoptosis stimulating agents

Our current range of anti-cancer drugs has been discovered by screening large numbers of chemicals and biologically-derived extracts on cell lines and then animal tumours. New approaches to screening using surrogate molecular end-points should allow the development of new compounds which may well have considerable effect on cell growth. Clinical trials are now just beginning with growth factor analogues, protein kinase inhibitors, and RAS function blockers, devised by these strategies (10).

3. Natural history of cancer

The clinical presentation of any cancer depends on the location and tissue type affected but usually involves an expanding tumour mass which causes symptoms through local invasion, local expansion, or the production of biologically active molecular products such as hormones or cytokines. Each tumour type has its own natural history which has been altered successfully by chemotherapy only in a few 'curable' malignancies such as certain germ cell tumours, leukaemias, and lymphomas.

In cellular terms, cancer represents a form of de-differentiation or, more generally, a disturbance of the normally differentiated state, that is associated with loss of growth control. Genetic changes or mutations in somatic cells of the body are the main initiating events and are responsible for tumour progression. It is clear also that changes in cell chromosomes either in number or organization are key events in tumorigenesis (see Chapter 1), and that the immune system plays a role in limiting or eliminating cancer to an extent through the recognition of novel antigens on cancer cells. There is considerable evidence that some cancers are caused by viruses either indirectly, by suppression of the host immune system and impaired elimination of tumour cells, or directly, by activation of oncogenes or the insertion of viral DNA into host chromosomes.

Under normal circumstances there is a balance between growth-promoting and growth-restraining signal transduction elements so that cellular proliferation only occurs as appropriate. There is an equilibrium between stem cells capable of replication and the cellular deficit resulting from natural cell loss. In specific circumstances this balance is capable of up-regulating in favour of a controlled increase in cell number such as during embryogenesis, wound repair, immune response, and in normal tissue turnover. Neoplastic growth, in contrast, is characterized by abnormalities in the activity of critical signalling molecules so that the balance is disrupted and abnormal cell growth ensues. Proteins encoded by overexpressed or mutant proto-oncogenes and loss of tumour suppressor gene products are important to this scenario. As a result, complex effector responses are initiated including ion transport, pinocytosis, glycolysis, changes in cytoskeletal architecture, and the synthesis of DNA and RNA. Deregulation of these events creates the biological framework driving aberrant cell proliferation, loss of differentiation, and the development of metastases.

As discussed in the following sections a number of characteristics have been used to describe how cancer cells behave differently from their normal counterparts.

3.1 Clonality

Genetic markers can be used to show that the vast majority of cancers are clonal (i.e. originating from a single stem cell). In addition to this clonality, there may be numerous epigenetic events to create an environment for abnormal cell division, such as chronic inflammation or persistent stimulation of the immune system. Virtually all solid tumours and a majority of haematological malignancies display abnormalities in the chromosomal karyotype which are inherited by the population of tumour cells. These may involve the translocation, deletion, or duplication of specific chromosomal segments (see Chapter 1).

Studies on tumours occurring in patients with glucose-6 phosphate dehydrogenase deficiency (G6PD) have demonstrated the clonal nature of certain cancers (11). This condition is common in Africa and is inherited in two forms, A and B, easily distinguished by electrophoresis. A female who is heterozygous for G6PD is a mosaic of cells, half of which express G6PD-A while the other half express G6PD-B. A tumour arising in such a female, if it is clonal, should not be a mosaic—all cells will arise from A or B. Tumours occurring in these individuals are always composed of either A or B cells but not both, so confirming clonal proliferation.

The observation of uniform karyotypic abnormalities in all cells in chronic myeloid leukaemia, which has the t(9;22) translocation (see Chapters 1 and 4), also provides strong evidence for clonality (12). Furthermore, since these types of translocation are never seen in normal cells, the chromosomal abnormalities may serve usefully as 'tumour markers' indicating the presence of a common malignant state in the individual; these changes should not be detectable after successful treatment and their subsequent detection may then be the first indication of disease relapse. The techniques currently available to the molecular geneticist allow clonal genetic abnormalities to be identified in non-dividing cells, including gene mutation, rearrangement, translocation, deletion, and amplification.

3.2 Anaplasia

Cancer cells may show some of the morphological characteristics of their normal counterparts, but the lack of normal cellular differentiation is a feature recognized readily by light microscopy. Anaplasia is a lack of normal co-ordinated cellular differentiation. The cells have large nuclei, increased nucleus to cytoplasmic ratio, with more apparent chromatin and prominent nucleoli. There may be increased numbers of mitotic cells, giant cells containing multiple nucleoli, and abnormal mitoses reflecting failure of karyokinesis. The presence of aneuploid cells as detected by techniques such as flow cytometry may have diagnostic and prognostic value. The process of anaplasia may be expressed either at a cellular level, with morphological derangement, loss of normal tissue architecture, invasiveness, destruction of normal tissue, pleomorphism, and a high mitotic rate, or at a biochemical level, with inappropriate and poorly controlled secretion of growth factors, hormones, or peptides (such as immunoglobulins). More recently correlations have been made to specific genetic alterations.

3.3 Autonomy

The many local and distant environmental factors which control normal cellular proliferation are circumvented when the process of malignant transformation occurs. This autonomy is usually relative and requires a minimal number of supporting factors such as platelet-derived growth factor (PDGF), epidermal growth factor (EGF), or insulin-like growth factors (IGFI, IGFII) (13). In certain circumstances, clonal proliferation results in further autonomy by the production of a growth-promoting factor by the tumour itself and this is termed autocrine stimulation (Chapter 2). The first molecule with the potential for autocrine stimulation was transforming growth factor-alpha (TGFα). Other mechanisms by which tumour cells show less dependence on growth factors is the expression of an increased number of receptors such as EGFR or ERBB2 on the cell surface (Chapter 3) or they may activate an internal biochemical process such as a protein tyrosine kinase ordinarily dependent upon binding of a specific growth factor to a cell surface receptor, thereby completely bypassing the need for exposure to the growth-promoting agent.

3.4 Metastasis

Dissemination of cancer occurs through the process of contiguous spread and metastasis. Cells lose their adherence and restrained position within an organized tissue, develop the capacity to invade, and become capable of proliferating in unnatural locations and tissue environments. These changes in growth patterns are accompanied by biochemical changes which may promote the metastic process. The first step probably involves the attachment to the extracellular matrix via binding to receptors on the cell membrane that bind specifically to glycoproteins such as fibronectin and laminin. The tumour then progresses from a homogeneous proliferating clone to a group of heterogeneous subpopulations of cells, some of which have progressively accumulated the entire array of surface molecules and enzymes required for metastasis, such as collagenases, and lysosomal hydrolases.

4. Genetic basis of cancer

Chromosomal analysis of human cancer cells has yielded a huge amount of information about the nature and incidence of chromosomal abnormalities in malignant cells (Chapter 1). Certain abnormalities have diagnostic and prognostic significance in both haematological and solid malignancies. Although there are a wide variety of cancer-related cytogenetic abnormalities, these are relatively small in number and non-randomly distributed throughout the genome. The types of aberration observed may be due to:

- deletions of part of or whole chromosomes
- translocations
- gain of chromosomal material

Chromosome aberrations may be primarily related to the formation of a specific tumour and may be the only genetic abnormality present (14). Secondary aberrations are not random, are rarely the only phenomenon, and occur in the presence of the primary change; they may be epiphenomena or they may determine the biological behaviour of the tumour including invasion, metastasis, and response to treatment. Primary aberrations would be expected to occur early in tumorigenesis whereas secondary changes would become more frequent in the later stages.

As discussed in Chapter 10, a number of constitutional chromosomal abnormalities are associated with predisposition to cancer. These may be associated with numerical or structural abnormalities of chromosomes or chromosome breakage syndromes. In some cases the molecular pathology of the chromosome rearrangement has been delineated and a translocation or deletion has been demonstrated to inactivate a tumour suppressor gene as in del(11p13) and the Wilms' tumour gene (*WT1*) (15). In adenomatous polyposis coli (APC), which predisposes to colon cancer, all individuals have a specific chromosomal deletion at 5q21 (16). This can now be readily detected and genetic analysis has been shown to facilitate diagnosis and screening.

Other situations in which there is a systemic inherited susceptibility to tumorigenesis include disorders characterized by genomic instability which can be recognized by increased spontaneous chromosome breakage in cultured cells. The pattern of this breakage is specific for each disorder. Conditions predisposing to cancer in this way include Xeroderma pigmentosa, in which there is extreme sensitivity to the effects of sunlight and carcinogens due to reduced ability to repair damaged DNA; Blooms' syndrome, in which there is a defect in a gene encoding a DNA ligase leading to inefficient joining of nucleotides; Ataxia telangiectasia (Chapter 10), and Fanconi anaemia. The genes involved in these syndromes have been identified and tests devised for heterozygotes, so making genetic counselling more precise.

Certain carcinogens increase the risk of developing cancer by increasing the mutation frequency or by interfering with chromosome organization. Some may act as tumour promotors so that the possibility of developing cancer after some initiating event increases significantly. Variation in the metabolism of certain carcinogens has been shown to have a genetic basis. There are inherited differences in the ability to metabolize drugs such as debrisoquine. 10% of the population are poor metabolizers in the homozygous state and this is associated with increased toxicity when the drug is administered in normal doses. Studies have shown that there is a sixfold reduced frequency of lung cancer in slow metabolizers suggesting a link between debrisoquine and carcinogen metabolism (17).

5. Colorectal cancer

The clinical presentation of colorectal tumours depends to a large degree on the location and rate of growth of the primary tumour. Features common to all sites of tumour include anorexia, malaise, and weight loss but, more specifically, as pain, mucorrhoea, chronic blood loss leading to iron-deficient anaemia, and a change in bowel habit occasionally with the classical symptoms of alternating constipation and diarrhoea. Right-sided lesions may be very insidious in nature, and often present as vague abdominal pain or sometimes mimicking cholecystitis or peptic ulcer disease. Left-sided colonic lesions are more often circumferential and, therefore, may present as partial or total obstruction; they are more likely to present with blood visibly mixed in the stool (18).

5.1 Screening

The natural history of colorectal carcinoma suggests that it may be amenable to intervention through screening. The prognosis is related to the depth of invasion of the cancer and, since surgery cures approximately 90% of cancers limited to the mucosa and submucosa, early diagnosis could improve survival. Since colorectal carcinoma usually arises in adenomas, removing adenomas should prevent most cases of cancer. Population screening studies using faecal occult blood tests have shown that a higher proportion of cancers at an early stage are detected in groups offered screening compared to unscreened controls (19). These tests are low in cost but to date have been found to have disappointing uptake and poor yield. Despite the increased facilities to perform flexible sigmoidoscopic examination in recent years, no randomized clinical trial has yet demonstrated that screening by sigmoidoscopy improves survival in patients with colorectal carcinoma. The main evidence for reduced mortality from any type of screening comes from case-control studies.

5.2 Mechanisms of colorectal tumorigenesis

The development of colorectal cancer results from an interplay of environmental factors on the genetic background of the individual. The risk of colorectal tumorigenesis has been related to a number of factors. Like all cancers, colorectal carcinoma, whether sporadic or secondary to a genetic predisposition, is a consequence of a series of poorly understood changes in the genome of the normal cells. It is an excellent model for understanding the sequential molecular changes that occur during the development of malignancy.

The multistep process of colorectal carcinogenesis involves the formation of adenomas from either hyperplastic epithelium or from polyps, with subsequent progression to carcinoma. Recognition of this sequence has allowed the study of molecular events along each stage of eventual tumour formation. 98% of colorectal cancers are adenocarcinomas and it is likely that such carcinomas arise in a small number of pre-existing adenomatous polyps. The evidence for a sequential change from adenoma to carcinoma comes from a number of observations. Minute adeno-carcinomas generally arise within adenomatous polyps and removal of polyps diminishes the incidence of cancer in those patients. Adenomas coexist with carcino-mas in over a third of patients. Foci of cancer may be detected within large dysplastic adenomas, or a residual region of adenoma can often be noted at the margins of a carcinoma specimen. A markedly increased frequency of cancer is seen in the familial polyposis syndromes, and oncogene and tumour suppressor gene abnormalities are seen in both adenomas and carcinomas (20). This process of tumour initiation and progression is likely to be continuous and probably occurs over a period measured in years or decades. In particular, the study of relatively common forms of inherited colorectal cancer have been extremely useful; they have been well described and analyses of large family cohorts have been possible. A summary of a possible genetic model for colorectal carcinoma is shown in Fig. 1; providing an excellent example of several genetic alterations of the types discussed in the preceding chapters in this book.

5.3 Screening based on molecular genetics

In addition to identifying individuals with an inherited predisposition to colorectal carcinoma, mutation analysis is a potential method of screening for sporadic cancer. A recent study of stool samples from colorectal carcinoma patients found that *K-RAS* mutations could be identified in stool samples in eight of nine patients in whom the

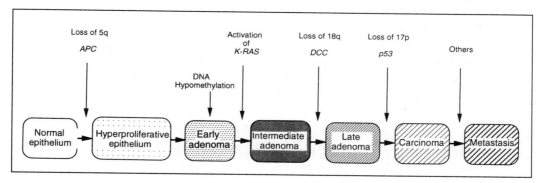

Fig. 1 Molecular progression of the normal colon epithelion to colon cancer. A series of 5–6 genetic changes are necessary to convert the normal epithelial cell to a metastatic carcinoma.

mutations were present in the tumour (36). Although *K-RAS* mutations are only present in 40% of colorectal tumours, they are present at the pre-malignant stage and so facilitate the early identification of an adenoma or of a recurrent carcinoma.

6. Potential therapies based on molecular genetics

Colorectal cancer is clearly a disease caused by defective somatic cell genetics. Genetic therapy strategies therefore seem an appropriate avenue for further research. The main problem facing the gene therapist is how to incorporate new genes into every tumour cell. If this cannot be achieved, then any malignant cells that remain unaffected will emerge as a resistant clone. Presently we do not have ideal vectors. Despite this drawback, there are already over 100 protocols accepted for clinical trial in cancer patients world-wide, the majority in the USA. The ethical issues are fairly straightforward with oncology providing some of the highest possible benefit/risk ratios. There are several strategies currently under investigation.

6.1 Genetic tagging

There are several situations where the use of a genetic marker to tag tumour cells may help in making decisions on the optimal treatment for an individual patient. The insertion of a foreign marker gene into cells from a tumour biopsy and replacing the marked cells into the patient prior to treatment can provide a sensitive new indicator of minimal residual disease after chemotherapy. The commonest marker is the gene for neomycin phosphotransferase (*neoR*), an enzyme which metabolizes the aminoglycoside antibiotic G418. This gene, when inserted into an appropriate retroviral vector, can be stably incorporated into the host cell's genome. Originally detected by antibiotic resistance, it can now be picked up by the more sensitively polymerase chain reaction. In this way, as few as one tumour cell among one million normal cells can be identified. This procedure can help in the design of aggressive chemotherapy protocols.

A particularly elegant use of this strategy has been the analysis of the reasons of failure in autologous bone marrow transplantation for childhood acute myeloblastic leukaemia (21). Failure can be due to inadequate chemotherapy or to reinfusion of viable tumour cells in the stored marrow. Reinfused marrow was labelled with *neoR* and recurrent tumour analysed for the presence of this gene. In the majority of cases, tumour cells contain the marker indicating a failure of the purging process. Similar studies are now in progress for neuroblastoma as well as chronic myeloid and acute lymphoid leukaemia. So far no marking protocols for colorectal cancer have been developed.

6.2 Enhancing tumour immunogenicity

The presence of an immune response to cancer has been recognized for many years. The problem is that human tumours seem to be predominantly weakly immunogenic. If ways could be found to elicit a more powerful immune stimulus then effective immunotherapy could become a reality. Several observations from murine tumours indicate that one reason for weak immunogenicity of certain tumours is the failure to elicit a T-helper cell response. This in turn releases the necessary cytokines to stimulate the production of cytolytic T cells which can destroy tumours. The expression of cytokine genes such as interleukin-2 (IL-2), tumour necrosis factor (TNF), and interferon in tumour cells has been shown to bypass the need for T-helper cells in mice. Similar clinical experiments are now in progress (22). Melanoma cells have been prepared from biopsies and infected with retrovirus containing the *IL-2* gene. These cells are being used as a vaccine to elicit a more powerful immune response. Many tumours express low amounts of the products of the major histocompatibility complex (MHC). These molecules are necessary for antigen presentation and their absence may help tumours evade immune scrutiny. There are now several examples of mouse model systems where tumour cells transfected with MHC class II genes can be used to not only prevent tumour spread when given as a prophylactic vaccine but also to induce remission of established leukaemias, lymphomas, carcinomas, and sarcomas. Clinical experiments involving the direct intratumoral injection of foreign HLA genes are currently in progress for several tumour types including colorectal carcinoma.

6.3 Vectoring cytokines to tumours

Cytokines such as the interferons and interleukins have been actively explored for their tumoricidal properties. Although there is evidence of cytotoxicity, their side effects are profound so limiting the dose that can safely be administered. It is possible to insert cytokine genes into cells that can potentially home in on tumours so releasing a high concentration of their protein product locally. TNF genes have been inserted into tumour-infiltrating lymphocytes from patients with melanoma and given systemically (23). These experiments are controversial for two reasons. First, it appears from *in vitro* studies that the amount of TNF expressed from such cells was unlikely to be sufficient to cause a significant cytotoxic effect and secondly the insertion of a foreign gene limits the ability of the lymphocyte to target into tumour masses.

6.4 Inserting drug activating genes

The main problem with existing chemotherapy is its lack of selectivity. If drug activating genes could be inserted which would only be expressed in cancer cells then the administration of an appropriate prodrug could be highly selective. There are now many examples of genes preferentially expressed in tumours (24). In some cases their promoters have been isolated and coupled to drug activating enzymes. Examples include, carcino-embryonic antigen (CEA) in colorectal carcinoma, alphafoetoprotein in hepatoma, prostate-specific antigen in prostate cancer, and *ERBB2* in breast cancer. Such promoters can be coupled to enzymes such as cytosine deaminase or thymidine kinase so producing unique retroviral vectors which are able to infect all cells but whose encoded gene product can only be expressed in tumour cells. These suicide or

Trojan horse vectors may not have absolute tumour specificity but this may not be essential—it may be possible to perform a genetic prostatectomy or mastectomy—so effectively destroying all tumour cells. Much work is currently in progress to develop both the promoter systems which rely on differential transcription control and also the design of the drug activating systems. Cytosine deaminase for example converts the relatively non-toxic anti-fungal drug 5-flourocytosine to the cytotoxic 5-fluorouracil. Both drugs are already in clinical use and provide a useful system for further development. Other drug activating systems are being explored which release even more potent toxins. An example is the enzyme linamarase, which converts amygdalin to cyanide. Clinical trials using genetically activated prodrugs are anticipated shortly in hepatoma, melanoma, pancreatic, and breast cancer.

6.5 Suppressing oncogene expression

The down-regulation of abnormal oncogene expression has been shown to revert to malignant phenotype in a variety of *in vitro* tumour lines. It is possible to develop *in vivo* systems such as the insertion of genes coding for complementary (antisense) mRNA to that produced by the oncogene (25). Such anti-genes specifically switch off the production of the abnormal protein product. The mutant form of the *RAS* oncogene is an obvious target for this approach. Clearly the major problem is to ensure that every single tumour cell becomes infected. Any cell which escapes will have a survival advantage and produce a clone of resistant tumour cells. For this reason, it may be that future treatment schedules will require the repetitive administration of vectors in a similar way to fractionated radiotherapy or chemotherapy.

6.6 Replacing defective tumour suppressor genes

In cell culture malignant properties can often be reversed by the insertion of normal tumour suppressor genes such as *RB*, *p53*, and *DCC*. Although tumour suppressor genes were often identified in rare tumour types, abnormalities in their expression and function are abundant in common human cancers. Defects in p53 occur in up to 60% of colorectal carcinomas. As with anti-gene therapy, the difficulty in this approach lies in the delivery of actively expressed vectors to every single tumour cell *in vivo*. Nevertheless, clinical experiments are in progress in non-small cell lung cancer where retroviruses which encode wild-type p53 are being administered bronchoscopically (26). No results are as yet reported. Perhaps the biggest risk from gene manipulation *in vivo* is the possibility of insertional mutagenesis and the activation of oncogenes leading to neoplasia (Chapter 1). Such risks are clearly important factors in the consideration of the ethical basis for gene therapy for disorders such as cystic fibrosis, haemophilia, and the haemoglobinopathies. For patients with metastatic cancer the risks are low. Such patients are often desperate for some form of treatment and are already searching for the gene therapy programmes described in the media. Therapies with even minimal potential benefit will be avidly considered. In this situation the biggest problem is offering false hope. It is unrealistic to expect such new strategies to be effective immediately. The first patients entering trials will provide much information for little personal benefit. This must be recognized by both the investigator and patient to reduce the 'breakthrough' mentality that surrounds novel cancer treatments.

There have been remarkable advances in our understanding of the molecular biology of cancer. Interventional genetics is now poised to provide new selective tumour destruction mechanisms for patients with widespread cancer. But there are many hurdles still to overcome: how to transfer efficiently and stably genes into tumour cells *in vivo*; how to ensure safety for both patient and staff; and how best to place genetic approaches alongside more familiar therapies. We are witnessing the beginnings of molecular therapy. 50 years ago the first alkylating agents were discovered and were about to enter clinical trial as systemic chemotherapy. None of our predecessors could have predicted the successes and disappointments that have led to the practice of modern medical oncology. We are now leaving an era of empiricism and entering an age when our knowledge of genetics and logical molecular design is likely to radically change the future face of cancer treatment.

References

1. National Research Council. (1988) Committee on the Biological Effects of Ionising Radiations. Health risks of radon and other internally deposited alpha emitters. Washington National Academy Press.
2. Rothman, N., Poirier, M. C., Baser, M. E., Hansen, J. A., Genilte, C., Bowman, E. D., *et al.* (1990) Formation of polycyclic aromatic hydrocarbon DNA adducts in peripheral blood cells during consumption of charcoal broiled beef. *Carcinogenesis*, **11**, 1241.
3. Hennikens, C. II, Stampfer, M. J., and Willett, W. C. (1994) Micronutrients and cancer prevention. *Cancer Prev. Detect.*, **7**, 147.
4. Wald, N., Cuckle, H., and Frost, C. (1991) Breast cancer screening: the current position. *Br. Med. J.*, **302**, 845.
5. Pandah, H., Waxman, J., and Sikora, K. (1994) Tumour markers. *Br. J. Hosp. Med.*, **51**, 297.
6. Sidransky, D., Tokino, T., Hamilton, S. R., Kinzler, K. W., Levin, B., Frost, P., *et al.* (1992) Identification of *ras* oncogene mutations in the stool of patients with curable colorectal tumors. *Science*, **256**, 102.
7. Leung, H. Y. and Lemoine, N. R. (1994) Pancreatic cancer. In *Cancer: a molecular approach*, (ed. N. R. Lemoine, J Neoptolomos, and T. Cooke), pp. 105–15. Blackwell Scientific, Oxford.
8. Paris, J. R., Morrow, M., and Bonnadonna, G. (1993) Cancer of the breast. In *Cancer: principles and practice of oncology* 4th edn (ed. V. De Vita, S. Hellman, and S. Rosenberg), pp. 1264–332. J. B. Lippencott & Company, Philadelphia, PA.
9. Moertal, C. G., Fleming, T. R., MacDonald, J. S., Haller, D. G., Laurie, J. A., Goodman, P. J., *et al.* (1990) Levamisole and Fluorouracil for adjuvant therapy of resected colon carcinoma. *N Engl. J. Med*, **322**, 352.
10. Kohl, N. E., Omer, C. A., Conner, M. W., Anthony, N. J., Davide, J. P., DeSolms, S. J., *et al.* (1995) Inhibition of farnesyl transferase induces regression of mammary and salivary carcinomas in *ras* transgenic mice. *Nature Med.*, **1**, 792.

11. Vogelstein, B., Feron, F. R., and Hamilton, S. R. (1987) Clonal analysis using recombinant DNA probes from the X chromosome. *Cancer Res.*, **47**, 4806.

12. Tkachuk, D. C., Westbrook, C. A., Andreeff, M., Donlon, T. A., Cleary, M. L., Suryanarayan, K., *et al.* (1990) Detection of *bcr-abl* fusion in chronic mylogenous leukemia by *in situ* hybridisation. *Science*, **250**, 559.

13. Lambert, S., Collette, J., Gillis, J., Franchimont, P., Desaive, C., and Gol-Winkler, R. (1991) Tumor IGFII content in a patient with a colon adenocarcinoma correlates with abnormal expression of the gene. *Int. J. Cancer*, **48**, 826.

14. Knudson, A. (1971) Mutation and cancer. A statistical study of retinoblastoma. *Proc. Natl. Acad. Sci. USA*, **68**, 820.

15. Huff, V., Miwa, H., Haber, D. A., Call, K. M., Housman, D., Strong, L. C., *et al.* (1991) Evidence for WT1 as a Wilms tumor (WT) gene: intragenic germinal deletion in bilateral WT. *Am. J. Hum. Genet*, **48**, 997.

16. Nishisho, I., Nakamura, Y., Miyoshi, Y., Miki, Y., Ando, H., Horii, A., *et al.* (1991) Mutations of chromosome 5q21 genes in FAP and colorectal cancer patients. *Science*, **253**, 665.

17. Ayesh, R., Idle, J. R., Ritchie, J. C., Crothers, M. J., and Hetzel, M. R. (1984) Metabolic oxidation phenotypes as markers for susceptibility to lung cancer. *Nature*, **312**, 169.

18. Eisenberg, B., Decosse, J. J., Harford, F., and Michalek, J. (1982) Carcinoma of the colon and rectum: the natural history reviewed in 1704 patients. *Cancer*, **49**, 1131.

19. Flehinger, B. J., Winawer, S., and Schorrenfield, D. (1993) Screening for colorectal cancer with faecal occult blood and sigmoidoscopy. *J. Natl. Cancer Inst.*, **85**, 311.

20. Vogelstein, B., Fearon, E. R., Hamilton, S. R., Kern, S. E., Preisinger, A. C., Leppert, M., *et al.* (1988) Genetic alteration during colorectal-tumor development. *N. Engl. J. Med.*, **319**, 525.

21. Brenner, M. K., Rill, D. R., Moen, R. C., Krance, R. A., Mirro, J. Jr., Anderson, W. F., *et al.* (1993) Gene marking to trace origin or relapse after autologous bone-marrow transplantation. *Lancet*, **341**, 85.

22. Dalgleish, A. (1994) The role of IL2 in gene therapy. *Gene Ther.*, **1**, 83.

23. Rosenburg, S. A. (1992) Gene therapy for cancer. *J. Am. Med. Assoc.*, **268**, 246.

24. Sikora, K. (1994) Genes, dreams and cancer. *Br. Med. J.*, **308**, 1217.

25. Skuse, G. and Ludlow, J. W. (1995) Tumour suppressor genes in disease and therapy. *Lancet*, **345**, 902.

26. Roth, J. A. (1994) Clinical protocol for modification of oncogene and tumour suppressor gene expression in non-small cell lung cancer. *Cancer Gene Ther.*, **1**, 78.

Index